PATHOLOGY ANNUAL
PART 1
1977

PATHOLOGY ANNUAL

PART 1

VOLUME 12

1977

 APPLETON-CENTURY-CROFTS/New York

77 78 79 80 81 / 10 9 8 7 6 5 4 3 2 1

Library of Congress Catalog Card Number: 66-20355

Prentice-Hall International, Inc., London
Prentice-Hall of Australia, Pty. Ltd., Sydney
Prentice-Hall of India Private Limited, New Delhi
Prentice-Hall of Japan, Inc., Tokyo
Prentice-Hall of Southeast Asia (Pte.) Ltd., Singapore
Whitehall Books Ltd., Wellington, New Zealand

PRINTED IN THE UNITED STATES OF AMERICA
0-8385-7748-2

CONTRIBUTORS

Richard D. Bell, Ph.D.

Department of Pathology, Veterans Administration Hospital, Oklahoma City, Oklahoma

William A. Blanc, M.D.

Attending Pathologist, Columbia-Presbyterian Medical Center, New York, New York; Director, Division of Developmental Pathology at Babies Hospital, New York, New York; Professor, Department of Pathology, Columbia University College of Physicians and Surgeons, New York, New York

J.A.H. Campbell, M.Med.(Path.), F.R.C.Path.

Senior Specialist, Department of Pathology, University of Cape Town and Groote Schuur Hospital, Cape Town, South Africa

Bernard Czernobilsky

Chief, Department of Pathology, Kaplan Hospital, Rehovot, Israel; Associate Professor, Department of Pathology, Medical School of the Hebrew University and Hadassah, Jerusalem, Israel

Ettore DeGirolami, M.D.

Pathologist, South Miami Hospital, Miami, Florida; Associate Professor, Department of Pathology, University of Massachusetts School of Medicine, Worcester, Massachusetts (Formerly Chief Pathologist, Worcester Hahnemann Hospital, Worcester, Massachusetts)

Rolando G. Estrada, M.D.

Assistant Professor, Department of Pathology, Baylor College of Medicine, Houston, Texas; Assistant Professor, Department of Pathology, Ben Taub General Hospital, Houston, Texas

Robert E. Fechner, M.D.

Professor, Department of Pathology, Baylor College of Medicine, Houston, Texas; Associate Chief of Anatomic Pathology, The Methodist Hospital, Houston, Texas

Cecilia M. Fenoglio, M.D.

Assistant Professor, Department of Pathology, and Associate Director, Division of Obstetric and Gynecologic Pathology, Sloane Hospital for Women, New York, New York; Director, Central Tissue Facility of Cancer Research Center, Columbia-Presbyterian Medical Center, New York, New York

Judith D. Goldberg, S.M., Sc.D.

Assistant Professor, Biostatistics, The Mount Sinai School of Medicine of the City University of New York, New York, New York

Joel E. Haas, M.D.

Associate Pathologist, Children's Orthopedic Hospital and Medical Center, Seattle, Washington

Yoshie Hashida, M.D.

Assistant Professor, Department of Clinical Pathology, Children's Hospital of Pittsburgh, Pittsburgh, Pennsylvania

Theodore C. Iancu, M.D.

Head, Department of Pediatrics, Carmel Hospital, Haifa, Israel; Formerly Research Fellow, Pediatric Pathology and Electron Microscopy, Department of Pathology, Children's Hospital of Los Angeles, Los Angeles, California, and University of Southern California School of Medicine, Los Angeles, California

Gordon I. Kaye, M.D.

Professor and Chairman, Department of Anatomy, Albany Medical College, Albany, New York

Paul E. Lacy, M.D., Ph.D.

Professor and Chairman, Department of Pathology, Washington University Medical School, St. Louis, Missouri

Benjamin H. Landing, M.D.

Professor of Pathology and Pediatrics, Department of Pathology, Children's Hospital of Los Angeles, Los Angeles, California; Professor, Department of Pathology and Pediatrics, University of Southern California School of Medicine, Los Angeles, California

Nathan Lane, M.D.

Professor of Pathology and Surgical Pathology, Columbia-Presbyterian College of Physicians and Surgeons, New York, New York

Robert D. Lindeman, M.D., F.A.C.P.

Chief, Section of Nephrology, Veterans Administration Hospital, Oklahoma City, Oklahoma; Professor of Medicine, University of Oklahoma College of Medicine, Oklahoma City, Oklahoma

Anil K. Mandal, M.D., F.A.C.P.

Research Associate, Veterans Administration Career Development Program, and Director, Renal Electron Microscopy Laboratory, Veterans Administration Hospital, Oklahoma City, Oklahoma; Associate Professor of Medicine, University of Oklahoma College of Medicine, Oklahoma City, Oklahoma

Harry B. Neustein, M.D.

Director of Electron Microscopy and Professor, Department of Pathology, Children's Hospital of Los Angeles, Los Angeles, California; Professor, University of Southern California School of Medicine, Los Angeles, California

John A. Nordquist, M.S.

Electron Microscopist, Veterans Administration Hospital, Oklahoma City, Oklahoma

Luciano Ozzello, M.D.

Professor and Chairman, Department of Pathology, University of Lausanne Medical School, Lausanne, Switzerland

José Pardo, M.D.

Associate Chief Orthopedic Surgeon, Department of Orthopedics and Traumatology, La Fé Medical Center, Valencia, Spain

Robert R. Pascal, M.D.

Associate Professor, Department of Pathology, University of South Florida College of Medicine, Tampa, Florida; Chief Anatomic Pathologist, Veterans Administration Hospital, Tampa, Florida

Benoît Roethlisberger, M.D.

Chief Resident, Department of Otorhinolaryngology, University of Lausanne Medical School, Lausanne, Switzerland

Marcel Savary, M.D.

Professor and Chairman, Department of Otorhinolaryngology, University of Lausanne Medical School, Lausanne, Switzerland

Harlan J. Spjut, M.D.

Professor, Department of Pathology, Baylor College of Medicine, Houston, Texas; Surgical Pathologist, St. Luke's Episcopal Hospital, Houston, Texas

Luís V. Tamarit, M.D.

Head, Department of Pathology, La Fé Medical Center, Valencia, Spain

Cyril Toker, M.D.

Professor and Head, Division of Surgical Pathology, Department of Pathology, The University of Maryland School of Medicine, Baltimore, Maryland

Marie A. Valdes-Dapena, M.D.

Professor, Departments of Pathology and Pediatrics, University of Miami School of Medicine, Miami, Florida; Director, Division of Pediatric Pathology, Jackson Memorial Hospital, University of Miami Medical Center, Miami, Florida; Consultant in Pediatric Pathology, Office of the Medical Examiner, Dade County, Florida; Vice-President and Chairman of the Medical Board, National Sudden Infant Death Syndrome Foundation, Chicago, Illinois

H. Joachim Wigger, M.D.

Associate Attending Pathologist, Columbia-Presbyterian Medical Center, New York, New York; Associate Professor of Clinical Pediatric Pathology, Columbia University College of Physicians and Surgeons, New York, New York

Eduardo J. Yunis, M.D.

Professor, Department of Pathology, University of Pittsburgh School of Medicine, Pittsburgh, Pennsylvania; Director of Laboratories, Children's Hospital of Pittsburgh, Pittsburgh, Pennsylvania

CONTENTS

PATHOLOGY ANNUAL
PART 1
1977

ISLET CELL FUNCTIONAL PATHOLOGY

PAUL E. LACY

During the past few years, a new, exciting, and challenging era has been opened with respect to the functional pathology of the islets of Langerhans. New hormones have been identified and localized to the islets of Langerhans; new basic information has been provided on the intracellular events of hormone secretion by the islet cells; new information has been obtained on the possible role of genetics, viruses, and autoimmunity in the etiology of diabetes; isolated islets have been transplanted into diabetic animals with a resultant cure of the diabetic state; in vitro procedures have been developed for studies on the structure and function of normal and abnormal human islet cells. The tremendous breadth of this topic prohibits a detailed discussion and documentation of all the findings. Thus, this review represents my assessment of the present status of the functional pathology of the islets of Langerhans, with sufficient general references provided to permit the reader to explore in greater depth areas of particular interest.

Abnormal functions of the islets of Langerhans can be classified into two categories—hypersecretion and hyposecretion. Functioning islet cell tumors represent examples of hypersecretion, and diabetes mellitus represents hyposecretion or inappropriate secretion of hormones from the islet cells. These two topics will be considered as well as the function of normal islets transplanted into an abnormal location.

Diseases of Islet Cell Hypersecretion

Types of Human Islet Cells and Hormones Stored

Islets of Langerhans are scattered throughout the pancreas, with a greater number present in the tail than in the body or head. They comprise approximately 1 to 2 percent of the wet weight of the adult human pancreas. The number of islets per pancreas is estimated to be between 500,000 and 1 million.[1] The different

Supported in part by Grants #AM01226, AM03373, AM06181.

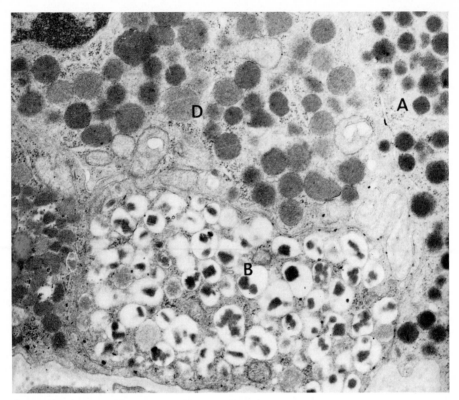

Fig. 1. Electron micrograph of portions of an alpha (A), beta (B), and delta (D) cell of a normal human islet. × 28,900. (Courtesy of Dr. Marie Greider, Washington University.)

types of cells present within normal human islets are alpha, beta, and delta cells, with additional types that have not been clearly identified at the present time. Human pancreatic polypeptide and gastrin are two hormones which have been recently localized to human islets; however, the specific cell types containing these hormones have not been established. The alpha, beta, and delta cells have been identified by using special staining techniques, electron microscopy, and immunochemical techniques for the identification of specific hormones in these cells.

Normal Alpha Cells

Alpha cells comprise approximately 20 to 25 percent of the islet cell population. In man, alpha cells are scattered throughout the islet, whereas in other species, such as the rat and mouse, they form a rim at the periphery of the islet. Ultrastructurally, these cells can be differentiated from other types of islet cells on the basis of the appearance of their secretory granules. The alpha granules are round with a closely applied membranous sac, and the center of the granule is extremely electron dense with a less dense area surrounding it (Fig. 1). Alpha cells contain glucagon as demonstrated by the fluorescent antibody technique.[2]

Normal Beta Cells

Beta cells comprise approximately 75 to 80 percent of the islet cell population in the adult pancreas and can be stained specifically with aldehyde fuchsin or aldehyde thionin.[3] Ultrastructurally, the beta cells of man contain characteristic secretory granules with rectangular profiles (Fig. 1) and have a crystalline matrix containing lines of repeating periodicity of approximately 50 Å. The secretory granules of the beta cells contain insulin, which has been demonstrated by the immunoperoxidase technique for electron microscopy [4] as well as by subcellular fractionation of the islets.[5]

Normal Delta Cells

The delta cell was first identified in human islets by Bloom in 1931,[6] using the Mallory–Heidenhain stain, which imparted a blue color to the cytoplasm of the delta cell. Unfortunately, this staining procedure is not specific, and it is difficult to obtain reproducible results. Silver staining procedures have been used for the identification of delta cells,[7] but these procedures also do not provide uniform reproducible staining. Delta cells can be identified specifically and reproducibly with electron microscopy. The basis of the identification is the secretory granules, which are large, pale, and different in structure than either alpha or beta granules in the human islet (Fig. 1). Immunochemical ultrastructural studies have localized somatostatin to the delta cell of the rat pancreas.[8] Fluorescent antibody studies on the human pancreas have also revealed somatostatin-containing cells in the islets, which are presumably delta cells.[9] The presence of this hormone in human islets is extremely interesting. From a functional standpoint, somatostatin suppresses glucagon and insulin release with a greater effect on glucagon.[10] The possible role of a hormone that would affect both alpha and beta cell secretion is unknown at the present time. It has been suggested that somatostatin may have a local control over the release of glucagon from alpha cells.[11]

Gastrin in Normal Islets

Gastrin has been localized by light and electron microscopic, immunochemical techniques to the G cell in the gastric mucosa.[12] This cell contains small, round, homogenous granules enclosed in smooth membranous sacs. Studies on human islets with the fluorescent antibody technique have demonstrated gastrin-containing cells within the islets.[13] These cells comprise approximately 5 percent of the islet cell population. Ultrastructurally, a cell resembling the G cell of the gastric mucosa is present in the normal human islet. At the present time, specific identification of this cell as the one containing gastrin has not been accomplished.

Human Pancreatic Polypeptide in Normal Islets

A new hormone that contains 36 amino acids has been isolated from the chicken pancreas.[14] A peptide that appears to be homologous to avian pancreatic polypeptide has been isolated from human pancreas. The biologic activity of human pancreatic peptide is essentially unknown at the present time. The administration of avian pancreatic polypeptide to chickens stimulates gastric acid secretion, accelerates glycogenolysis in the liver without altering blood glucose levels, and depresses triglyceride levels in the bloodstream.[15] Human pancreatic polypeptide has been localized with the fluorescent antibody technique to cells within human islets and in scattered individual cells in the exocrine parenchyma of the pancreas.[16] The localization of this new hormone to the human pancreas is a most interesting observation, and detailed studies are needed to determine the biologic activity of this hormone in man as well as the factors controlling the secretion of the hormone.

Functioning Islet Cell Tumors

Several different types of islet cell tumors occur in the pancreas and produce specific hormones. These neoplasms cannot be differentiated on the basis of their morphologic appearance using ordinary light microscopic procedures. Special stains, electron microscopy, and immunoassay of the tumor for specific hormones are required to establish the specific identity of the particular tumor.

Alpha Cell Tumors

Islet cell tumors composed only of alpha cells are a rare neoplasm. Histologically, the neoplasms have a gyriform pattern with ribbons and columns of alpha cells passing between the vascular channels within the tumor.[17, 18] Ultrastructurally, identification of these neoplasms is based upon the appearance of the secretory granules within the tumor cells. The granules are round with an extremely dense core, have a diameter of 225 to 425 nm and appear identical to the secretory granules in normal alpha cells. The neoplasms contain glucagon, and usually the level of circulating glucagon in the patient is markedly elevated.

Beta Cell Tumors

The rate of release of insulin from normal beta cells is dependent upon the level of the circulating blood glucose. When the concentration of glucose is increased above 100 mg percent, insulin secretion is stimulated. In contrast, neoplastic beta cells no longer respond to the level of blood sugar, with a resultant uncontrolled release of insulin and repeated attacks of hypoglycemia. Histologically, the neoplasms usually have a gyriform pattern similar to alpha cell tumors.[18] Staining of the neoplasms with aldehyde fuchsin may or may not reveal beta granules within the neoplasm. Ultrastructurally, the neoplasm can be identified as a beta cell tumor if secretory granules are found which have a rectangular crystalline appearance similar to the granules present in normal beta cells.

Ulcerogenic Tumors of the Pancreas

Zollinger and Ellison[19] described a diagnostic triad that consisted of a fulminating peptic ulcer diathesis, marked gastric acid hypersecretion, and the presence of a non–beta cell tumor in the pancreas. The level of circulating gastrin in these patients is usually increased. Histologically, the neoplasms are composed of large solid nests of cells containing glandular structures, and the tumors do not have the gyriform pattern observed in alpha and beta cell tumors. Ultrastructurally, the neoplastic cells contain secretory granules which are of two types.[18] In type I, the granules are round and homogeneous with a diameter ranging from 150 to 200 nm. In type II, the granules have a pleomorphic shape with diameters ranging up to 350 nm. Both types of granules may be present in the same neoplasm.

Diarrheogenic Tumors of the Pancreas

Verner and Morrison [20] described a second type of syndrome associated with non–beta cell tumors of the pancreas. In this syndrome, the patients had profuse diarrhea with hypokalemia and achlorhydria. Histologically and ultrastructurally, these neoplasms are similar to the ulcerogenic tumors. The neoplastic cells are arranged as large solid nests that contain glandular structures, and the secretory granules within the neoplastic cells resemble the type I and type II granules observed in ulcerogenic tumors. The hormone produced by these tumors has not been identified with certainty. It has been suggested that the neoplasms may contain a secretin-like substance of a gastric inhibitory polypeptide, which would compete with gastrin for receptor sites of the gastric parietal cell with the resultant production of achlorhydria.[21] At the present time, the identity of this particular islet cell tumor can be established only by the process of exclusion, since neither the hormone produced by the tumor nor the islet cell of origin has been identified.

Syndromes for the Future

As indicated earlier, human pancreatic polypeptide and somatostatin have been demonstrated in the human pancreas and localized to islet cells. These two hormones have only recently been isolated from the human pancreas, thus no information is available concerning their role in normal metabolism. When this information becomes available, undoubtedly, new endocrine syndromes will be identified in which there is either hypersecretion or hyposecretion of these hormones.

Diabetes Mellitus

During the past few years, several lines of evidence have accumulated which indicate that the primary defect in diabetes mellitus may reside in islet cells. The evidence is as follows:

1. Sulfonylurea compounds, such as tolbutamide, stimulate the release of insulin from beta cells. In certain diabetic subjects, sulfonylurea compounds will maintain normoglycemia. These observations indicate that sulfonylurea compounds are able to stimulate insulin release from beta cells, whereas the hyperglycemia of these diabetic patients is incapable of stimulating sufficient insulin secretion.
2. The pattern of insulin release following glucose stimulation in a normal subject

is biphasic in nature, with the first phase of secretion reaching a peak approximately five minutes after raising the level of blood sugar. In maturity-onset diabetics and in the early stages of juvenile diabetes, the release of insulin is delayed with a resultant absence or marked diminution of the first phase of insulin secretion.[22] These findings indicate a possible defect in the beta cell with respect to glucose-induced insulin release.

3. Recent studies have shown an elevated level of circulating glucagon in diabetic patients.[23] In a normal subject, an elevation of the blood glucose results in an inhibition of glucagon secretion with a resultant lowering of the circulating glucagon levels. Apparently, this inhibitory effect of glucose does not occur in the diabetic subject. These observations have formed the basis for suggesting the presence of a possible defect in the alpha cell in diabetes.[24]

4. Transplantation of the entire normal pancreas into diabetic patients has been attempted,[25] and in those instances in which the transplants survived, normoglycemia was maintained without the use of exogenous insulin therapy. Thus, the transplanted normal islets replaced the apparently defective islets of the diabetic.

These four lines of evidence indicate that the primary lesion in diabetes mellitus is in the islet cells and probably involves the secretory mechanisms of beta and alpha cells. In this section, the normal and possible abnormal mechanisms of hormone secretion by beta and alpha cells will be reviewed, as well as the possible factors in the etiology and pathogenesis of diabetes mellitus.

Beta Cell Secretion

During the past few years, a tremendous amount of new information has been obtained concerning the mechanisms by which glucose brings about the release of insulin from the beta cell. Based upon this information, a model for insulin secretion is illustrated in Figure 2. Further basic information will, of course, be needed to establish the validity of certain aspects of this model.

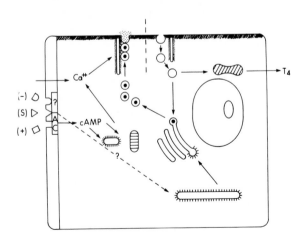

Fig. 2. Model of beta cell secretion. (From Lacy: Am J Pathol 79:170, 1975)

Glucose is the primary signal for the stimulation of insulin release in man. Indirect evidence indicates that glucose may be interacting with a specific gluco-receptor on the beta cell membrane, thereby initiating a chain of events leading to insulin secretion.[26, 27] The specific identity of this receptor has not as yet been established. As a result of the interaction of glucose with the beta cell membrane, cyclic AMP levels are increased in the beta cell, and a change in membrane permeability to calcium occurs with the resultant accumulation of calcium within the cells.[28] Following glucose stimulation, intracellular movement of beta granules is stimulated,[29] and we have proposed that the microtubular–microfilamentous system is responsible for the movement of columns of beta granules to the surface of the cell and that calcium may serve as the trigger for the initiation of this movement.[30] It is unknown whether the propelling force for the movement of the granules is provided by a change in conformation of the microtubules or whether it is due to a contraction of microfilaments or another contractile element associated with the microtubules.[31] Under the latter condition, the microtubules would simply serve as rods for guiding the movement of the granules to the cell surface. The role of cyclic AMP in these intracellular events is probably a modulating one in which cyclic AMP may release bound calcium from intracellular depots or stimulate the formation of new microtubules from microtubulin. The granules transported to the cell surface are released by emiocytosis. Following emiocytosis, recycling of the plasma membrane occurs with conveyance of the membrane either to the Golgi complex or to the lysosomes where it would be destroyed.[32]

This model for insulin secretion could also explain the biphasic pattern of insulin release from the beta cells. Following glucose stimulation, granules associated with the microtubular–microfilamentous system would be released initially, forming the first phase of insulin secretion. The second phase of release could be due to the association of other stored and newly-formed granules with the microtubular–microfilamentous system.

In comparing this mechanism of insulin release with secretion by other endocrine glands, it is interesting that the microtubular–microfilamentous system is involved in thyroid secretion.[31] The colloid within a single follicle can be visualized as a huge secretory granule. Following stimulation with thyrotrophic hormone, portions of the granule are pinched off and conveyed to the lysosomes where thyroxin is released. The microtubular–microfilamentous system is involved in the pinocytotic removal of the colloid and in the conveyance of the colloid droplets to the lysosomes.[33] Thus, as a general concept, it would appear that secretion of thyroxin involves only the membrane-recycling portion of insulin secretion.

Glucose also stimulates the new formation of insulin in the beta cell. Following glucose stimulation, proinsulin production is initiated in the endoplasmic reticulum.[34, 35] The precise biochemical events linking glucose stimulation with proinsulin production have not been delineated. It would appear that glucose causes an increased translation of messenger RNA for proinsulin production in the endoplasmic reticulum. Proinsulin is transported to the Golgi complex by an energy-requiring mechanism, and in the Golgi sacs, the C-peptide of proinsulin is apparently removed leaving insulin. The enzyme or enzyme systems for the removal of the C-peptide have not been identified. Insulin is then packaged into granules within the Golgi system and is ejected into the cytoplasm of the beta cell. At some point in this journey, zinc enters the secretory granules, complexes with insulin, and forms microcrystals of zinc insulin. Isolated beta granules have been examined with electron microscopy in negatively stained preparations, and lines of repeating periodicity 50 Å in diameter have been demonstrated. This distance is consistent with the size of the hexameric form of a zinc insulin crystal.

The preceding description of the mechanisms involved in the formation, storage, and release of insulin forms a basis for considering possible defects in this system in diabetes mellitus. As indicated earlier, the primary defect in diabetes appears to involve the release of insulin from the beta cell, with a sluggish response of the beta cell to glucose stimulation. This impaired response could be due to a defect involving glucoreceptors on the beta cell membrane, calcium transport, the adenylate cyclase system, or the microtubular–microfilamentous system. An animal model of diabetes exists which resembles diabetes in man. The spiny mouse (*Acomys cahirinus*) has a delayed insulin response to glucose stimulation with resultant diabetes. In vitro studies of islets from these animals have demonstrated a deficiency of microtubules [32] and a delayed and diminished formation of cyclic AMP following glucose stimulation.[36] A similar deficiency in insulin release can be produced by fasting rats for 48 hours [37] or by maintaining islets in vitro for 4 days in the presence of low concentrations of glucose.[38] In both of these conditions, adenylate cyclase activity and cyclic AMP within the islets are diminished. A deficiency in microtubules has also been demonstrated in the islets of the fasted rat.[39] These findings suggest a direct association between the adenylate cyclase system and the microtubular system, which in turn is associated with.an impaired insulin release. Human islets are needed in order to accomplish similar in vitro studies. The establishment of a Clinical Unit for Recent Expirations (CURE unit) in our institution has now made it feasible to obtain normal human islets from transplant donors, since the CURE unit encompasses a transplantation and autopsy suite. As this program is developed further, it is hoped that islets can also be obtained from diabetic patients in order to determine the intracellular defect or defects involving insulin release.

Alpha Cell Secretion

Relatively little information is available concerning the intracellular events involved in the release of glucagon from alpha cells. The primary stimulus for glucagon secretion appears to be amino acids. As indicated earlier, glucose causes an inhibition of glucagon release from normal alpha cells. It has been suggested that receptors for glucose may exist on the alpha cell, which in this case would initiate a series of events that would inhibit glucagon release in contrast to the stimulation of insulin release from beta cells. The release of glucagon from alpha cells has been shown to be biphasic in nature, similar to beta cell secretion.[40] The role of the microtubular–microfilamentous system in glucagon secretion has not been clearly established. Since circulating levels of glucagon are significantly elevated in diabetic subjects and cannot be suppressed with glucose following treatment with insulin, it has been suggested that a defect may also exist in the alpha cell.[24] This is an interesting hypothesis; however, it is possible that the lack of responsiveness of the alpha cell is simply an adaptational change to prolonged, recurrent exposure to elevated levels of glucose. In an insulin-dependent diabetic, it is not possible to maintain normoglycemia throughout a 24-hour interval; thus, the alpha cells are not exposed to normal levels of blood glucose for any long intervals of time during insulin therapy.

Etiology of Diabetes

Epidemiologic studies clearly indicate that diabetes is genetically determined. In maturity-onset diabetes, studies on identical twins have demonstrated a 90 percent chance that both of the individuals will become diabetic.[41] In contrast, in juvenile diabetes, the chance of both members of identical twins becoming diabetic is less than 50 percent.[42] These studies clearly indicate a genetic basis for maturity-onset diabetes. Recent studies on histocompatibility antigens in juvenile diabetics have demonstrated a significantly higher incidence of HLA-8 and W15 antigens in juvenile diabetics as compared to maturity-onset diabetics and the normal population.[43] Thus, juvenile diabetes would appear also to have a genetic basis that is probably different from maturity-onset diabetes.

Diabetes has been produced in certain strains of mice by infection with encephalomyocarditis virus.[44] The viral infection involves the islets with a resultant inflammatory reaction and destruction of islet tissue. The susceptibility to infection by this virus with the production of diabetes is genetically determined, since certain strains of mice are resistant to the development of diabetes. These experimental findings have, of course, led to the speculation that certain juvenile diabetics may be genetically susceptible to a viral infection that specifically affects the endocrine pancreas.

Circulating antibodies to normal human islet tissue have been demonstrated in juvenile diabetics during the initial two to three years of the disease.[45] The antigen participating in the reaction is apparently not insulin but is some other component of the islets. The antibody reacts with normal beta cells, but it is not certain whether other types of islet cells are also reacting. Experimentally, diabetes has been produced in the rabbit by repeated immunization with crystalline beef insulin.[46] Repeated immunization with homogenates of isolated rat islets produced fibrosis and deposition of hemosiderin in the islets of the immunized rats, but the animals did not become diabetic.[47]

In recent ultrastructural studies,[48] peculiar perinuclear inclusions were observed in ductal, acinar, and a few islet cells in juvenile diabetics and children with idiopathic hypoglycemia and islet hyperplasia (Fig. 3). The inclusions resemble the tubular type of network that has been reported in glomerular endothelial cells of patients with lupus erythematosis. The inclusions may be incomplete viruses or they may represent an unusual reaction of the cells to a specific injury. Ultrastructural studies are in progress on the pancreases of maturity-onset diabetics, neonatal deaths of offspring of diabetic mothers, and patients with beta cell tumors. The finding is intriguing, but it cannot be interpreted until these additional ultrastructural studies are completed and the perinuclear inclusions are isolated and identified.

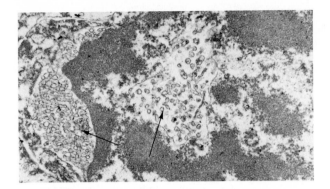

Fig. 3. Perinuclear and intranuclear inclusions in pancreatic duct cell of a juvenile diabetic. × 20,000. (Courtesy of Dr. Marie Greider, Washington University)

On the basis of circumstantial evidence, it could be suggested that the etiology of certain forms of juvenile diabetes may be due to a genetic susceptibility to infection of the pancreas by a specific virus, with resultant islet damage and the subsequent production of autoantibodies to the islets. In the maturity-onset diabetic, a genetic defect may exist in beta cells involving the secretion of insulin which coupled with an additional environmental stress such as obesity, would result in overt diabetes mellitus. The evidence is purely circumstantial—the concepts are simply speculations at the present time. Basic information is needed on the normal and abnormal structure and function of human islets. This information can only be obtained by in vitro, biochemical, metabolic, functional, and ultrastructural studies of islets obtained from recent expirations.

Transplantation of the Islets of Langerhans

While the basic investigations on the mechanism of insulin secretion and the search for the etiology and pathogenesis of diabetes mellitus are in progress, other approaches are being sought to attempt to prevent the complications of diabetes mellitus. The question that is of vital importance to these alternate approaches is the following: Are the complications of diabetes mellitus secondary to the altered metabolic state of the individual or are they due to a separate genetic defect? The classic studies of Kilo et al [49] and Williamson et al [50] on the thickness of the basement membrane of muscle capillaries of the lower extremities in normal and diabetic subjects have demonstrated the following: (a) In nondiabetic subjects, the capillary basement membrane increases in thickness with age. In the male, the increase in thickness is linear, whereas, in the female the increase in thickness reaches a plateau from age 30 to 60 and then increases again. (b) A significant increase in thickness of the basement membrane occurs in diabetic patients. (c) The incidence and amount of thickening in diabetic patients increases with the duration of the disease. (d) The thickness of the basement membrane is normal at the onset of juvenile diabetes. (e) In prediabetics, the thickness of the membrane is normal. (f) Significant thickening of the capillary basement membrane correlates with the clinical evidence of either diabetic retinopathy or glomerulonephropathy in diabetic patients. These findings clearly indicate that the microvascular changes in diabetes are truly complications of diabetes and are not due to separate genetic defects. Experimentally, microaneurysms of retinal vessels and intraretinal hemorrhage have been demonstrated in dogs with alloxan diabetes of five-years duration.[51] Studies on the effect of the control of the diabetic state in these animals indicate that the incidence of the retinal changes was decreased when the diabetic state was well controlled by insulin therapy. The production of diabetic retinopathy experimentally provides further evidence for the microvascular lesions being complications of diabetes, as well as indicating a relationship of the severity of the changes to the degree of control of the diabetes. These findings provide the impetus for devising a means of replacing the defective islet cells of diabetes with normal islet cells with the hope of preventing or arresting the complications of diabetes.

Transplantation of the whole pancreas has been attempted in 47 patients since 1966. In July, 1975, the transplanted pancreas in four of these patients was still functioning from 10 to 37 months after transplantation. Because of the complexity of this procedure and the risk of surgical complications, other means have been sought which would make it possible to transplant only the needed tissues—the islets of Langerhans.

The development in our laboratory of a simple procedure for the isolation of intact islets from the rat pancreas made it possible to attempt to transplant normal islets into inbred strains of rats with experimentally induced diabetes.[52, 53] Initially, the islets were transplanted into the abdominal cavity of the recipients, which produced a partial amelioration of the diabetic state. After trying several other implantation sites, we decided to inject the islets directly into the portal vein with the hope that the islets would be retained in the portal tract. This approach resulted in a complete reversion of the diabetic state to normal, and the animals remained normoglycemic for 1.5 years.[54] Allografts of islets injected into the portal vein also maintained normoglycemia when immunosuppressive agents were used.

Morphologic studies on the implanted islets in the liver demonstrated marked degranulation of the beta cells during the first few days after injection.[55] The islets became regranulated and reached a normal degree of beta granulation when the blood sugar remained normal (Fig. 4). Alpha, beta, and D cells could be demonstrated in the implanted islets. The implanted islets derived their vascular supply from both the arterial and portal venous system, as demonstrated by vascular injection techniques. The double vascular supply to the liver and to the islets was probably one of the major reasons for the success of this approach. Ultrastructural studies revealed a thick capillary endothelium during revascularization of the islets. Subsequently, the endothelium appeared fenestrated and resembled the capillaries of normal islets. It was of interest that desmosomes could be demonstrated between individual liver cells and islet cells.

The effect of islet transplantation on experimentally induced glomerular lesions in diabetic rats has been studied.[56] In diabetic animals, gamma globulin and other proteins were demonstrated by the fluorescent antibody technique in the mesangial area of the glomerulus, with a slight increase in thickness of the mesangium. The glomerular lesions disappeared following the establishment of normoglycemia in the diabetic animals by islet transplantation.

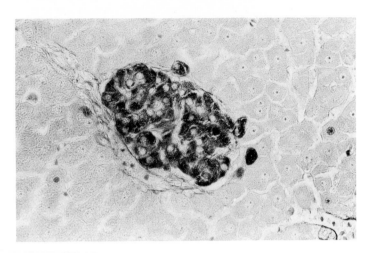

Fig. 4. Photomicrograph of an islet in the portal tract of the liver, 5 weeks after transplanting islets via portal vein injection into a diabetic rat. The rat was normoglycemic, and beta granulation was normal in the transplanted islets. Aldehyde fuchsin stain. $\times$ 400.

Many problems remain to be resolved before islet transplantation can be attempted in the human diabetic patient. The first problem is to develop procedures for the mass isolation of islets from the human pancreas. Human islets can be isolated by the collagenase technique, but the yield per gram of pancreas is much less than in the rat. The site of transplantation is a second problem, since it would not appear appropriate to inject islets into the entire vascular system of the liver. Studies in the rat indicate that islets can be injected via the portal vein into one lobe of the liver with a resultant establishment of normoglycemia in the diabetic animals. Normoglycemia can be attained by injecting the islets into the spleen of diabetic rats, but larger numbers of islets are required as compared to implanting the islets in the liver. When the technical problems are resolved and the optimum and safest site of implantation is determined, then it may be feasible to attempt islet transplantation into diabetic patients who are also receiving a renal transplant and are already receiving immunosuppressive agents. In order to evaluate the possible effectiveness of islet transplantation in arresting the complications of diabetes mellitus, it will be necessary to accomplish extensive, detailed investigations of the status of these complications prior to and following transplantation.

The Future

The exciting advances in the last few years provide a firm foundation for future exploration of the normal structure and function of the islet cells and the delineation of specific abnormalities of these cells in certain diseases in man. The recent recognition of new hormones in the islands of Langerhans will undoubtedly lead to the identification of new endocrine syndromes in man. Until a few years ago, diabetes was considered simply as a disease of insulin deficiency. It is now apparent that diabetes is a complex entity and most probably is not due to a single etiologic factor. Within the foreseeable future, the etiology of a segment of the diabetic population may well be determined, and definitive insight will be gained as to the etiology and pathogenesis of the remaining portion of diabetic patients.

Within a few years, islet cell transplantation will be accomplished in certain diabetic patients, and the question will be answered as to whether replacement of defective islet cells with normal islets will halt the progression of the microvascular and macrovascular complications of diabetes. From the standpoint of transplantation immunology, islet cell transplantation provides a superb model for attempting to alter the antigenic recognition of foreign cells by the host. Finally, this descriptive chronicle of the attainment of basic information on the normal structure and function of one endocrine gland, the translation of this information into devising new approaches for the therapy of diabetic patients, and the utilization of this information in the search for the etiology and pathogenesis of diseases involving the islands of Langerhans serve as one of many examples of the exciting challenge of amalgamating basic sciences with clinical sciences in the field of pathology.

References

1. Clark E: The number of islands of Langerhans in the human pancreas. Anat Anz 43:81, 1913
2. Bussolati G, Capella C, Vassallo G, Solcia E: Histochemical and ultrastructural studies on pancreatic A cells. Evidence for glucagon and nonglucagon components of the alpha granules. Diabetologia 7:181, 1971
3. Gomori G: Aldehyde-fuchsin: A stain for elastic tissues. Am J Clin Pathol 20:665, 1950
4. Misugi K, Howell SL, Greider MH, Lacy PE, Sorenson GD: The pancreatic beta cell. Demonstration of peroxidase-labeled antibody technique. Arch Pathol 89:97, 1970
5. Howell SL, Young DA, Lacy PE: Isolation and properties of secretory granules from rat islets of Langerhans. III. Biochemical studies of the isolated beta granules. J Cell Biol 41:167, 1969
6. Bloom W: A new type of granular cell in the islets of Langerhans of man. Anat Rec 49:363, 1931
7. Grimelius L: A silver nitrate stain for A_2 cells in human pancreatic islets. Acta Soc Med Ups 73:243, 1968
8. Pelletier G, LeClerc R, Arimura A, Schally AV: Immunohistochemical localization of somatostatin in the rat pancreas. J Histochem Cytochem 23:699, 1975
9. Dubois MP: Immunoreactive somatostatin is present in discrete cells of the endocrine pancreas. Proc Natl Acad Sci USA 72:1340, 1975
10. Gerich JE, Lorenzi M, Hane S, et al: Evidence for a physiologic role of pancreatic glucagon in human glucose homeostasis: Studies with somatostatin. Metabolism 24:175, 1975
11. Orci L, Unger RH: Functional subdivision of islets of Langerhans and possible role of D cells. Lancet 2:1243, 1975
12. Greider MH, Steinberg V, McGuigan JE: Electron microscopic identification of the gastrin cell of the human antral mucosa by means of immunocytochemistry. Gastroenterology 63:572, 1972
13. Greider MH, McGuigan JE: Cellular localization of gastrin in the human pancreas. Diabetes 20:389, 1971
14. Kimmel JR, Pollock HG, Hazelwood RL: A new polypeptide hormone. Fed Proc 30:1318, 1971
15. Hazelwood RL, Turner SD, Kimmel JR, Pollock HG: Spectrum effects of a new

polypeptide (third hormone?) isolated from the chicken pancreas. Gen Comp Endocrinol 21:485, 1973

16. Larsson LI, Sundler F, Hakanson R: Immunochemical localization of human pancreatic polypeptide (HPP) to a population of islet cells. Cell Tissue Res 156:167, 1975

17. McGavran MH, Unger RH, Recant L, et al: A glucagon-secreting-alpha-cell carcinoma of the pancreas. N Engl J Med 274:1408, 1966

18. Greider MH, Rosai J, McGuigan JE: The human pancreatic islet cells and their tumors. II. Ulcerogenic and diarrheogenic tumors. Cancer 33:1423, 1974

19. Zollinger RM, Ellison EH: Primary peptic ulcerations of the jejunum associated with islet cell tumors of the pancreas. Ann Surg 142:709, 1955

20. Verner JV, Morrison AG: Islet cell tumor and a syndrome of refractory watery diarrhea and hypokalemia. Am J Med 25:374, 1958

21. Sircus W, Brunt PW, Walker RJ, et al: Two cases of "pancreatic cholera" with features of peptide-secreting adenomatosis of the pancreas. Gut 11:197, 1970

22. Cerasi E, Luft R: The plasma insulin response to glucose infusion in healthy subjects and in diabetes mellitus. Acta Endocrinol (Kobenhavn) 55:278, 1967

23. Unger RH, Aguilar-Parada E, Muller WA, Eisentraut AM: Studies of pancreatic alpha cell function in normal and diabetic subjects. J Clin Invest 49:837, 1970

24. Unger RH, Orci L: The essential role of glucagon in the pathogenesis of diabetes mellitus. Lancet 1:14, 1975

25. Kelly WD, Lillehei RC, Merkel FK, Idezuki Y, Goetz FC: Allotransplantation of pancreas and duodenum along with kidney in diabetic nephropathy. Surgery 61:827, 1967

26. Matschinsky FM, Ellermann JE, Krzanowski J, et al: The dual function of glucose in islets of Langerhans. J Biol Chem 246:1007, 1971

27. Tomita T, Lacy PE, Matschinsky FM, McDaniel ML: Effect of alloxan on insulin secretion in isolated rat islet perfused in vitro. Diabetes 23:517, 1974

28. Malaisse-Lagae F, Malaisse WJ: The stimulus-secretion coupling of glucose-induced insulin release. III. Uptake of 45-calcium by isolated islets of Langerhans. Endocrinology 88:72, 1971

29. Lacy PE, Finke EH, Codilla RC: Cinemicrographic studies on beta granule movement in monolayer culture of islet cells. Lab Invest 33 (5):570, 1975

30. Lacy PE: Beta cell secretion—from the standpoint of a pathobiologist. Banting Memorial Lecture. Diabetes 19 (12):895, 1970

31. Lacy PE: Endocrine secretory mechanisms. Am J Pathol 79 (1):170, 1975

32. Orci L: A portrait of the pancreatic B cell. The Minkowski Award Lecture, 1973. Diabetologia 10:163, 1974

33. Williams JA, Wolff J: Possible role of microtubules in thyroid secretion. Proc Natl Acad Sci USA 67:1901, 1970

34. Bauer GE, Lindall AW, Dixit PK, Lester G, Lazarow A: Studies of insulin biosynthesis. Subcellular distribution of leucine-H^3 radioactivity during incubation of goosefish islet tissue. J Cell Biol 28:413, 1966

35. Howell SL, Kostianovsky M, Lacy PE: Beta granule formation in isolated islets of Langerhans: A study by electron microscopic radioautography. J Cell Biol 42:695, 1969

36. Cerasi E, Grill V, Rabinovitch A: Cyclic AMP in pancreatic B cells: Key role for insulin secretion. Frontiers of Internal Medicine. 12th Int Congr Internal Med, Tel Aviv, 1974. Karger, Basel, 1975, pp 115–19

37. Howell SL, Green IC, Montague W: A possible role of adenylate cyclase in the long-term dietary regulation of insulin secretion from rat islets of Langerhans. Biochem J 136:343, 1973

38. Lacy PE, Finke EH, Conant S, Naber S: Long-term perifusion of isolated rat islets in vitro. Diabetes 25:484, 1976

39. Pipeleers DG, Pipeleers-Marichal MA, Kipnis DM: Microtubule assembly and the

intracellular transport of secretory granules in pancreatic islets. Science 191:88, 1976

40. Norfleet WT, Pagliara AS, Haymond MW, Matschinsky F: Comparison of alpha and beta cell secretory responses in islets isolated with collagenase and in the isolated perfused pancreas of rats. Diabetes 24:961, 1975

41. Gottlieb MS, Root HF: Diabetes mellitus in twins. Diabetes 17:693, 1968

42. Tattersall RB, Pyke DA: Diabetes in identical twins. Lancet 2:1120, 1972

43. Nerup J, Platz P, Andersen OO, et al: HL-A antigens and diabetes mellitus. Lancet 2:864, 1974

44. Craighead JE, Stinke J: Diabetes mellitus-like syndrome in mice infected with encephalomyocarditis virus. Am J Pathol 63:119, 1971

45. Lendrum R, Walker G, Gamble DR: Islet cell antibodies in juvenile diabetes mellitus of recent onset. Lancet 1:880, 1975

46. Toreson WE, Lee JC, Grodsky GM: The histopathology of immune diabetes in the rabbit. Am J Pathol 52:1099, 1968

47. Heydinger DK, Lacy PE: Islet cell changes in the rat following injection of homogenized islets. Diabetes 23:579, 1974

48. Greider MH, Lacy PE, Kissane JM: Pancreatic perinuclear inclusions and idiopathic hypoglycemia. (submitted to Diabetes)

49. Kilo C, Vogler N, Williamson JR: Muscle capillary basement membrane changes related to aging and to diabetes mellitus. Diabetes 21:881, 1972

50. Williamson JR, Vogler N, Kilo C: Basement membrane thickening in muscle capillaries. Observations on diabetics and non-diabetics with both parents diabetic. In Scow RO (ed): Proceedings of the IV International Congress of Endocrinology. Amsterdam, Excerpta Medica, 1973, pp 1122–28

51. Engerman RL, Bloodworth JMB: Role of diabetes control in microvascular disease. Excerpta Medica, International Congress Series 280:188, 1973

52. Lacy PE, Kostianovsky M: A method for the isolation of intact islets of Langerhans from the rat pancreas. Diabetes 16:35, 1967

53. Ballinger WF, Lacy PE: Transplantation of intact pancreatic islets in rats. Surgery 72:175, 1972

54. Kemp CB, Knight MG, Scharp DW, Ballinger WF, Lacy PE: Transplantation of isolated pancreatic islets into the portal vein of diabetic rats. Nature 244:447, 1973

55. Griffith R, Scharp DW, Hartman B, Ballinger WF, Lacy PE: A morphologic study of the intraportal islet isograft. Diabetes 26:201, 1977

56. Mauer SM, Sutherland DER, Steffes MW, et al: Pancreatic islet transplantation. Effects on the glomerular lesions of experimental diabetes in the rat. Diabetes 23:748, 1975

THE PRUNE BELLY SYNDROME

H. JOACHIM WIGGER AND WILLIAM A. BLANC

The prune belly syndrome (PBS), classically described as the triad of absence or hypoplasia of abdominal muscles, urinary tract abnormalities, and cryptorchidism, is a rare but well-described entity. Anomalies of other organ systems may be associated with the syndrome, especially those of the intestinal tract and the skeletal system. This chapter reviews the cases autopsied at the Babies Hospital and previously published instances that fulfill the criteria for the full syndrome.[1-70] Conveniently, cases of PBS may be divided into those who die in the perinatal period, those who die in infancy and childhood, usually of chronic renal disease, and those who survive. Death from the syndrome in the neonatal period has generally been considered to be due to severe urinary tract involvement. In a significant number of cases, however, respiratory distress from pulmonary hypoplasia as part of the oligohydramnios syndrome may well have been the primary cause of death. In this instance, anuria or oliguria is associated with oligohydramnios. This is, in turn, complicated by amnion nodosum, pulmonary hypoplasia, Potter's facies, microgastria, and frequently, clubbed feet.[51, 71-74]

In view of the importance of the urinary tract pathology for the prognosis of patients with PBS, the relationship between renal pathology and lower urinary tract obstruction is of special significance. Some authors have played down the incidence and importance of obstruction, while others have emphasized it.[46, 49] A better understanding of the relationship between lower urinary tract obstruction and renal development, dysplasia, and cyst formation would be helpful in shedding light on this problem.

The abdominal muscle involvement has been believed to be a localized muscle agenesis or hypoplasia, related to the urinary tract malfunction.[62] In fact, abdominal muscle defects occur also as an isolated anomaly[75, 76] or in association with other neuromuscular syndromes like arthrogryposis[32, 45, 77] and the pterygium syndrome.[78] Our histologic findings suggest a myopathic or dysplastic process.

17

Material and Results

The data are summarized in Tables 1 through 4. The cases were collected over a period of 21 years.

In contrast to many of the previous studies, this chapter deals only with autopsied cases. Thus, it is not surprising that it includes mostly young patients with severe lesions. All of the 14 patients were infants and 12 died in the perinatal period, one was stillborn; only three of the patients were premature by weight, and two patients survived for 2 and 6 months, respectively. The fact that 13 of the 14 patients were male reflects the predominance of boys that has been noted in the literature. Our single female patient had both abdominal muscle defects and urinary tract malformations (Table 1).

TABLE 1. Babies Hospital
Cases of Prune Belly Syndrome

Total Number		*14 **
Sex	Male	13
	Female	1
Birth	Term	11
	Premature	3
Death	Perinatal	12
	Infancy	2

* Material for one of these cases was kindly made available by Drs. E. Dawson, R. Carnes, and F. d'Esposito of St. Michael's Medical Center, Newark, N.J.

The degree of abdominal muscle deficiency was difficult to evaluate in the older cases because of incomplete dissection and sampling. In the 4 most recent cases, a detailed evaluation was made which included controls (Table 2).

Complete absence of the transverse abdominal muscle was seen in 2 cases, that of the rectus in 1. The other muscles were either hypoplastic, normal, or showed focal aplasia. The individual fibers in the involved muscles varied from severe atrophy to marked hypertrophy. Vessels and nerves appeared normal (Figs. 1 and 2).

There was no grouping of muscle fibers by size as seen in neurogenic atrophy. In 3 cases the entire spinal cords were sampled histologically but failed to show any appreciable variation from the usual. In some sections, the whole muscle thinned out within the fascia, in others the muscle seemed replaced by thick bundles of wavy collagen surrounded by the fascia, containing cartilage or fragments of muscle fibers (Figs. 3 and 4). Muscle spindles were frequently seen in the hypoplastic muscles, suggesting secondary muscular atrophy. Isolated muscle bundles demonstrated widened spacing of Z bands and fragmentation. The most hypertrophied muscle fibers, at times, had central cavities. Occasional fibers showed a condensation of sarcolemmal nuclei.

TABLE 2. Abdominal Muscle Deficiency in Four Cases

Case Number	Transverse Abdominal		Internal Oblique		External Oblique		Rectus	
BA 10,237	Ø	Ø	(+)	(+)	(+)	(+)	(+)	(+)
	Ø	Ø	Ø	Ø	Ø	(+)	(+)	Ø
BA 10,253	Ø	Ø	(+)	Ø	(+)	(+)	(+)	Ø
	Ø	Ø	(+)	Ø	(+)	Ø	(+)	(+)
BA 10,600	(+)	(+)	(+)	(+)	(+)	(+)	Ø	Ø
	(+)	Ø	(+)	(+)	(+)	(+)	Ø	Ø

Medial Portion of IO, EO, and T Absent

BA 10, 958	(+)	(+)	+	+	(+)	(+)	+	(+)
	(+)	(+)	+	(+)	(+)	(+)	+	+

φ, absence of muscle; (+), hypoplasia of muscle; +, normal muscle mass.

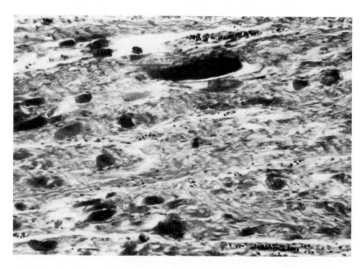

Fig. 1. Rudimentary skeletal muscle fibers are surrounded by wavy fibrous tissue. H&E. × 230.

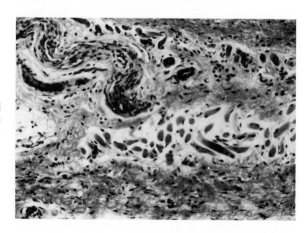

Fig. 2. Fibrous tissue and fragments of muscle with nerve and blood vessels. H&E. × 120.

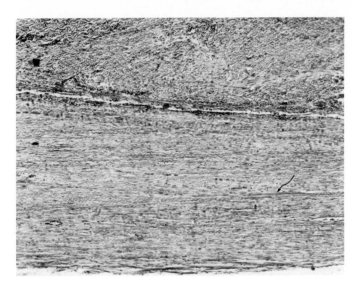

Fig. 3. Layers of wavy collagen take the place of skeletal muscle; only a solitary muscle fiber is present (arrow). H&E. × 63.

Bladder and ureters were abnormal in all cases (Table 3). Megacystis was impressive in some cases, in others, the hypertrophy was more evident than the dilatation (Fig. 5). The more distended bladders also had diverticula. Draining of a persistent urachus at the navel was associated with a relatively small but hypertrophied bladder. The thickening of the bladder wall was due to increase in smooth muscle. Fibrosis was only seen in the urachus.

Hypoplasia of the prostate made the organ appear flatter than normal; a decreased number of tubules was observed in 4 of 6 cases in which enough material

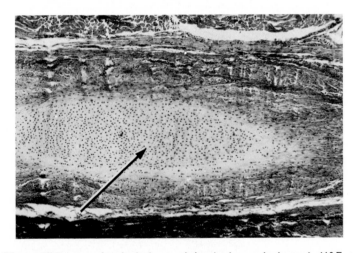

Fig. 4. Fibrocartilagenous dysplasia in an abdominal muscle (arrow). H&E. × 63.

TABLE 3. Findings at Autopsy:
Genitourinary Tract

Bladder	
Megacystis	14/14
Diverticulum	4/14
Urachus	
Patent	8/14
Draining	4/14
Prostate, hypoplasia	4/13
Urethra	
Atresia	3/14
Valve	4/14
Stenosis	4/14
Proximal dilatation	8/14
Phimosis	3/12
Penis, hypoplasia	2/13
Ureters	
Megaureter	14/14
Stenosis	4/14
Atresia	2/14
Kidney	
Hypoplasia	3/14
Dysplasia	11/14
Hydronephrosis	8/14
Pyelonephritis	5/14

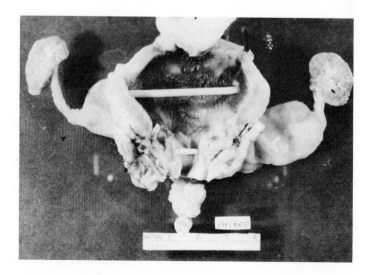

Fig. 5. Megacystis, megaureters, and bilateral renal hypoplasia and dysplasia of a newborn. The anterior urethra was atretic, the proximal urethra dilated, and the urachus patent. The lungs showed hyaline membrane disease.

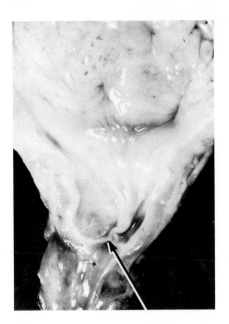

Fig. 6. Posterior urethral valve (arrow) in a full-term newborn with oligohydramnios syndrome, hyaline membrane disease, pneumothorax, and pneumomediastinum. The kidneys revealed only subcapsular cysts.

was available for study. One other prostate was not only flat but also extended posteriorly into the bladder wall.

Obstruction of the urethra anywhere from the bladder neck to the prepuce was observed in 8 of the 14 cases. Each type, atresia, valve, or stenosis, was seen in about the same frequency (Table 3). In 1 case, the entire anterior urethra was

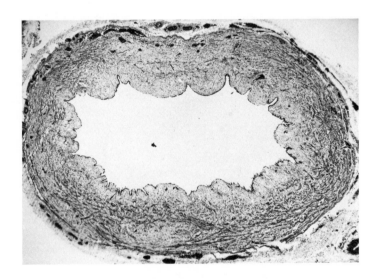

Fig. 7. Partial ureteral fibrosis in a megaureter. H&E. $\times$ 25.

absent (Fig. 6). The penis was found to be hypoplastic twice, but any sign of defective closure of the anterior abdominal wall—epispadias, exstrophy, or omphalocele—was not detected.

The ureters were all found to be dilated and at least somewhat tortuous (Fig. 5). Stenosis of the ureters was found 3 times at the ureteropelvic junction, and only once at the ureterovesical junction. One of the atretic ureters was partially forked. Focal fibrosis of the wall was seen in 3 of 8 cases (Fig. 7). None of the 4 cases of ureteral obstruction were associated with hydronephrosis because of insufficient urine production by the dysplastic kidneys.

The association of a distal obstruction with renal cystic dysplasia deserves special emphasis. All 11 cases with dysplasia were accompanied by some form of obstruction of either ureter or urethra or both. Two cases had ureteral atresia alone, 2 had associated urethral atresia, 1 of these with stenosis at the ureteropelvic junction, and 4 cases had associated urethral obstruction due to valves. Three types of dysplasia were distinguished in the kidneys, none associated with congenital hepatic fibrosis:

1. A severe cystic dysplasia with marked disorganization of the parenchyma, reduction in nephrons, metaplastic cartilage formation, and an increase in loose mesenchyme (Fig. 8). This picture was seen in 5 cases, 1 of which had virtually no renal parenchyma at all (Fig. 9). Two of these were associated with urethral atresia, 1 with urethral stenosis, and 1 with ureteral atresia. This type of cystic dysplasia corresponds to Potter type II cystic kidney (failure of nephron induction).[72]
2. Three cases had changes of Potter type IV cystic kidney (dysplasia secondary

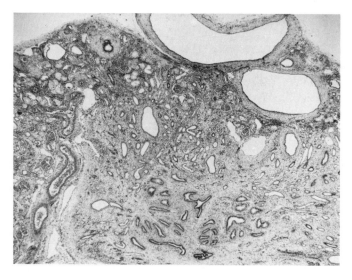

Fig. 8. Disorganization and deficient nephron formation in a dysplastic cystic kidney. H&E. × 25.

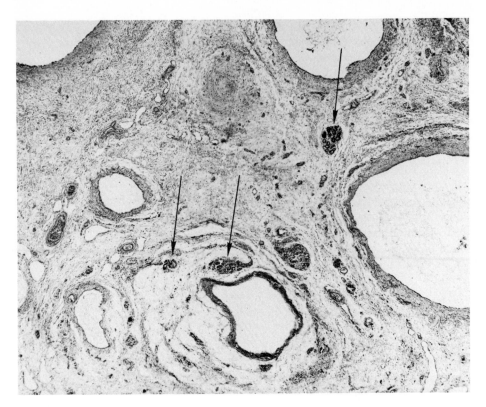

Fig. 9. Renal agenesis. Tissue from the expected site of the kidney contains a few cysts and rudimentary tubules. H&E. × 18.

to obstruction) with subcapsular cortical cysts and good preservation of renal parenchyma (Fig. 10); all were associated with urethral valves.[72]

3. Two cases demonstrated renal changes that fell somewhere between the two previous groups. In this mixed category, type IV alterations were prevalent throughout the kidneys; however, at least one segment revealed architectural disorganization with findings of cystic dysplasia of type II (Potter), such as reduction in nephrons, increase in loose mesenchymal tissue, and abnormal tubular elements, as well as occasional fibrous-walled cysts. The lower urinary tract obstruction associated with this type of renal change was a urethral valve in one instance and a ureteral atresia in the other.

Hypoplasia of the kidneys in the absence of dysplasia was found bilaterally twice, and unilaterally once; in the bilateral hypoplasia there was, however, preponderance of the hypoplasia on one side. Hydronephrosis was bilateral in all but one case. The development of pyelonephritis may be related to the coexistence of obstruction and dysplasia.

Cryptorchidism was present in 12 of the 13 males of this series. The reason for the testicular descent in the single exception was not evident; all other features were typical of the PBS.

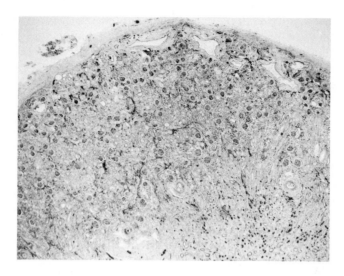

Fig. 10. Subcapsular cysts (Potter type IV). H&E. $\times$ 25.

Some form of malrotation of the bowel was the most frequent associated intestinal anomaly (Table 4). Jejunal atresia, imperforate anus, and rectovesical fistula were encountered once, all in the same patient. Ileal stenosis occurred in another case; this infant was also the only one with a single umbilical artery in the group.

Deformity of thorax and extremities were the most commonly observed

**TABLE 4. Associated Malformations
at Autopsy**

Malrotation	6/14
Ileum, stenosis	1/14
Jejunum, atresia	1/14
Anus imperforate	1/14
Fistula, rectovesical	1/14
Spleen, cyst	1/14
Foramen ovale, fenestrated	1/14
Ductus arteriosus, dilatation	1/14
Ductus venosus, dilatation	2/14
Ductus venosus, stenosis	1/14
Vertebral artery, left absence	1/14
Single umbilical artery	1/14
Lung, hypoplasia	5/14
Lung, accessory lobe	1/14
Thorax, deformity	5/14
Palate, arched	1/14
Neck, short	1/14
Digit, hypoplasia	2/14
Varus deformity, feet and knees	8/14
Joints, thickening	1/14
Potter's facies	5/14

skeletal anomalies. Five patients had a deformity of the chest. These included pectus excavatum or pigeon chest (3), poor development of the sternum (1), shortening of the rib cage (1), and asymmetry (2). The flaring of the rib cages is considered to be secondary to the absence of abdominal muscles.

Pulmonary pathology was a striking and unusual finding encountered in six patients. In five of these, pulmonary hypoplasia was present as part of the oligohydramnios syndrome. Two of these patients developed hyaline membrane disease in spite of being full-term infants. One of the premature infants also had hyaline membrane disease. The presence of Potter's facies is related to the oligohydramnios syndrome; it is characterized by a flattened and crooked nose, abnormally shaped ears, receding chin, and prominent palpebral folds. Clubbed feet have been believed to be the result of oligohydramnios as well, but in this series, they were also seen in 6 cases without evidence of the oligohydramnios syndrome at birth. An empty, hypoplastic stomach accompanied one case of pulmonary hypoplasia and was also secondary to oligohydramnios. Since little or no amniotic fluid was available for swallowing by the fetus, the stomach remained relatively empty and small.

The opposite occurred with polyhydramnios in the case of jejunal atresia. Little amniotic fluid was absorbed by the short fetal intestine proximal to the obstruction. This led to an increase in fluid in the amniotic cavity and to distention of the stomach with amniotic fluid.

Discussion

Muscle

The term "prune belly" is particularly descriptive of the appearance of the abdominal wall in the newborn with deficient abdominal musculature (Fig. 11). Because of its colorful and distinctive character, this sign has frequently been used as label for the whole syndrome. One should, however, keep in mind that mild deficiency of abdominal muscles might not give the characteristic picture or that a markedly distended bladder may mask it. Also, the appearance of the abdominal wall will change with age from wrinkled and wizened, thin and crisscrossed with creases in the newborn, to more like a potbelly when the abdominal panniculus adiposus increases.[58] If only the recti are absent, a midline vertical ridgelike protrusion of the abdominal contents may develop.[62] * Occasionally, the abdominal distention in PBS has been thought to be responsible for dystocia during delivery.[47] Infants with uremia from severe congenital urethral obstruction may have flabby muscle and a distended abdomen possibly from an enlarged bladder, but not true abdominal muscle deficiency.[58]

It should also be noted that both in males and females abdominal muscle deficiency may occur alone or in association with anomalies that are usually not part of the PBS, such as fibrocystic disease of the pancreas (B.H. case), arthrogryposis multiplex,[32, 77] or the pterygium syndrome.[78] Therefore, we would like to

* See Babies Hospital case 9.

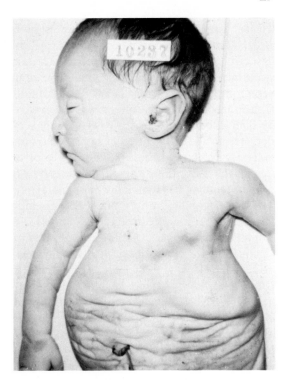

Fig. 11. Newborn infant with "prune belly," flaring and asymmetry of thorax, and Potter's facies. This patient also had pulmonary hypoplasia and hyaline membrane disease.

define the term "prune belly syndrome" as the obligatory association of abdominal muscle deficiency with urinary tract abnormalities with or without anomalies of other organs. In this form, the syndrome was first described by Parker in 1895.[1] Since then, about 265 cases have been reported in the literature.[1-70]

Previous reports agree that the lower abdominal muscles are usually more severely affected than the upper ones.[49, 58] In most cases, the muscles are present near the costal margins and the flanks, and occasionally only one side may be affected.[62] Housden [19] gives the incidence of deficiency of the individual muscles as follows: transverse abdominal × 25, rectus below navel × 24, internal oblique × 23, external oblique × 21, and rectus above navel × 12.

Older theories on the etiology of the abdominal muscle deficiency included intrauterine poliomyelitis, congenital syphilis, and deficiency of intramural nerve plexus, as well as atrophy secondary to pressure from an enlarged bladder.[4, 19, 26, 44, 80] None have been proven to be applicable in all instances.[46, 84] Primary aplasia or hypoplasia has been favored and is supported by the reported absence of fascia and nerves in some cases.[62] Recent studies concur with some of our findings and suggest a focal congenital muscular dystrophy.[69] The presence of apparently normal anterior horn cells argues against a neurogenic atrophy (three B.H. cases).[26]

The possibility of a neurogenic or primary myopathy is suggested in some cases by an arthrogryposislike picture with flexion deformity and genu valgum.[83] Three apparently classic cases of arthrogryposis were indeed found to be associated with absence of abdominal muscles.[32, 45, 77] Another case of abdominal muscle deficiency was complicated by weakness of muscles of the shoulder and pelvic girdle and pterygium formation; this was believed to fit the pterygoarthromyelodysplasia of Rossi.[78] The contractures in this case were not deformative, and cranial and spinal nerves were normal. Extensive contractures might be inferred from the picture in the report of Ráliš and Forbes,[64] although the massively dilated bladder of their macerated male infant was believed to have exerted enough pressure on the iliac arteries to lead to uneven atrophy of muscle and gangrene of the right foot. There had been no evidence to suspect an amniotic band as cause of this pathology. Whether or not the hypoplasia of the iliac arteries was due to the compression or was primary is difficult to say. The lower extremities were described to be in semiflexion, semiabduction, and external rotation at the hip joints. A case with single umbilical artery and PBS was also associated with hypoplasia of one iliac artery, but muscle atrophy had not occurred.[60]

At this point one should consider deformative changes due to longstanding oligohydramnios. One of our cases exhibited an arthrogryposislike picture with stiffness and thickening of joints and reduced mobility probably from contractures; there was definite evidence of oligohydramnios with pulmonary and gastric hypoplasia as well as clubbed feet. The other reports of arthrogryposis with absence of abdominal muscles failed to comment on the amniotic fluid volume and the lesions associated with it.[32, 45, 77] Clubfeet are believed, at least at times, to be due to this condition. A transient oligohydramnios may explain the development of clubfeet and the absence of oligohydramnios at birth.

The predominant involvement of abdominal muscles in the medial and lower regions and the dysplastic changes observed in our material suggest an interference with normal development and differentiation of somitic mesenchyme to striated muscle. In the somitic embryo, one finds the paraxial mesoderm divided into a medial segmental component, the somites, and an unsegmented lateral plate mesoderm bridged by the nephrogenic cord (Fig. 12). Formation of the coelomic cavity splits the lateral plate mesoderm into a visceral layer (origin of muscular and serosal coats of primitive gut and derivatives) and a parietal or somatic layer which contributes to the body wall. Exempted is the most caudal part of the

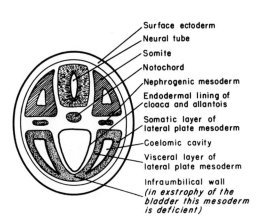

Surface ectoderm
Neural tube
Somite
Notochord
Nephrogenic mesoderm
Endodermal lining of cloaca and allantois
Somatic layer of lateral plate mesoderm
Coelomic cavity
Visceral layer of lateral plate mesoderm
Infraumbilical wall (in exstrophy of the bladder this mesoderm is deficient)

Fig. 12. Schematic cross section through the infraumbilical part of a somite embryo. (After Glenister).[92]

embryo, to which the coelom does not extend and where an undivided lateral plate mesoderm extends around cloaca and allantois, joining in the middle and thus separating these organs from the infraabdominal ectoderm. The deeper portion of this lateral plate mesoderm gives rise to the musculature of cloaca and allantois and later forms the bladder wall. The abdominal muscle does not, however, develop from lateral plate mesoderm, but from lower thoracic somites.[91] Their ventral extensions or buds migrate into the lateral plate mesoderm lateromedially and craniocaudally, and differentiate in a craniocaudal sequence. This process of somitic bud formation seems to take place in embryos from 5 to 9 mm in length; at this stage, the mesoblast changes to secondary mesenchyme and myoblasts, the differentiating cells showing a high RNA content. Gradually, the muscle will extend to the ventral midline.[91, 92]

The integrity of the abdominal wall is not affected in PBS, and neither omphalocele, exstrophy of the bladder, nor epispadias occur. These are defects of the lower lateral plate mesoderm which fails to meet in midline; a contact between endoderm and ectoderm persists along the midline until this infraumbilical membrane breaks down and exposes the lumen of cloaca and allantois or later the urogenital sinus. The thoracic somites, however, are not affected, explaining why the abdominal muscle can migrate as far as the margin of the cleft.[92]

In PBS, a noxious insult probably occurs when the lateral plate mesoderm has already extended to the midline. Then the somitic buds either fail to differentiate into myoblasts, or the myoblasts fail to continue their ventral and caudal migration, or already formed abdominal muscle undergoes degeneration. The presence of fibrous tissue enclosed by the fascia that should surround muscle suggests faulty differentiation (Fig. 1). The total absence of muscle in the central portion of the abdomen may imply deficient migration or complete absence of a mesenchymal development (Fig. 12). The dystrophic and sporadic appearance of muscle in the wall speaks for a haphazard differentiation, incomplete migration, or a partial degeneration of already formed muscle.

Bladder

One of the most common findings reported with the PBS are enlargement and hypertrophy of the urinary bladder. It was seen in about 60 percent of cases reported and in all of the Babies Hospital cases. These changes are easily understood when distal obstruction is obvious. Duration and degree of obstruction are clearly determinants of the severity of the bladder pathology. Thus, in cases of urethral atresia, the megacystis syndrome presents its classic picture. With such severe and longstanding obstruction, the bladders are largest and thickest unless outflow of urine is provided via a patent urachus. When the ureters are also obstructed, one might assume that this was a relatively late event, which occurred after the bladder had already had time to react to another more distal obstruction. If, however, no adequate evidence for obstruction distal to the bladder can be detected, the cause is very difficult to determine. Aganglionosis or deficient innervation have been blamed by some.[33] The discovery of intestinal aganglionosis and associated dilatation of the urinary tract initially supported this possibility and so did the report of simultaneous occurrence of the PBS with megacolon by Blasi.[82] Unfortunately, he did not have any pathologic confirmation of the diagnosis of aganglionosis in the urinary or the intestinal tract and, in fact, did not present evidence of urinary tract pathology at all. Later reports demonstrated ample nerves and ganglion cells around the bladder in PBS.[48, 58, 59] Of interest is the single female case in our series in whom a segment of ileum was found at autopsy to be hypoganglionic. It is impossible to be certain whether this decrease in ganglion cells was a primary deficiency or secondary to anoxia; the patient had undergone previous surgery for ileal stenosis and developed peritonitis and sepsis. Other investigators found focal patchy fibrosis and absence of smooth muscle in the bladder, which might lead to poor and uneven contraction.[49, 58] The only fibrosis seen in any of our cases was present in the transition zone between bladder and urachus and the urachus itself.

Also of interest are the results of electromanometric pressure tests used in addition to contrast studies. Nunn and Stephens[49] found their three survivors with dilated urinary tracts to have normal voiding pressure in the bladder and normal pressure gradients, although the bladder capacity was greater than normal and detrusor action was uneven. The latter resulted in an hourglass effect because the lower portion of the bladder contracted better than the superior portion. One wonders whether or not this poorly contracting portion was part of the urachus.

Both the smooth muscle hypertrophy and the fibrosis of the bladder may be due to the same noxious insult that could have interfered with the growth and differentiation of the abdominal muscles. At approximately the same time as these develop, the visceral layer of the lateral plate mesoderm contributes smooth muscle to the urinary tract. Interference with this normal process would explain the megacystis in the absence of distal obstruction.

Urethra

There has been a great variation in the literature about the frequency and significance of urethral obstruction. Lattimer judged the incidence to be 85 percent, while others made a strong point for dilatation without obstruction.[19, 24, 49, 62] The overall incidence of urethral obstruction of the reported and reviewed cases is about 32 percent. Most of these (23 percent) showed stenosis. Atresia, valve, diaphragm, diverticulum, and phimosis were much less common. It must, however, be mentioned that in many reports, detailed information was missing, and the true incidence of mechanical obstruction may be higher.

In our series, it occurred in 8 of 14 cases, an obviously slanted incidence because all cases were fatal. At times, a distinct obstruction may not be evident, but the entire anterior urethra may be narrowed.[49] This is usually associated with hypoplasia of the prostate and dilatation of the prostatic urethra. Prostatic hypoplasia was mentioned in the literature not infrequently (29 times). Which of the two lesions, prostatic hypoplasia or dilatation of the prostatic urethra, is cause and which effect is difficult to say. Some authors believed that faulty development of the prostate, especially of the smooth muscle component, was concomitant with muscle deficiency in the bladder.[62] A decrease or absence of the prostatic epithelium may also occur.[49] The defect of the smooth muscle layer in the anterior urethra gave rise to a congenital diverticulum in one case.[50] Rising pressure in the urethra has led to reflux into the utriculus.[49] However, dilatation of the bladder may occur in the absence of urethral obstruction, as well as in fibrosis with muscle defects of the bladder as one of the Babies Hospital cases demonstrates. One wonders about the influence of hormones on these structures, especially during their development. Injections of large amounts of estrogen into mice have been known to produce a marked dilatation of the urethra and the urinary bladder, sometimes associated with megaureter and hydronephrosis. If the male animals were so treated prior to testicular descent, they remained cryptorchid.[85] There were no comments in the maternal records of our cases as to hormonal therapy.

Two possibilities for a temporary exacerbation or relief of obstruction remain to be mentioned. In PBS, a megacystis, when filled, may prolapse anteriorly and thus produce kinking with hindrance of the urinary outflow [45]; it has been suggested, in turn, that an increase in pressure proximal to an obstruction may become sufficiently high to overcome the obstacle.[47]

For most cases, however, it appears more reasonable to assume again an interference with mesenchymal growth and differentiation as cause of urethral malformations, as already suggested by Boissonnat and Duhamel.[50] This interference may take the form of absence or hypoplasia of smooth muscle with or without fibrosis beginning in the prostate. It may also lead to abnormal development of the mesenchyme designed to form the urethral fold, eg, failure of formation of a lumen for the endodermal urethral plate in the penile urethra (Fig. 2).

Ureter

Megaureters seem to be even more common with PBS than enlargement and thickening of the bladder. It was reported in 81 percent of all cases published and demonstrable in all of the Babies Hospital cases. Mural fibrosis and muscle deficiency have been observed in the ureters, as in the other portions of the lower urinary tract. Atresia, stenosis, and ureterocele were rarely recorded in the literature. Yet, dilatation has definitely been found in the absence of distal obstruction.[58] Nunn and Stephens were struck by the remarkable variation in ureteral size and contour from case to case and from one side to the other. While general elongation and enlargement of gross proportions with tortuosity occurred, focal gigantism or focal narrowing were seen more commonly. The ureteral orifices were all patent, except for one stenosis.[49, 58] Vesicoureteral reflux was not uncommon in older patients studied roentgenologically and might account for some of the ureteral dilatation.[26, 48, 53, 58, 61] Functionally, such megaureters have shown atony.[49, 59] Radiographically, peristalsis was not evident; ureteral pressure studies in one child confirmed these observations. Thus with or without obstruction or reflux, these ureters seem to be inefficient urinary conduits.[62]

A cause for this poor function has been sought in a deficiency of ganglion cells or nerves. Some authors have claimed to have seen ganglion cells in the ureteral wall, others have come to the conclusion that ganglion cells are not present.[86, 87] A considerable autonomic innervation, however, is not in doubt, but it is believed that ureteric peristalsis cannot be coordinated by this nerve net, as it is too sparsely distributed and devoid of ganglion cells. It is presumed to be able to influence ureteric activity only by way of the efferent nerves observed. The co-ordinated wave of ureteral contractions is passed along the ureter by transmission of the excitation from smooth muscle cell to smooth muscle cell through their nexus.[87] It is conceivable that multiple areas of fibrosis as seen with the PBS may interfere with a normal propagation of the wave of contraction. This could then represent the initial handicap in function followed by dilatation and tortuosity exacerbating the poor urinary flow. Deficiency of smooth muscle, fibrosis, stenosis, and atresia could again be explained best as in the case of urethra, bladder, and abdominal muscles, namely, by a disturbance of growth and differentiation of mesenchyme derived from the visceral layer of the lateral plate mesoderm.

Kidney

The renal involvement in the PBS may be severe or mild, or may be considered either primary or secondary to distal obstruction and to infection. The variation in the pathology has been considerable and confusing. The most severe and also primary defect of the kidney with PBS is unilateral agenesis; it occurred three times in more than 200 cases. Hypoplasia was recorded in 10 percent of cases. In our experience and in one other report, hypoplasia has a tendency to be unilateral or, if bilateral, to be more severe on one side.[2] At times, the opposite kidney was enlarged. Other anomalies, such as horseshoe kidney (once), ectopy (twice), or duplication of pelvis and ureter (once) were extremely rare. A single instance of nephrolithiasis was reported in a 4-year-old boy with a long history of renal disease, including infection and ureteral stenosis on the side of the nephrolithiasis.[56]

Renal dysplasia was reported in 25 of the 265 previously published cases, but its type cannot be evaluated from the descriptions. In contrast, we found dysplasia and cyst formation in the kidneys of 11 of our 14 autopsies. Dysplasia is here understood in its widest sense as any disorganization of renal parenchyma during development with or without cyst formation or metaplasia. All our cases were associated with some degree of distal obstructive malformation. The severest dysplasia involved both entire kidneys and would seem to be incompatible with normal renal function and life. Potter [79] found such cases reminiscent of her type II cystic kidneys. Their small size and the associated ureteral abnormalities support this interpretation. Most likely, these kidneys were damaged much before significant numbers of nephrons were formed, ie, at the stage of ampullary development. The severe disorganization, impaired nephron induction, and increase in connective tissue support this view. Most of the cysts may be either terminal portions of collecting tubules or greatly enlarged primitive nephrons of early generations. What the relationship of this teratogenic event is to the lower urinary tract obstruction and to abdominal muscle deficiency is still in the realm of speculation, but it seems more likely that both are the result of the same teratogenic injury rather than that the kidney lesions are secondary to the distal malformation. From this point of view, it is not surprising that severe renal dysplasia is also associated with severe ureteral or urethral malformations.

In case of the mixed form of dysplasia, ie, focal type II and generalized type IV cystic kidneys (Potter), the organs seem to have escaped severe injury during their early development and are capable of producing urine. Since only in the last half of intrauterine life is urine output appreciable, cystic changes of type IV can develop following distal obstruction.

The same argument holds true for purely type IV cystic kidneys in PBS. The structures responsible for intrinsic development are normal, especially the ureteral-bud ampulla and its divisions. Cysts are found in the subcapsular cortex and the columns of Bertin. They are formed by late generations of nephrons still in S form. Collecting tubules are usually normal or only slightly distended. Maturation of older nephrons is normal. The extent of the cystic change is determined by the degree of obstruction and the length of time it has been present. The reason that only late generation nephrons are affected, according to Potter, lies in their direct alignment with the collecting tubules; the older nephrons are protected by virtue of their acutely angulated takeoff from the collecting tubules. Thus the great mass of renal parenchyma is normal, assuring adequate renal function, if the distal urinary tract obstruction can be relieved.

The incidence of hydronephrosis in our series was smaller than that of dysplastic and cystic malformations. The cause may be in part the incompleteness of the obstruction and in part the reduction in urine output from severely malformed kidneys. In addition, such kidneys have usually also poorly formed papillae and calyces making diagnosis of a mild or moderate hydronephrosis quite difficult. One would most likely expect hydronephrosis with kidneys that have near normal urine output and obstruction below the renal pelvis. Such information cannot be gleaned from the literature in which the total incidence of recorded hydronephrosis in PBS is about 50 percent. The incidence of 17 percent for pyelonephritis does not appear high when one considers that poor urinary flow and dysplasia are likely to lead to urinary tract infection.[62]

Testes

One of the most constant findings in PBS is cryptorchidism. In only 2.5 percent of all cases reported and reviewed had the testes descended into the scrotum. When intraabdominal, the testes were often lifted off the posterior abdominal wall by the enlarged ureters. If not located near the inguinal ring, they were most often found near the ureterovesical junction, or attached to the midportion of the ureters.[46, 49] The gubernaculum may be long, short, or absent.[49, 58] The histology of testis, epididymis, and vas deferens was normal for prepuberal age.[49, 62] Chromosomal abnormalities were found only twice.[52, 62, 66] These isolated cases of chromosomal mosaicism (45/XY, 16–46/XY) occurred in two siblings with classic PBS.[66] The infertility of the male patients with PBS is most likely due to the progressive disappearance of spermatogonia in cryptorchid testes after the age of 6 to 7 years. In PBS, the testicular descent has been believed to have been hindered by the megacystis and megaureters.[26, 34] Yet Helbig's patient with Fröhlich's syndrome (abdominal muscle deficiency) had cryptorchid testes in the absence of any urinary tract pathology.[76] It seems more likely that either hormonal factors are responsible, or failure of formation of the inguinal canal or the gubernaculum testis.[58, 62]

Associated Anomalies

Gastrointestinal anomalies are associated with the PBS in about 25 percent of cases in some series.[48, 60] In our series, the frequency was about 20 percent. The most common anomaly is malrotation. It has been explained as the result of the urinary tract malformation, but it is more likely to be secondary to the enlargement of the abdominal cavity and a dilatation of the embryonal umbilical orifice, both being due to deficiency of the abdominal muscles.[52] The return of small and large bowel into the abdominal cavity may thus happen in a disorderly sequence and lead to failure of normal attachment.[26, 80, 81] Imperforate anus, small bowel atresia, and stenosis, as well as atresia of extrahepatic bile ducts, were extremely rare.

Skeletal anomalies were quite common in PBS. In our series, they were reported in 16 percent of cases. Other reports gave a higher incidence, eg, 29 to 41 percent, for anomalies of the lower extremities only.[46, 48, 62] Aside from chest deformities (pigeon chest, Harrison groove), scoliosis, spina bifida, hip dislocation, and club feet have been noted. Hypoplasia of digits and portions of a lower extremity were also occasionally seen. One wonders about the possible relationship between single umbilical artery, hypoplasia of iliac vessels, and underdevelopment of an extremity (B.H. case).[60] Positional malformation could certainly be related to oligohydramnios, and amniotic bands could result in hypoplasia, gangrene, or amputation of all or a portion of an extremity. Torticollis and micrognathia were seen only in an isolated instance.[59]

Cardiovascular malformations were mentioned only in 15 instances and, as in our cases, affected mainly the ductus arteriosus and the foramen ovale with two exceptions, one cor triatriatum with coarctation of the aorta and one tetralogy. Central nervous system malformations were extremely rare; hydrocephalus and macrogyria each were noted only once.[32, 64]

Insufficient emphasis has been given the pulmonary hypoplasia in PBS.[51] While the lungs may be inflated to some degree, overzealous artificial ventilation may lead to rupture of air spaces and exacerbation of the respiratory distress by interstitial emphysema, pneumomediastinum, and pneumothorax. Even if fatal pneumothorax does not occur, an air block syndrome may lead to the infant's demise.[89] The coexistence of hypoplasia and hyaline membrane disease in the lung of term infants should also be considered when a baby with PBS exhibits respiratory distress. All newborn infants with PBS ought to be suspected of having pulmonary hypoplasia until proven otherwise. The presence of Potter's facies and amnion nodosum would make the diagnosis almost certain. Unless there had been chronic leakage of amniotic fluid, this would imply that the baby had either severe renal disease preventing urine formation or a severe urinary tract obstruction or both.

Conclusion

The great variety of anomalies in the PBS has been puzzling. The major and obligatory components of the syndrome, ie, abdominal muscle deficiency and urinary tract anomalies, may well be explained as the result of a teratogenic insult in embryonic life to the somitic myoblasts and the mesoderm, which forms the mesenchyme for the development of urinary tract smooth muscle and connective tissue, as well as ureteral bud and urethral fold. The renal malformations may be secondary to ureteral-bud ampulla abnormalities (Potter type II cystic kidney) or to urinary retention (Potter type IV cystic kidney). Poor urinary flow is also likely to be secondary to abnormalities of ureteral smooth muscle distribution. These explanations de-emphasize the importance of distal mechanical urinary tract obstruction in the pathogenesis of proximal disease.

Unexplained is still the high incidence of the PBS in boys. Chromosomal anomalies are exceptional, and a genetic mechanism has not been found. Only in one family were there three cases of PBS, two of which occurred in twins, and another two siblings were detected in a second family.[56, 60] On the other hand, the presence of the PBS in only one of twins and one of homozygous triplets was also noted.[69, 90] There is no knowledge as to the teratogenetic agent or agents that might be responsible for the PBS.

In terms of management, several important points need to be remembered.

1. In the neonate, pulmonary hypoplasia and insufficiency must be suspected to avoid complications (air block syndrome, pneumothorax) from ventilatory assistance. In spite of term birth, hyaline membrane disease should be considered as a cause of respiratory distress. An examination of the placenta and the appearance of the fetus as well as roentgenograms of the chest should be helpful.
2. The urine flow must be evaluated. It may be deficient because (a) there is little urine production (severe renal dysplasia), (b) there is mechanical obstruction (atresia, stenosis, valve, diverticulum), or (c) there is functionally inefficient propulsion of urine (atony, reflux). In case of (a), little can be done short of a renal transplant. For (b) and (c), failure to relieve a significant urine retention is likely to result in hydronephrotic damage to the renal parenchyma and risk of infection.
3. The possibility of serious intestinal malformations should be kept in mind, ie, atresia, stenosis, and malrotation with volvulus as the dangerous sequelae.
4. The skeletal system should be checked in order to institute timely correction.

If these abnormalities and complications are either absent, minimal, or correctible, the prognosis for survival and health would seem good. Improvement in the statistics of mortality and morbidity are, therefore, dependent on a thorough and informed evaluation of the neonate with PBS at the time of birth, by a team of physicians consisting of an obstetrician, a pediatrician, a urologist, a radiologist, and a pathologist.

Acknowledgments

The authors would like to thank Miss Kathleen Edwards and Mrs. Ida Nathan for their photographic assistance and Mrs. Beryl Meikle for clerical assistance.

References

1. Parker RW: Absence of the abdominal muscles in an infant. Lancet 1:1252, 1895
2. Guthrie L: Case of congenital deficiency of the abdominal muscles with dilatation and hypertrophy of the bladder and ureters. Tr Path Soc London 47:139, 1896
3. Osler W: Congenital absence of the abdominal muscles, with distended and hypertrophied urinary bladder. Bull Johns Hopkins Hosp 12:331, 1901
4. Stumme EG: Ueber die symmetrischen kongenitalen Bauchmuskeldefekte und ueber die Kombination derselben mit anderen Bildungsanomalien des Rumpfes. Mitt Grenzgeb Med Chir 11:548, 1903
5. Garrod AE, Davies LW: On a group of associated congenital malformations, including almost complete absence of the abdominal wall, and abnormalities of the genito-urinary apparatus. Med Chir Tr 88:363, 1905
6. Bolton C: Congenital absence of lateral abdominal muscles with enlargement of bladder and ureters. Tr Clin Soc London 38:247, 1905
7. Hall G: Two cases of congenital deficiency of the muscles of the abdominal wall associated with pathological changes in the genito-urinary organs. Lancet 2:1672, 1907
8. Pels-Leusden F: Ueber den sogenannten congenitalen Defect der Bauchmuskulatur, zugleich ein Beitrag zur Physiologie der Bauchmuskel und der Zwerchfellsfunktion und zum Descensus testiculorum. Arch klin Chir Berlin 85:392, 1908
9. Thatcher L: Case of congenital defect of abdominal muscles, with anomaly of urinary apparatus. Edinburgh Med J 11:127, 1913
10. Eckhoff NL: Congenital deficiency of abdominal muscles, with postmortem report. Guys Hosp Rep 73:490, 1923
11. Carstens JHG: Aangeboren Atrophie der Buikspieren met Dilatatie en Hypertrophie van Blaas, Ureteren en Nierenbekken. Nederl Maandschr Geneesk, Leiden, 13:483, 1926
12. Ikeda K, Stoesser AV: Congenital defect in the musculature of the abdominal wall: Case. Am J Dis Child 33:286, 1927
13. Poli A: Comportamento dei dislivelli del dorso negli scoliotici in stazione eretta ed in flessione anteriore del tronco. Arch ortop 45:775, 1929
14. Moncrieff A: Specimens from a case of congenital deficiency in abdominal muscles. Brit J Child Dis 28:220, 1931
15. Molossi C, Gelli G: L'agenesia dei muscoli addominali. Lattante (Parma) 2:101, 1931
16. Friedley RS: Cited in Silverman and Huang[26]
17. McClendon SJ: Agenesia of the abdominal muscles. Arch Pediat 51:673, 1934
18. Gibbens J: Specimen of complete genito-urinary tract from a case of congenital absence of abdominal muscles. Brit J Child Dis 31:43, 1934
19. Housden LG: Congenital absence of the abdominal muscles. Arch Dis Child 9:219, 1934
20. Lichtenstein BW: Congenital absence of the abdominal musculature: Associated changes in genito-urinary tract and in spinal cord. Am J Dis Child 58:339, 1939
21. Howard PJ: Congenital absence of the abdominal muscles and genito-urinary malformation: Report of 2 cases. Am J Dis Child 60:669, 1940
22. Aldrich CA: Report of a case of congenital absence of abdominal muscles, case report. Child Mem Hosp, Chicago 1:13, 1942

23. Daut RV, Emmett JL, Kennedy RLJ: Congenital deficiency of abdominal musculature with urologic complications; report on patient successfully treated. Proc Staff Meet, Mayo Clin 22:8, 1947
24. Irvin GE, Kraus JE: Congenital megaloureter and hydroureter: Pathogenesis and classification. Arch Pathol 45:752, 1948
25. Obrinsky W: Agenesis of abdominal muscles with associated malformation of the genito-urinary tract. Am J Dis Child 77:362, 1949
26. Silverman FN, Huang N: Congenital absence of the abdominal muscles associated with malformations of genito-urinary and alimentary tracts; reports of cases and review of literature. Am J Dis Child 80:91, 1950
27. Bruton OC: Agenesis of abnormal musculature with genito-urinary and gastrointestinal tract anomalies. J Urol 66:607, 1951
28. Cadilla A, Irezarry-Bulls E, Isales LM: Agenesis of abdominal muscles in an infant. Bol Asoc Med PR 43:118, 1951
29. Bjerrum J: Medfødt mangel pa bugmuskulatur ledsaget af forandringer i urogenitalsystemet. Nord Med 46:1274, 1951
30. Martischnig E: Kongenitale Aplasie der Bauchmuskulatur (zugleich kritische Eroerterung der Genese). Wien klin Wschr 64:116, 1952
31. Greene LF, Emmett JL, Culp OS, Kennedy RL Jr: Urologic abnormalities with congenital absence or deficiency of abdominal musculature. J Urol 68:217, 1952
32. Mathieu BJ, Goldowsky S, Chaset N, Mathieu PL Jr: Congenital deficiency of the abdominal muscles (with associated multiple anomalies). J Pediatr 42:92, 1953
33. Henley WL, Hyman A: Absent abdominal musculature, genito-urinary anomalies and deficiency in pelvic autonomic nervous system. Am J Dis Child 86:795, 1953
34. Torres HR, Milan E, Curbelo PG: Congenital absence of abdominal wall musculature; case report. Bol Asoc Med PR 45:393, 1953
35. Stephenson KL: New approach to the treatment of abdominal muscular agenesis. Plast Reconstr Surg 12:413, 1953
36. Verger P, Conteau, Pery: Aplasie de la musculature abdominale et malformations urinaires. Arch Fr Pediatr 10:604, 1953
37. Kaijser K: Congenital deficiency of abdominal musculature with associated genito-urinary abnormalities. Ann Paediatr 181:173, 1953
38. Culp DA, Flocks RH: Congenital absence of abdominal musculature: Report of 2 cases. J Iowa Med Soc 44:155, 1954
39. Sansone G, Sardini G: Su di un caso inconsueto di ipoplasia dei muscoli della parete addominale associata a multiple complesse malformazioni. Minerva Pediatr 6:109, 1954
40. Riparetti PP, Ahaanock DA: Urological problems in agenesis of abdominal wall musculature. Tr West Sect Am Urol A 20:57, 1954
41. Luginbuhl WH: Hypoplasia of abdominal muscles; case report. Child Mem Hosp, Chicago 13:1, 1955
42. Jameson SG, Cooper JO: Agenesis of abdominal musculature with ectopic ureteral orifice and congenital absence of opposite kidney and ureter. J Pediatr 47:489, 1955
43. Roberts P: Congenital absence of the abdominal muscles with associated abnormalities of the genito-urinary tract. Arch Dis Child 31:236, 1956
44. Metrick S, Brown RH, Rosenblum A: Congenital absence of the abdominal musculature and associated anomalies. Pediatrics 19:1043, 1957
45. Parkkulainen KV: Congenital deficiency of the abdominal muscles; a series of eleven cases. Acta Paediatr Scand [Suppl] 118:151, 1958
46. Lattimer JK: Congenital deficiency of the abdominal musculature and associated genito-urinary anomalies: A report of 22 cases. J Urol 79:343, 1958
47. Begg NC: Congenital deficiency of abdominal muscles in males. NZ Med J 58:154, 1959

48. McGovern JH, Marshall VF: Congenital deficiency of the abdominal muscula-
     ture and obstructive uropathy. Surg Gynecol Obst 108:289, 1959
49. Nunn IN, Stephens FD: The triad syndrome: A composite anomaly of the ab-
     dominal wall, urinary system and testes. J Urol 86:782, 1961
50. Boisonnat P, Duhamel B: Congenital diverticulum of the anterior urethra asso-
     ciated with aplasia of the abdominal muscles in a male infant. Br J Urol 34:59,
     1962
51. Brierre JT: Congenital abnormalities of the genito-urinary tract: Abdominal
     muscle dysplasia and choanal atresia. Pediatrics 31:290, 1963
52. Andren L, Bjersing L, Lagergren J: Congenital aplasia of the abdominal muscles
     with urogenital malformations. Acta Radiol [Diagn] (Stockh) 2:298, 1964
53. Spence H, Allen T: Congenital absence of abdominal musculature—urologic
     aspects. JAMA 187:814, 1964
54. Kroh G: Beitrag zum Krankheitsbild des angeborenen Bauchmuskeldefektes und
     der mit ihm verbundenen Anomalien im Bereich des Urogenital- und Darmtraktes.
     Urologe [A] 4:191, 1965
55. Jaeger J: Kasuistische Mitteilungen und Schrifttumsübersicht zum kongenitalen
     Bauchmuskeldefektsyndrom. Paediatr Grenzgeb 5:307, 1966
56. von Sladzyk E: Das gehäufte familiäre Auftreten des angeborenen Bauchmuskel-
     wanddefektes. Zbl Chir 92:426, 1967
57. Bourne CW, Cerny JC: Congenital absence of the abdominal muscles: Report
     of 6 cases. J Urol 98:252, 1967
58. Williams DI, Burkholder GV: The prune belly syndrome. J Urol 98:244, 1967
59. Burke EC, Shin MH, Kelalis PP: Prune-belly syndrome. Am J Dis Child 117:668,
     1969
60. O'Kell KT: Embryonic abdominal musculature associated with anomalies of the
     genito-urinary and gastrointestinal systems. Am J Obstet Gynecol 105:1283,
     1969
61. Waldbaum RS, Marshall VF: The prune belly syndrome: A diagnostic therapeutic
     plan. J Urol 103:668, 1970
62. Burkholder GV, Harper RC, Beach PD: Congenital absence of the abdominal
     muscles. Am J Clin Pathol 53:602, 1970
63. Ruprecht KW, Treske U: Das Bauchdeckenaplasie Syndrom. Dtsch Med Wochen-
     schr 95:327, 1970
64. Ráliš Z, Forbes M: Intrauterine atrophy and gangrene of the lower extremity of
     the foetus caused by megacystis due to urethral atresia. J Pathol 104:31, 1971
65. Cremin BJ: The urinary tract anomalies associated with agenesis of the abdominal
     walls. Br J Radiol 44:767, 1971
66. Harley LM, Chen Y, Rattner WH: Prune belly syndrome. J Urol 108:174, 1972
67. Petersen DS, Fish L, Cass AS: Twins with congenital deficiency of abdominal
     musculature. J Urol 107:670, 1972
68. Rogers LW, Ostrow PT: The prune belly syndrome. J Pediatr 83:786, 1973
69. Welch KJ, Kearney GP: Abdominal muscular deficiency syndrome: Prune belly. J
     Urol 111:693, 1974
70. Palmer JM, Tesluk H: Ureteral pathology in the prune belly syndrome. J Urol
     111:701, 1974
71. Bain AD, Scott JS: Renal agenesis and severe urinary tract dysplasia; a review of
     50 cases with particular reference to the associated anomalies. Br Med J 1:841,
     1960
72. Blanc WA, Apperson JW, McNally J: Pathology of the newborn and of the
     placenta in oligohydramnios. Bull Sloane Hosp Women 8:51, 1962
73. Perlman M, Levin M: Fetal pulmonary hypoplasia, anuria, and oligohydramnios:
     Clinicopathologic observations and review of literature. Am J Obstet Gynecol
     118:1119, 1974

74. Déglon P, Blanc WA: Fetal and placental lesions in 100 cases of oligohydramnios. Pediatr Res 6:408 (abstract), 1972
75. Froehlich F: Der Mangel der Muskeln, insbesondere der Seitenbauchmuskeln. Dissertation, Würzburg. CA Zurn, 1839
76. Helbig G: Zum Krankheitsbild des angeborenen Bauchmuskeldefektes. Arch Kinderheilk 165:68, 1961
77. Mogens Hansen O, Zachariae L: Arthrogryposis multiplex congenita mit sekundärer Skoliose infolge Bauchmuskelhypoplasie. Ann Paediat 192:306, 1956
78. Stanga E: Über multiple Abartungen mit Flughautbildungen (Pterygium-Syndrom) und kongenitaler Aplasie der Bauchdeckenmuskulatur. Ann Paediatr Basel 187:384, 1956
79. Potter EL: Normal and Abnormal Development of the Kidney. Chicago, Year Book, 1972, pp 209–221
80. von Ammon FA: Die angeborenen chirurgischen Krankheiten des Menschen in Abbildungen dargestellt und durch erläuternden Text erklärt. Berlin, Herbig, 1842; cited by Housden[19]
81. Henderson B: Congenital absence of abdominal muscles. Glasgow MJ 33:63, 1890
82. Blasi D: Mancanza congenita bilaterale die muscoli obbliqui dell'addome. Pediatria (Napoli) 35:720, 1927
83. Smith EB: Congenital absence of all abdominal muscles and other defects. Proc Soc Med 6:186, 1913
84. Eagle JF, Barrett GS: Congenital deficiency of abdominal musculature with associated genitourinary abnormalities: A syndrome. Report of 9 cases. Pediatrics 6:721, 1950
85. Gardner WU: Sexual dimorphism of pelvis of mouse, effect of estrogen hormones upon pelvis and upon development of scrotal hernias. Am J Anat 59:459, 1936
86. Forbes M, Underwood J, Emery JL: The intrinsic nerve plexus of the human ureter. Br J Urol 42:158, 1970
87. Notley RG: The musculature of the human ureter. Br J Urol 42:724, 1970
88. Dott NM: Anomalies of intestinal rotation: Their embryology and surgical aspects. Br J Surg 11:251, 1923
89. Renert WA, Berdon WE, Baker DH, Rose JS: Obstructive urologic malformations of the fetus and infant—relation to neonatal pneumomediastinum and pneumothorax (air block). Radiology 105:97, 1972
90. Accordi V, Barbareschi G: Aplasia dei muscoli della parete addominale associata a megauretere e ad altre malformazione congenita (cistoureterimegalia leptolaparica). Riv Anat Pat Oncol 17:30, 1960
91. Theiler K: Über die Differenzierung der Rumpfmyotome beim Menschen und die Herkunft der Bauchwandmuskeln. Acta Anat (Basel) 30:842, 1957
92. Glenister TW: A correlation of the normal and abnormal development of the penile urethra and of the infraumbilical abdominal wall. Br J Urol 30:117, 1958

COLUMNAR MUCOSA OF THE DISTAL ESOPHAGUS IN PATIENTS WITH GASTROESOPHAGEAL REFLUX

LUCIANO OZZELLO, MARCEL SAVARY, AND
BENOÎT ROETHLISBERGER

Many patients with persistent gastroesophageal reflux have a chronic nonspecific esophagitis of limited clinical consequence. Sometimes, however, this "reflux esophagitis" [5] progresses and may become complicated by peptic ulcerations and stenosis. In the more severe forms of the disease, the distal esophagus is frequently lined by secretory rather than stratified squamous epithelium which, as pointed out by Johnston,[31] makes this anomaly "look like esophagus on the outside and stomach on the inside."

The genesis and nature of this pathologic epithelium have been a matter of debate over many years. In 1957, Barrett [6] proposed the descriptive terminology of "lower esophagus lined by columnar epithelium." This terminology has gained wide acceptance, although it does not depict the full histologic picture of the lesion, which is characterized in the majority of cases by glands in addition to the columnar surface epithelium.

Although peptic lesions of the esophagus have been known since the last century, they evoked relatively little interest until 1929, when Jackson [29] reported to have found 88 cases (21 active ulcers and 67 scars probably secondary to peptic ulceration) in 4000 consecutive endoscopies, thus indicating that they were not as rare as generally thought. Since then, the number of cases recognized esophagoscopically has continued to increase as the esophagoscopic technique and the experience of endoscopists improved.[56] The clinical interest has been further stimulated by the high incidence of adenocarcinomas arising in this columnar epithelium, which can indeed be considered as a true precancerous lesion.

In this chapter, we propose to illustrate the esophagoscopic and structural aspects of this disease, and to discuss its pathogenesis and clinicopathologic implications.

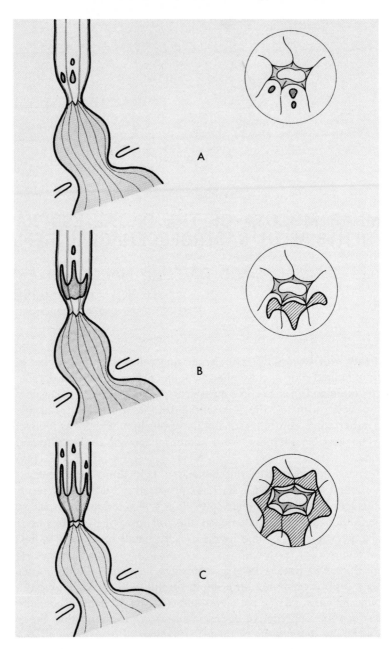

Fig. 1. Esophagoscopic staging of peptic esophagitis. Schematic representation of the anatomy (left) and of the corresponding esophagoscopic appearance (right) of stage 1 (A), stage 2 (B), and stage 3 (C). In stage 4, these lesions are complicated by chronic peptic ulcers or fibrotic alterations of the esophageal wall. The hiatal hernia shown in these diagrams is a frequent but not an obligatory component of the disease. The striated areas depict the superficial esophageal erosions; the dotted areas represent the gastric mucosa.

Esophagoscopic Observations

A rigid esophagoscope with Hopkins-type optics is used routinely in our endoscopy service. All lesions are photographed at multiple levels so that their architecture and extent can be precisely determined and their evolution accurately checked by subsequent examinations.[54] Selected lesions are recorded cinematographically.

Over a period of 12 years, 3193 patients suffering hiatal hernia or gastroesophageal reflux have been examined endoscopically. Of these, 1196 (37.4 percent) presented unequivocal evidence of peptic esophagitis with mucosal erosions. Experience has shown that such peptic injury to the esophageal lining can vary greatly from case to case and has led to the formulation of 4 esophagoscopic stages that reflect the evolution and the severity of the disease.[55]

Stage 1 (Fig. 1A) is characterized by one or more superficial erosions that are small and discrete. They are generally located on the longitudinal folds of the posterior wall of the esophagus, 1 to 2 cm proximal to the gastroesophageal junction.

Stage 2 (Fig. 1B) displays erosions that have become confluent and may be partly covered by pseudomembranes. They involve large portions of the esophageal lining, mostly on its posterior aspect, but not all of its circumference.

Stage 3 (Fig. 1C) shows a diffuse involvement of the entire circumference of the distal esophageal mucosa which is largely covered by a hemorrhagic and pseudomembranous exudate.

Stage 4 is reached when, in addition to the superficial erosions of any of the previous stages, there are complications such as deep ulcers, fibrous stiffening of the esophageal wall, stenosis, and brachyesophagus.

Foci of columnar epithelium can be found replacing the stratified squamous lining in the vicinity of the peptic lesions in any of the stages, but far more frequently in stage 4. Over a period of 12 years, these foci were recognized at esophagoscopy in 196 of our 335 patients in stage 4 (58.5 percent). It must be pointed out, however, that this percentage is deceptively low. In fact, these foci of columnar epithelium have been diagnosed esophagoscopically more and more frequently in recent years,[56] suggesting that many of them were previously overlooked.

The patches of columnar epithelium are sharply demarcated and can be readily recognized because of their tannish color and velvety appearance, which contrasts with the paler squamous epithelium. As illustrated diagrammatically in Figure 2, they can vary in extent and general configuration. In 55 percent of our cases, the columnar epithelium lined the entire circumference of the lower esophagus. For such cases, Lortat-Jacob[36] suggested the term *endo-brachy-oesophage*. In the remaining 45 percent of the cases, the involvement was localized and noncircumferential.

Microscopic Observations

The findings reported in this section are from the study of 27 patients selected on the basis of the following criteria.

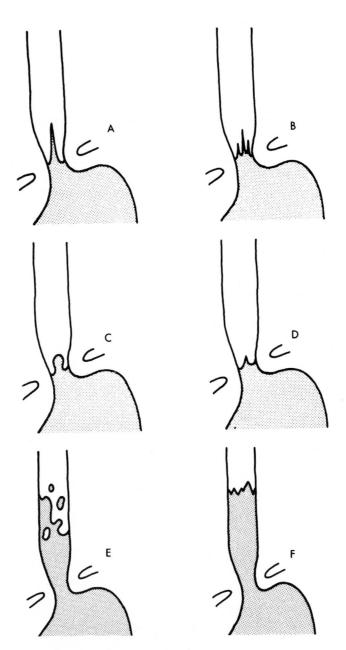

Fig. 2. Columnar replacement of the distal esophageal mucosa secondary to peptic esophagitis. Localized (A, B, C, D) and circumferential (E, F) involvement (dotted areas).

1. Clinical evidence of gastroesophageal reflux.
2. Esophagoscopic examination of the whole length of the esophagus permitting a thorough visual and photographic evaluation of the esophageal mucosa. Therefore, the cases in which the esophagoscope could not be passed beyond a stricture were excluded.
3. Precise localization of the biopsies performed under esophagoscopic control to ensure that the specimens were from the esophagus and not from the stomach.

The patients, 20 males and 7 females, ranged in age from 3 to 86 years when first seen. According to the esophagoscopic staging described previously, 21 patients were in stage 4, 1 in stage 3, 1 in stage 2, 3 in stage 1, and in 1, the stage was difficult to assess because of extensive neoplastic alterations. The involvement by columnar epithelium was circumferential in 26 patients and localized in 1. Hiatal hernia was present in 23 cases, annular stenosis in 12, chronic peptic ulceration in 5, and adenocarcinoma in 4.

Specimens for light microscopic examination were fixed in neutral formalin and embedded in paraffin. Serial sections were stained with hematoxylin and eosin, Masson's trichrome, the periodic acid–Schiff technique (PAS), alcian blue (AB) at pH 2.5 and pH 1.2, Masson-Fontana's technique for argentaffin cells, and Sevier-Munger's method for argyrophil cells.[58]

Biopsies from 8 patients were available for electron microscopy. They were fixed immediately in chilled glutaraldehyde (2.3 percent in cacodylate buffer, 0.2 M, pH 7.4) for 5 hours, repeatedly washed in the buffer, postfixed in osmium tetroxide (2 percent in cacodylate buffer) for 1 hour at 20C, and embedded in Epon 812. Thin sections (less than 1 μ) were stained with azure II-methylene blue for light microscopic control. In addition, selected sections were stained with PAS. Ultrathin sections were mounted on carbonized and parlodion-coated grids and stained with uranyl acetate and lead citrate for electron microscopic study.

Light and electron microscopic examination revealed that the diseased esophageal mucosa of all of these patients was characterized by a columnar epithelial lining associated or not with glandular structures in the underlying lamina propria. The architecture and cellular makeup of these mucous membranes presented considerable variability from case to case, and sometimes from one area to another of the same esophagus. Islands of stratified squamous epithelium were present next to the columnar lining in 5 cases.

Surface Epithelium

The surface columnar epithelium of all of the biopsies was largely composed of a single layer of mucus-secreting cells. The majority of them were tall and thin with a basilar portion containing the nucleus and an apical portion that on hematoxylin and eosin preparations appeared to be occupied by an elongated vacuole (Fig. 3). The vacuole was filled with granules that in all cases stained intensely with the PAS. Rarely did these cells contain granules that were also positive with the AB at pH 2.5. This reaction was faint to moderate in 18 cases and strong in 2 others. Some material giving a positive reaction with the AB at pH 1.2 was present on the

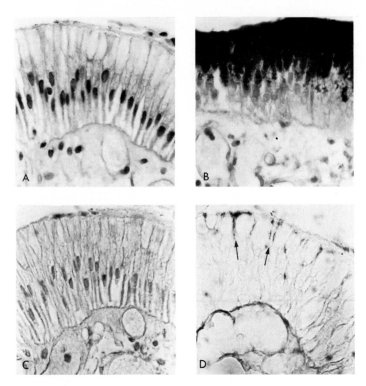

Fig. 3. Surface columnar mucous cells. The supranuclear mucin, appearing as empty vacuoles on H&E (A), is positive with PAS (B), and mostly negative with AB at pH 2.5 (C) and pH 1.2 (D). The cells of this biopsy are reminiscent of gastric surface mucous cells. Some granular material (glycoprotein surface coating?) stained with AB at pH 1.2 is present in the lateral intercellular spaces (arrows). × 325.

luminal surface and along the lateral intercellular spaces of many of these cells, but only rarely was it seen within the vacuoles themselves.

When examined with the electron microscope, these cells were highlighted by numerous round or oval mucus granules situated in the supranuclear portion of the cell (Fig. 4). Most of the granules were dark and uniformly dense, but some of them had a stippled appearance (Fig. 5). At the luminal surface, some granules bulged between microvilli as if they were being extruded, and an occasional one was seen lying free in the extracellular mucus (Fig. 6). Sometimes these cells contained uniformly pale granules (Fig. 7), and others displayed an admixture of granules of varying density (Fig. 8). The luminal surface of the cells presented a moderate number of microvilli (Figs. 4 to 8) coated by abundant glycocalyx. Between the microvilli, there were small round bodies (Figs. 8 and 9) composed of a moderately dense core surrounded by a trilaminar membrane. These structures, referred to in this laboratory as "glycocalyceal bodies" because of their uncertain nature and because of want of a better term, were present in all but two of our cases. They corresponded to those described by other authors in normal and pathologic digestive mucosae.[9, 15, 38, 43, 46, 49, 63]

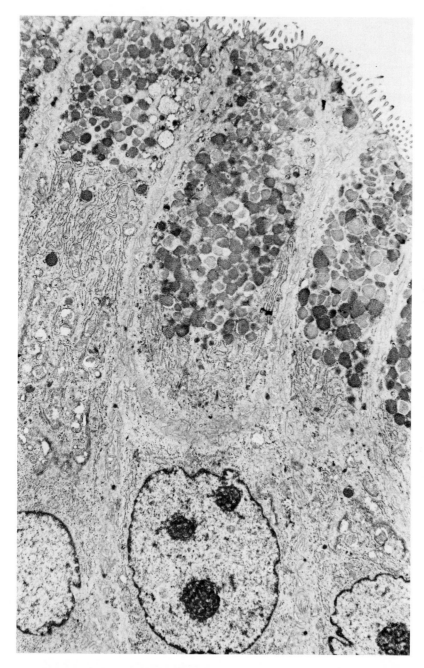

Fig. 4. Surface columnar mucous cells. Most mucin granules are dense and irregularly shaped. Surface microvilli are sparse. Well developed RER is present above the nuclei. × 6200.

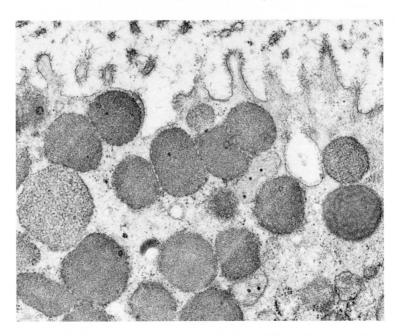

Fig. 5. Surface columnar mucous cells. Microvilli are stubby and covered by glycocalyx. Some mucin granules are lighter or stippled. Few small vesicles are visible. × 23,000.

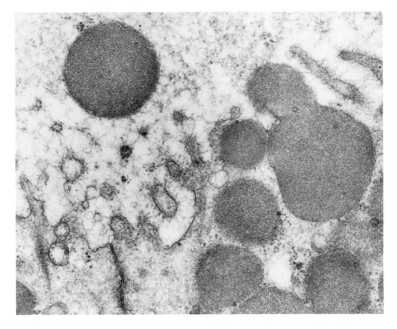

Fig. 6. Surface columnar mucous cells. Some mucin granules are bulging at the cell surface, and one of them is free in the lumen. × 29,500.

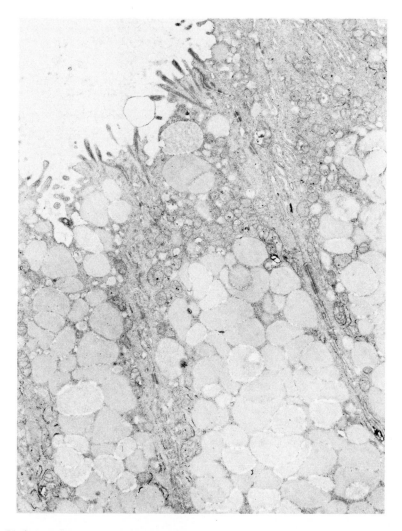

Fig. 7. Surface columnar mucous cells showing pale mucin granules and microvilli with long and deeply penetrating rootlets. These cells are different from those of Figures 5 and 6, although they are from the same biopsy. × 10,300.

The microvilli varied in length and were delimited by an unremarkable tri-laminar plasma membrane. Their central core was composed of longitudinally oriented filaments, which penetrated deeply into the apical cytoplasm in the form of long bundles (Figs. 7 and 8). No terminal web was ever seen in any of these cells. Golgi complexes and a moderate amount of rough endoplasmic reticulum (RER) were present between the nucleus and the secretory granules (Fig. 4). Mitochondria were inconspicuous and were sometimes closely related to the ergasto-plasmic membranes. Small vesicles were seen in some cells, mostly in their apical portion amidst the mucin granules (Figs. 5, 6, and 8). The basilar portion of these cells contained a moderate number of free ribosomes and infrequent deposits of

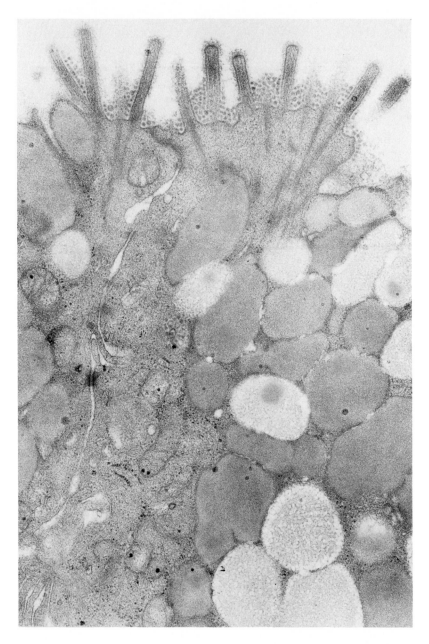

Fig. 8. Surface columnar mucous cells with mucin granules of variable density and some small vesicles. Microvilli are moderately long, sparse, and have long and deep filamentous rootlets. They are coated by glycocalyx. Numerous glycocalyceal bodies are well visible between the microvilli. × 24,200.

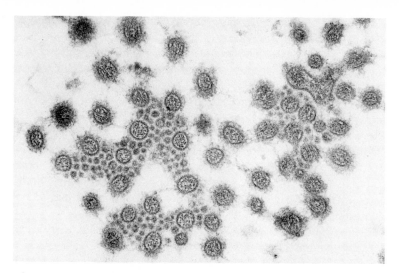

Fig. 9. Cross section of microvilli showing the trilaminar plasma membrane and the central filaments. These microvilli are sparse and fail to show the hexagonal arrangement of normal cells. Among them are numerous glycocalyceal bodies surrounded by a trilaminar membrane. × 38,600.

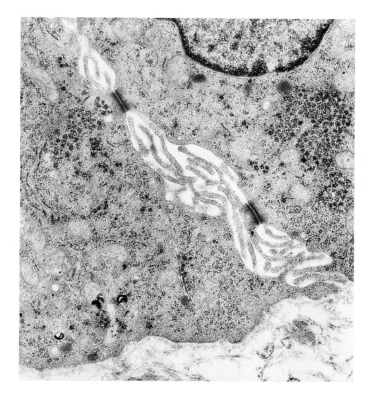

Fig. 10. Basilar portion of surface columnar mucous cells featuring a moderate number of free ribosomes and granular deposits appearing like glycogen. The dilated intercellular space with microvillous projections suggests fluid transport. × 14,000.

glycogen granules (Fig. 10). The lateral plasma membranes were mostly straight with some interdigitation between adjacent cells. The intracellular spaces were tight in the upper half of the cells where junctional complexes were well visible, whereas in the basilar portion, they were frequently dilated and presented numerous microvillous projections and rare desmosomes (Fig. 10).

Goblet cells were interspersed among the surface columnar cells in 15 cases (Fig. 11); in 5 cases, they were numerous. They were strongly positive with the PAS and with the AB at pH 2.5, whereas their reaction to AB at pH 1.2 varied from negative to strongly positive, thus resembling the goblet cells of both the small and the large intestines. Their ultrastructural features (Figs. 12 and 13) were typical of the intestinal goblet cells.[33, 43, 62, 64]

Surface non-mucus-secreting cells were difficult to evaluate with light optics, but were easily demonstrable with the electron microscope in 4 cases. They had long and straight microvilli that were irregularly spaced and never closely packed (Figs. 12 and 13). The microvilli were covered by glycocalyx in which glycocalyceal bodies were found in 3 cases, and featured long filamentous rootlets extending deeply into the apical cytoplasm. The latter was devoid of a terminal web. The lateral borders of these cells were mostly straight with some interdigitations and basilar dilatation (Fig. 12). Junctional complexes sometimes showed a greater

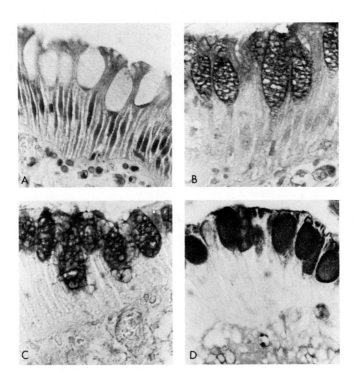

Fig. 11. Surface columnar epithelium with numerous goblet cells (A: H&E) whose mucin is strongly positive to PAS (B), to AB at pH 2.5 (C) and to AB at pH 1.2 (D). Compare with Figure 21. × 325.

number of desmosomes than usual (Fig. 14). Mitochondria were numerous and mostly concentrated in the apical cytoplasm (Figs. 12 and 13). Some of them had prominent matrical bodies (Fig. 14). Golgi complexes were predominantly supra-nuclear, as was the RER, which often appeared in juxtaposition to the mito-chondria. Many of these cells presented small vesicles, and less frequently few secretory granules, in the apical cytoplasm (Figs. 13 and 14). The granules varied in density from pale to dark, and some had a stippled appearance. Microfilaments were frequently prominent, especially in the apical portion of the cells (Fig. 14).

Pitlike Structures

As pitlike structures, we accepted those invaginations of the surface epithelium

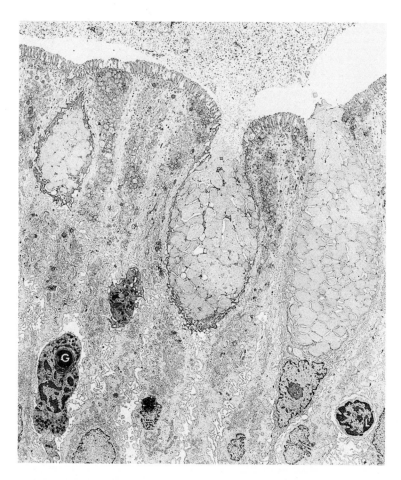

Fig. 12. Surface columnar epithelium composed of goblet cells and non-mucin-secreting cells. The latter are more easily detected in mucosae such as this one containing many goblet cells. A granulocyte (G) and a lymphocyte (L) are seen between epithelial cells. × 2250.

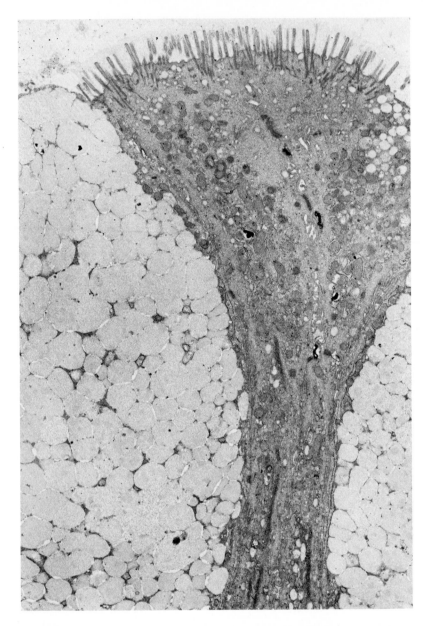

Fig. 13. Surface non-mucus-secreting cells with long and irregularly spaced microvilli whose filamentous rootlets penetrate deeply into the apical cytoplasm. There is no terminal web. The supranuclear cytoplasm contains longitudinally oriented Golgi complexes, scanty RER, apical concentration of mitochondria, and several vesicles. Few pale secretory granules are visible in the cell on the right. Goblet cells show the typical pale mucin granules. × 6200.

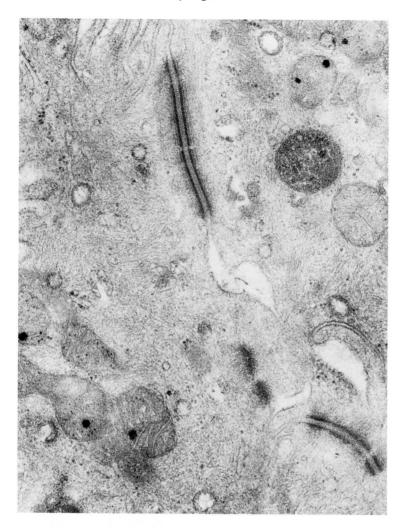

Fig. 14. Supernumerary and long desmosomes are often present in the apical portion of surface non-mucus-secreting cells. Small vesicles, mitochondria with prominent matrical bodies, and fine filaments are also visible. These features are frequently seen in immature gastrointestinal cells. × 38,600.

that showed a tubular configuration and could be differentiated from simple surface folds (Fig. 15). Such pitlike structures were present in all of our cases but one. They were lined by mucus-secreting cells that exhibited the same light microscopic features and the same reactivity to the PAS and to the AB as the columnar and goblet cells of the surface. Goblet cells, however, appeared to be more numerous than on the surface. Ultrastructurally, the columnar cells differed from the corresponding surface cells by being generally shorter and by featuring more irregular microvilli and fewer secretory granules. Some of the latter were stippled and contained dense areas (Fig. 16). The glycocalyx was present in variable quantity and

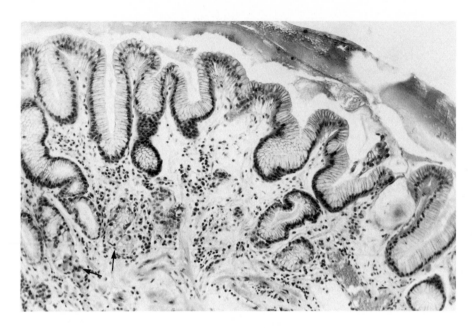

Fig. 15. Pitlike structures lined by columnar cells similar to the mucous surface cells. This mucous membrane is thin, but contains glands with parietal cells (arrows). × 130.

contained some glycocalyceal bodies. In one case, admixed to these cells, there were others containing very few mucin granules and prominent supranuclear ergastoplasm and Golgi complexes (Figs. 16 and 17).

Mitoses were found in the deep portion of pitlike structures in four cases. One of these mitoses was unquestionably in a mucus cell since mucin granules were well visible in the cytoplasm (Fig. 18).

Glands

Glands were found in the lamina propria of 18 patients (Figs. 19 to 21). They were predominantly composed of low cylindrical to cuboidal mucus-secreting cells with a pale cytoplasm and a basally located nucleus. These cells were moderately to strongly positive to the PAS, but generally less intensely so than the surface mucus cells. In 10 patients, a variable number of these cells stained faintly with AB at pH 2.5, while this reaction was strongly positive in some cells of 2 patients. With AB at pH 1.2, a strong reaction was noted in 1 case and a faint one in 9. Ultrastructurally (Fig. 22), the mucin granules were mostly pale and uniform, although in many cells, they were admixed with denser or stippled ones. The luminal microvilli were sparser and stubbier than those of the surface mucus cells. Other organelles, notably RER and Golgi complexes, were inconspicuous and located near the nucleus.

Tall cells with few or no secretory granules of variable density were found

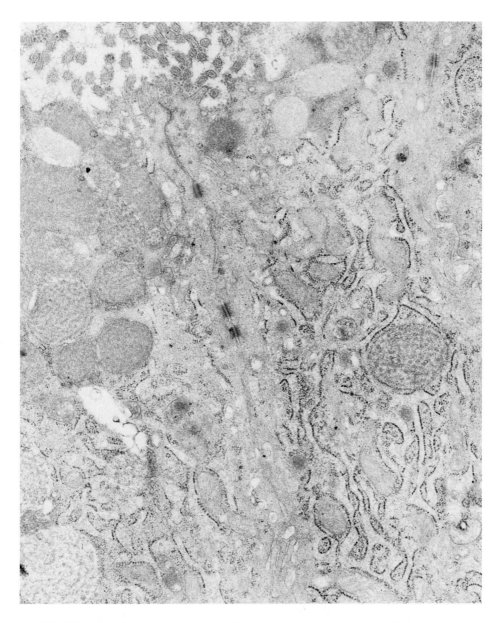

Fig. 16. Pitlike structure. A mucous cell with granules that are in part uniformly dense and in part stippled is flanked by an immature cell containing few mucin granules and prominent profiles of RER, some of which are in close relation to mitochondria. × 18,600.

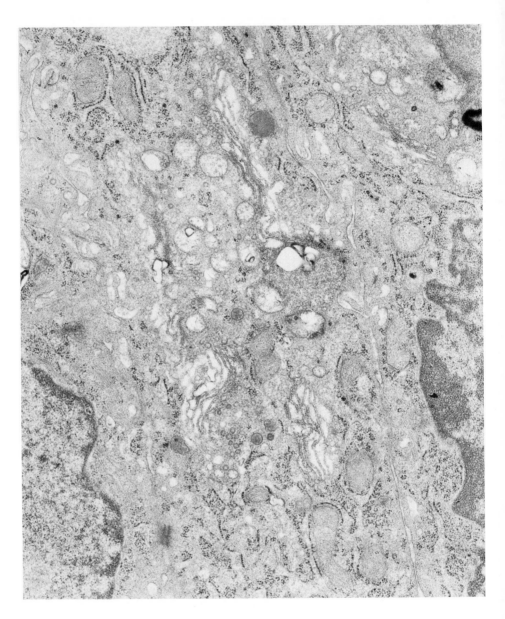

Fig. 17. Pitlike structure. Well-developed and longitudinally oriented Golgi complexes in an immature cell. RER is closely related to mitochondria. × 18,600.

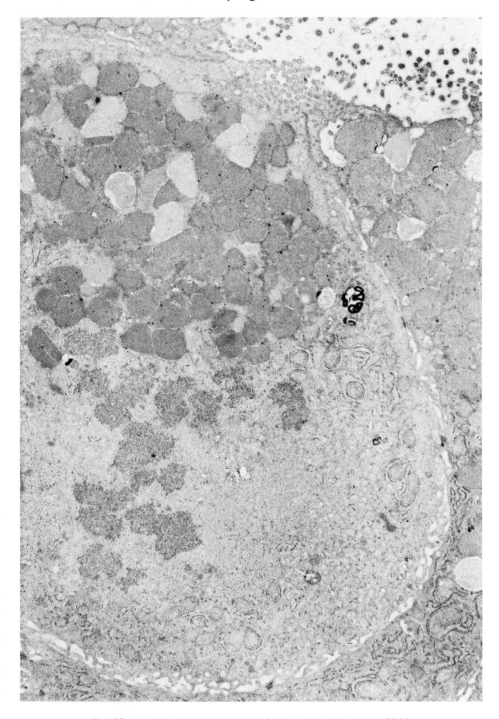

Fig. 18. Mitosis in a mucous cell of a pitlike structure. $\times$ 8900.

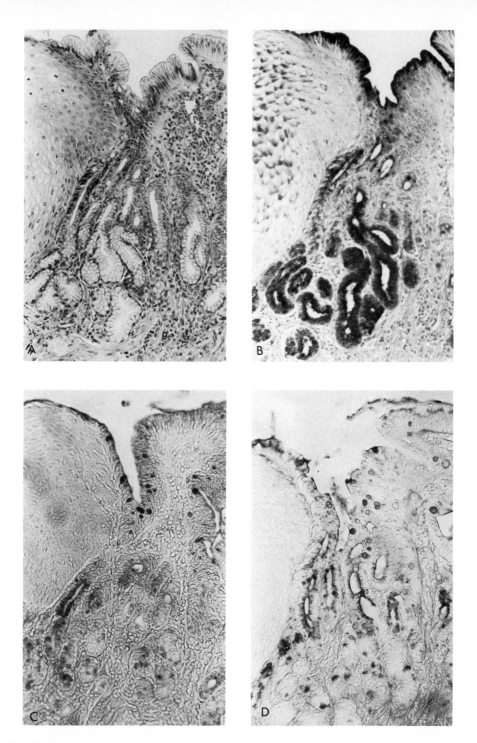

Fig. 19. These glands are mostly composed of cells resembling gastric mucous cells when stained with H&E (A) and with PAS (B). On the other hand, sulfated and nonsulfated acid mucins are more prominent than in normal gastric glands, as revealed by the AB at pH 2.5 (C) and at pH 1.2 (D). Goblet cells are best visualized by the AB stains. Note the sharp demarcation between the stratified squamous epithelium and the columnar lining. × 115.

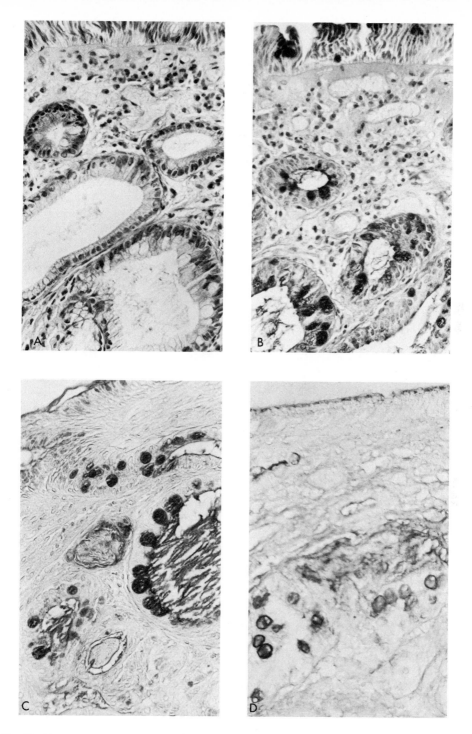

Fig. 20. Abnormal and dilated glands showing considerable staining variability. Goblet cells are numerous in some glands and absent on the surface. Some surface cells, however, are positive with AB at pH 2.5. A thin layer of material positive with AB at pH 1.2 covers the surface. A: H&E; B: PAS; C: AB at pH 2.5; D: AB at pH 1.2. × 230.

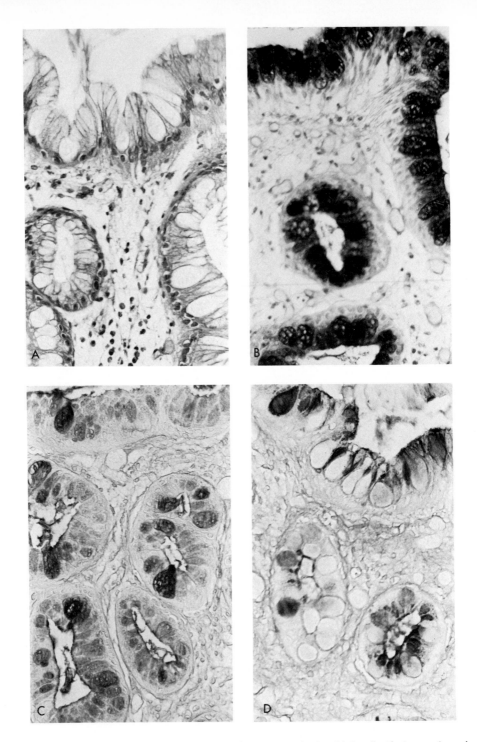

Fig. 21. Surface epithelium and glands largely composed of goblet cells that are strongly and uniformly positive with PAS. On the contrary, the reaction with AB varies from cell to cell, some of them staining as colonic goblet cells (positive with AB at pH 2.5 and at pH 1.2) and others as small intestinal goblet cells (positive with AB at pH 2.5 and negative with AB at pH 1.2). A: H&E; B: PAS; C: AB at pH 2.5; D: AB at pH 1.2. × 230.

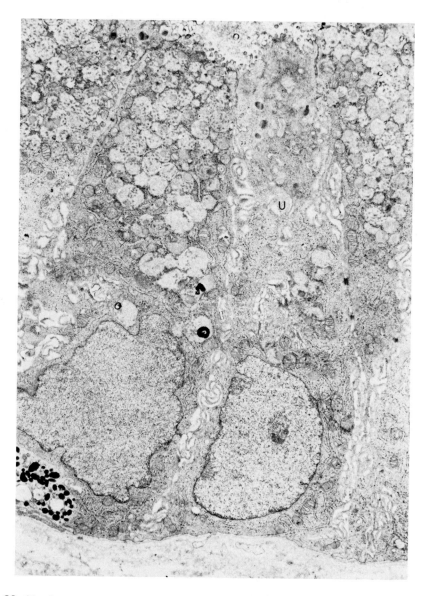

Fig. 22. Gland mucous cells containing granules of different density and in part stippled. An undifferentiated cell (U) shows a prominent supranuclear Golgi complex and inconspicuous secretory granules. Surface microvilli are rudimentary. Part of an endocrine cell with irregularly shaped dense secretory granules, probably an EC cell, is located below a mucous cell. × 6200.

amidst the mucus cells (Fig. 22). In some glands, they were the predominant cell type (Fig. 23). They had sparse and mostly rudimentary microvilli, apical vesicles, large mitochondria with numerous matrical bodies, scanty RER frequently in close relation to the mitochondria, and well-developed supranuclear Golgi complexes (Figs. 22 to 25). Centrioles were frequently seen. The intercellular spaces were mostly straight and narrow, although some dilatation and microvillous projections could be observed. Supernumerary cell-to-cell attachments could be seen in the apical portion of the intercellular spaces. They were frequently flanked by fine cytoplasmic filaments running parallel to the cell border (Fig. 26) and resembling the "lateral desmosomal bundles" described by Rubin and associates in human undifferentiated crypt cells.[52]

Goblet cells were found in the glands of 12 patients. They were numerous in 5 patients, in moderate number in 5 others, and rare in 2. Their light and electron microscopic features corresponded to those of the goblet cells described previously.

Few ciliated cells (Fig. 27) were present in the midst of the mucus cells of at least two glands of 1 case. Their cytoplasm was pale and contained a well-developed supranuclear Golgi, few ergastoplasmic profiles, scattered mitochondria, and some osmiophilic bodies. On their luminal surface, many cilia projected into the lumen among long microvilli. These cilia were delimited by a trilaminar ciliary membrane and were peculiar in that their axial filament complex featured 8 evenly spaced peripheral and 1 central doublet instead of the customary 9-plus-2 configuration.[16] Such an unusual axial complex was interpreted as a variation of the uncommon 9-plus-0 arrangement observed in other tissues.[14]

Parietal and chief cells were found in some of the glands of 3 patients (Fig. 15). In 1 patient, these cells were seen only in 1 of 2 simultaneous biopsies. In another patient, parietal and chief cells were found with the electron microscope, whereas, only parietal cells could be recognized with light optics. The light and electron microscopic features of these cells (Figs. 28 and 29) corresponded to those of normal mature parietal and chief gastric cells.[28, 35, 53]

Paneth cells were found with the electron microscope in 2 cases (Fig. 24). Their fine structure was typical,[62, 64] but in which portion of the glands they were located could not be determined.

Mitoses were found in the glands of 14 patients. They were mostly located in the upper portion of the glands and much less frequently in the deep portion. None were found at the base of the glands.

Submucosal glands with the characteristic features of normal esophageal glands were found in 1 case. They were readily distinguishable from the mucosal glands described previously because of their location and because their secretory portion was composed only of mucus cells that stained moderately with the PAS and very intensely with AB at pH 2.5 and 1.2. The excretory ducts were sometimes dilated and contained AB-positive mucin, but their lining cells did not stain with either the PAS or the AB (Fig. 30).

Endocrine Cells

Endocrine cells were found along a surface fold (or pitlike structure) of 1 case and in mucosal glands of 11. No endocrine cells were seen along the basal

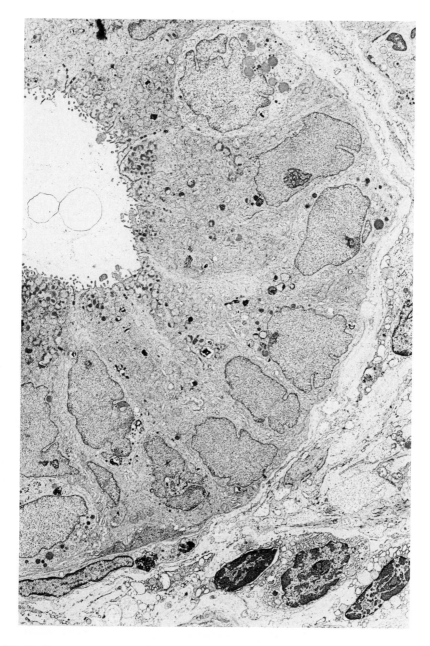

Fig. 23. Basilar portion of a gland. Some of the cells contain very few mucin granules. Microvilli are mostly sparse and rudimentary. Two endocrine cells of undetermined type are visible. The gland is surrounded by a thin basal lamina and in part by a closely apposed fibroblast. × 3500.

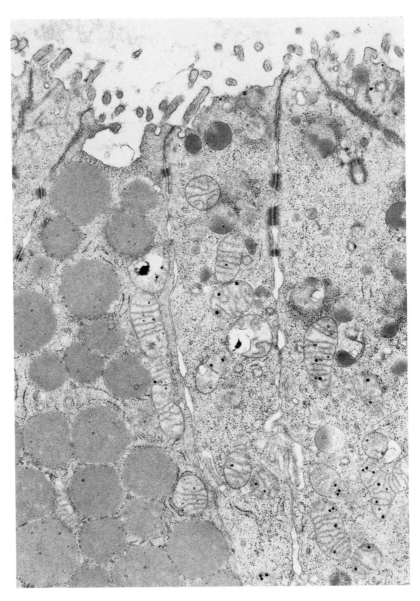

Fig. 24. Paneth cell next to immature cells featuring rudimentary microvilli, apical vesicles, few secretory granules, large mitochondria with matrical bodies, and a centriole. × 15,900.

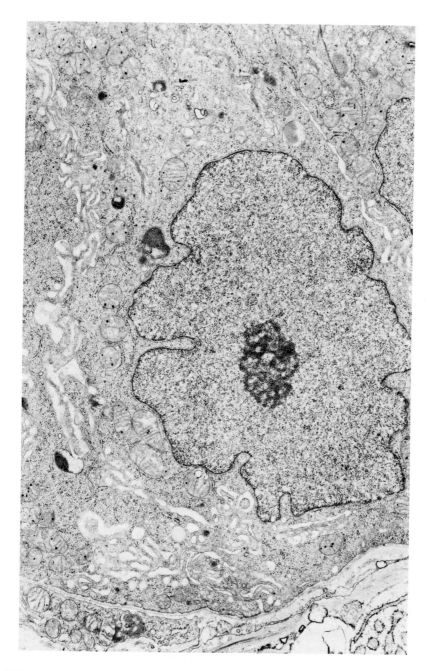

Fig. 25. Basilar portion of an undifferentiated cell containing large mitochondria with dense matrical bodies, double supranuclear Golgi complex, and rare profiles of RER. A thin basal lamina separates the epithelial cell and a juxtaposed fibroblast. × 11,000.

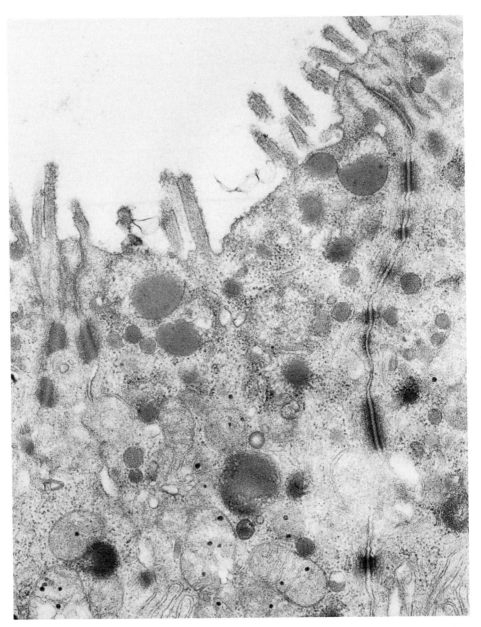

Fig. 26. Immature cells with few secretory granules of different size. The intercellular space is straight and presents supernumerary cell-to-cell junctions flanked by filaments running parallel to the cell membrane. × 28,750.

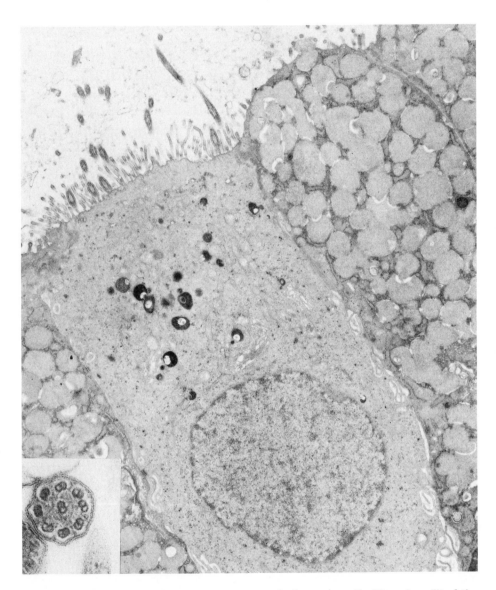

Fig. 27. Ciliated cell in a gland otherwise composed of mucous cells. The microvilli of the ciliated cell are particularly long and contrast with the rudimentary microvilli of the adjacent mucous cells. × 9000. Insert: The cilia are unusual in that they contain 8 peripheral and 1 central doublets. × 73,600.

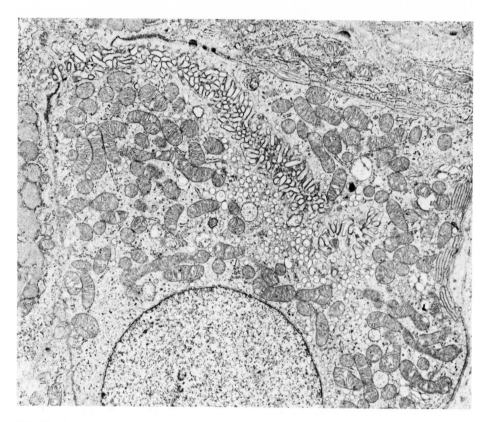

Fig. 28. Parietal cell showing a characteristic intracellular canaliculus emptying into the lumen, tubulovesicles, numerous mitochondria with tightly packed cristae, and interdigitating convolutions of the basilar plasma membrane. $\times$ 7400.

layer of the islands of stratified squamous epithelium.[60] The majority of these cells were situated along the basal lamina, and only a few of them appeared to reach the luminal surface. With the light microscope, they appeared to be argyrophilic (Fig. 31A). Argentaffin cells were much less numerous (Fig. 31B), but their distribution was patchy, and several of them could be seen in the same gland. With the electron microscope, these cells featured granules that for the most part were situated in the basilar part of the cytoplasm, but could be less frequently seen in the supranuclear portion especially when the cell extended up to the lumen. The most frequent granules were irregularly shaped, dense, and resembled those of enterochromaffin (EC) cells [45, 51] (Figs. 22 and 32). Other granules (Figs. 33 to 35) were round, but varied greatly in size and electron density. Their membranes were generally poorly visible. Golgi complexes, rough and smooth endoplasmic reticulum, mitochondria, and cytoplasmic filaments were the organelles most commonly visible in these cells, but their prominence varied from cell to cell. We found it difficult to determine with confidence the precise type of these endocrine cells on structural features alone. Furthermore, we found rare cells that contained an admixture of

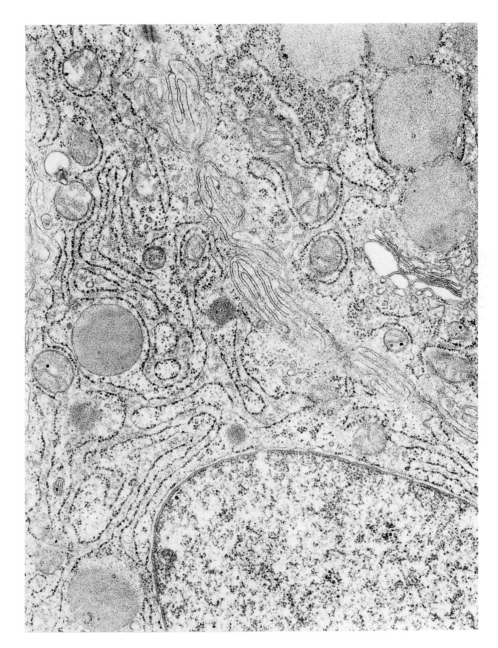

Fig. 29. Chief cells with typical zymogen granules, prominent RER and Golgi constituents. × 24,150.

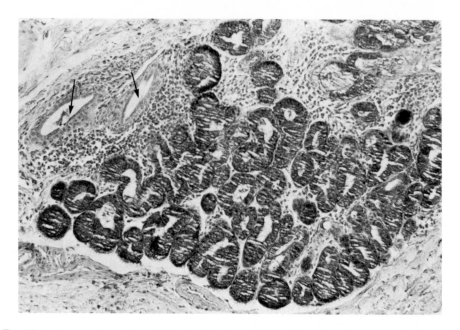

Fig. 30. Submucosal esophageal gland whose secretory cells stain intensely with AB at pH 2.5, whereas the cells lining the excretory ducts (arrows) do not. AB at pH 1.2 gives identical results. These glands are distinctly different from the metaplastic glands located in the lamina propria. × 130.

mucous granules and neurosecretory granules (Fig. 36) similar to those described in gastric carcinomas.[59]

Stroma

Surface epithelium, pitlike structures, and glands were separated from the stroma by an unremarkable basal lamina (Fig. 35). The stroma was loose and consisted essentially of fibroblasts and collagen fibers immersed in abundant ground substance. Some fibroblasts were closely apposed to the basal lamina surrounding some of the glands (Figs. 23 and 25) and were reminiscent of the pericryptal fibroblasts described by Kaye and collaborators, in the small and large intestine.[32, 44]

A moderate number of lymphocytes and plasma cells were always present in the lamina propria. An inflammatory reaction (Fig. 37), as judged by an unusually large number of these cells associated or not to an infiltration by granulocytes, was observed in 7 cases. Migration of inflammatory cells through the epithelium was also seen (Fig. 12). In some cases, there was edema of the lamina propria making the mucosal folds more prominent (Fig. 38). Fibrosis, as shown by the Masson's trichrome stain or on electron micrographs, was not unduly prominent.

Blood vessels were numerous, thin-walled, and often dilated. Their endothelium was frequently thin, fenestrated, and rich in pinocytotic vesicles (Fig. 35).

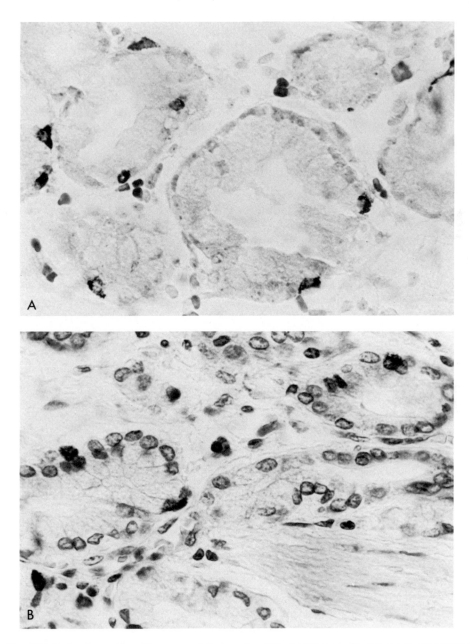

Fig. 31. Endocrine cells with argyrophil granules (Sevier-Munger, A) are more numerous than argentaffin cells (Masson-Fontana, B). × 600.

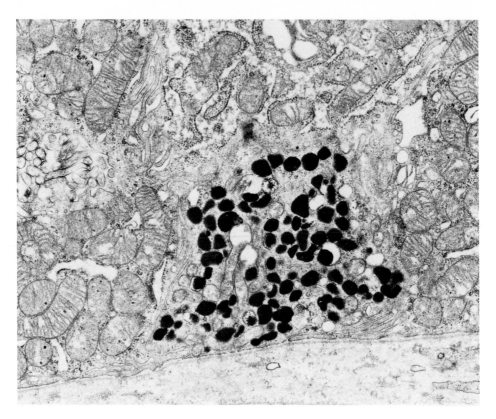

Fig. 32. Endocrine cell located along the basal lamina between two parietal cells. The secretory granules are uniformly dense, but vary in size and shape suggesting an EC cell. × 15,600.

Squamous Epithelium

No unusual findings were observed in the islands of stratified squamous epithelium within the columnar mucosa, nor in that lining the esophagus above the diseased segment. The demarcation between the squamous and the columnar epithelium was always sharp (Fig. 19); no gradual transition was ever seen.

Discussion

The difficulty in classifying the columnar and glandular lining of the esophagus in patients suffering reflux esophagitis is underscored by the variety of opinions reported in the literature. Most authors have regarded this lining as being gastric in type with or without parietal and chief cells,[1, 3, 4, 6, 11, 13, 20, 24-26, 31, 34, 36, 37, 39, 41] and sometimes displaying features of intestinal metaplasia.[1, 3, 20] Hayward[23] has suggested that this "gastric" epithelium in the esophagus is identical to what he calls "junctional esophageal epithelium" that, in his opinion, normally covers the esophagogastric junction and is different from the cardiac epithelium. Other authors

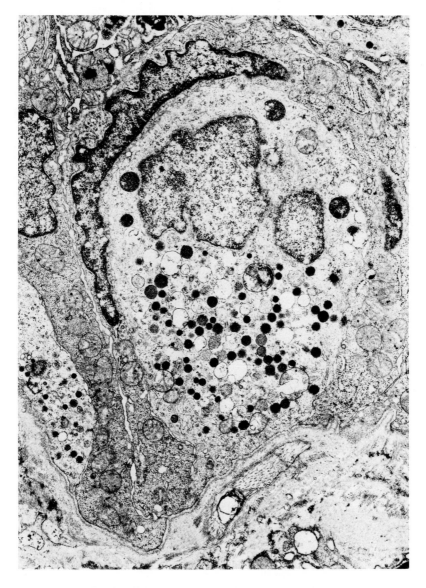

Fig. 33. Basally located endocrine cell "embedded" [50] in an epithelial cell. The pale cytoplasm contains round granules of variable density and several degranulated vesicles. This is probably an ECL cell. × 11,000.

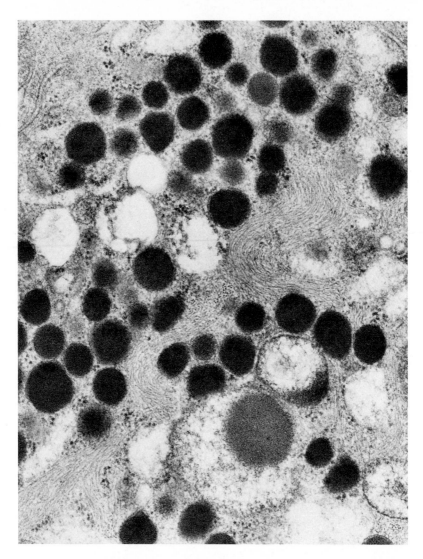

Fig. 34. Higher magnification of an endocrine cell along a surface fold or a pitlike structure. Most of the granules are dense and round with irregular membranes and others are larger with eccentric dense matrix. These granules and the prominent bundles of filaments are reminiscent of an ECL cell. × 41,350.

have preferred to describe this same kind of lining with the noncommittal term of columnar epithelium without characterizing it any further.[19, 40] More recently, Trier[63] studied 5 cases by light and electron microscopy and concluded that these esophagi were lined by a distinctive columnar secretory epithelium different from any other gastrointestinal epithelia, an opinion that has been subsequently shared by Berenson et al.[9]

In studying our material, we were struck by the differences in cellular mor-

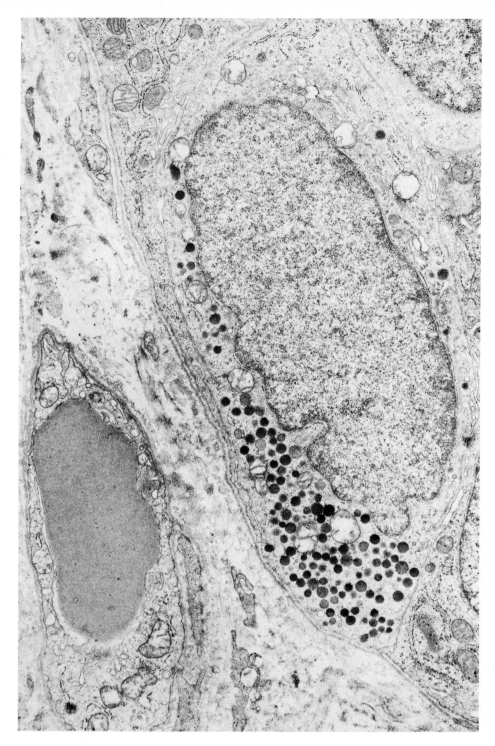

Fig. 35. Unclassified endocrine cell (ECL?) along the basal lamina of a gland. The adjacent blood vessel has fenestrated endothelial cells with numerous pinocytotic vesicles. × 12,900.

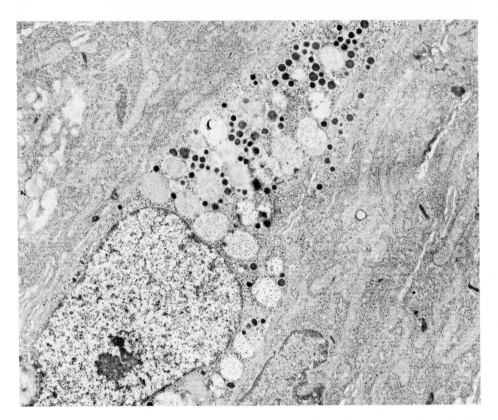

Fig. 36. Cell in columnar epithelium containing dense endocrine granules admixed with pale mucin granules. $\times$ 7400.

phology from case to case and even from area to area of the same case. This is, in part, the result of sampling by means of small biopsies. For instance, it was described previously that parietal and chief cells were found in 1 of 2 biopsies performed at the same time on the same patient. This also explains, at least in part, the seemingly contrasting findings reported in the literature.

In our material, some cells were recognizable because they displayed light and electron microscopic features typical of cells normally found in the stomach and in the intestines. These were all mature cells and included parietal, chief, Paneth, goblet, and some of the endocrine cells. Conversely, other cells had only some features in common with known gastric or intestinal cells and displayed or lacked others, which made them differ more or less profoundly.

Among the latter, the columnar mucus cells of the surface epithelium are a typical example. These cells correspond to those described by Trier [63] as "principal cells" and by Hage and Pedersen [20] as "mucus-producing columnar cells." Although reminiscent of the columnar epithelium surfacing the normal human gastric mucosa,[28, 35, 53] they differ from it in several respects. They secrete a mucin that

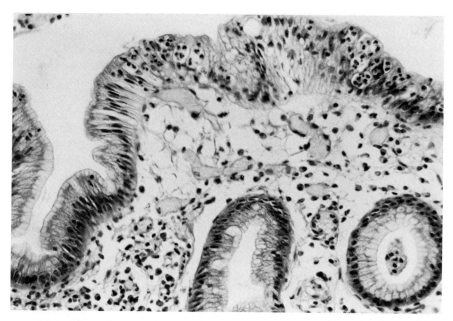

Fig. 37. Moderate inflammatory cell reaction in the lamina propria. Numerous granulocytes infiltrate focally the surface epithelium. H&E. × 260.

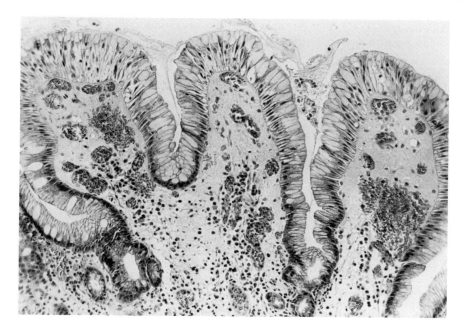

Fig. 38. Edema of the lamina propria can make the mucosal folds appear more prominent. Such edematous folds should not be misinterpreted as intestinal villi. H&E. × 130.

is mostly neutral (PAS-positive) as normal gastric surface mucus cells do,[17] but some of them contain material that stains also with AB indicative of nonsulfated (AB, pH 2.5) and of sulfated (AB, pH 1.2) acid mucopolysaccharides more typical of mucin of the small and large intestines.[17] These findings are similar to those of some authors,[1] but at variance with those of others,[20, 63] who described these cells as being PAS-positive and AB-negative (pH 2.5). With the electron microscope, the mucin granules of these cells vary from dark and stippled as seen in normal stomach, to pale like those of intestinal mucus cells. Furthermore, as compared with gastric surface mucus cells, these columnar esophageal cells have longer and more numerous microvilli, which frequently exhibit deeply penetrating micro-filamentous rootlets, and less frequent basilar deposits of glycogen. In similar fashion, these cells cannot be likened to the surface cells of the normal gastro-esophageal junction [63] nor to any mature or developing mucus-secreting cells of the intestine. Analogous observations can be made regarding the columnar mucus cells lining the pitlike structures.

The mucus cells present in the glands closely resemble the mucus cells of gastric glands. Their mucin, however, appears to be positive to AB at pH 2.5 and pH 1.2 more frequently and more intensely than generally seen in normal stomachs.[17]

Several types of partly differentiated cells were present in variable number at all levels of these mucus membranes. On the surface, they were seen especially in cases containing numerous goblet cells. Their ultrastructure, and in particular, the presence of vesicles and secretory granules, made them appear more similar to developing goblet cells than to other maturing gastrointestinal cells. The secretory granules, even though inconspicuous in some of them, made it unlikely that these cells might be related to developing absorptive cells. This is further supported by the fact that no mature absorptive cells with closely and uniformly spaced micro-villi and well-developed terminal web [33, 64] were ever seen in any of our specimens, nor were they described in any of the earlier ultrastructural studies.[9, 20, 63] The developing mucus cells found in some of the glands resembled the developing mucus cells of the neck of gastric glands, from which they differed, however, by being taller, richer in RER, and by displaying some long microvilli. Sometimes, cells could be recognized as being developing mucus cells, but whether they were of gastric or of intestinal type could not be determined. Likewise, rare cells appeared as undifferentiated because of rudimentary microvilli, large mitochondria with prominent matrical bodies, scanty RER, well-developed Golgi, frequent centrioles, supernumerary cell-to-cell junctions, and absence of secretory granules, but no finer recognition could be made. It should also be noted that transition forms between undifferentiated cells and parietal or zymogenic cells were sought for and not found.

As pointed out previously, we were unable to determine the type of many of the endocrine cells found in our material. Some cells could be recognized as EC and ECL (enterochromaffinlike) cells. Others, especially some of those reaching the lumen of the glands, were probably G (gastrin-secreting) cells. Hage and Pedersen,[20] using finer techniques, were able to demonstrate in 3 of their 5 esophageal biopsies G, D (equivalent to D pancreatic cells), and ECL cells, which so far have been found only in foregut derivatives, in addition to the ubiquitous EC cells.

If we consider how this heterogeneous cell population participates in the makeup of the mucosal lining of the distal esophagus, we are again struck by the varying degrees of architectural complexity ranging from simple columnar epithelium to glands containing highly differentiated cells. The classification of these mucosae is as difficult as that of the cells that compose them. The simple columnar epithelium resembles that of the normal gastric surface, but at the same time differs from it because of the features of the mucus-secreting cells and the presence of goblet cells and immature cells. Similarly, many of the glandular structures are evocative of gastric glands, albeit incompletely formed. This is particularly true where one can envision a pit, a neck with mucus cells in mitosis, and a deeper glandular portion containing parietal and chief cells next to mucus cells. Nevertheless, at close scrutiny, the histochemical and ultrastructural characteristics in some of their cells point out several differences between these esophageal glands and those of the stomach. Furthermore, although we observed mitotic activity only in the upper portion of the glands, Trier [63] found mitoses at the base of "crypt-like glands" as well. Some glands, especially those containing many goblet cells and occasional Paneth cells, suggest intestinal crypts, but none of them show all the typical features. It is also important to remark that in our material we never observed structures recognizable as intestinal villi. The presence of rare and abnormal ciliated cells in some of the glands adds to the complexity of these structures. To our knowledge, ciliated epithelium is normally found in the esophagus during embryonal life [30] and has been seen in the distal esophagus of newborns [48] and of one adult,[47] but only in the superficial lining and not in glands.

From a functional point of view this epithelium has been shown to secrete hydrochloric acid following histamine stimulation [25] and to contain fundal type pepsinogens by agar gel electrophoresis zymograms,[31] both suggestive of gastric secretory type of activities. As to intestinal functions, Trier [63] did not find any light and electron microscopic evidence suggesting a lipid absorptive capacity of this epithelium after esophageal perfusion with a micellar solution of oleic acid, monoolein, and sodium taurocholate. Further, the absence of mature intestinal absorptive cells in this epithelium has already been pointed out. On the other hand, Berenson et al [9] showed that columnar esophageal epithelium lacked disaccharidase activity, and that alkaline and acid phosphatases, glucose-6-phosphatase, leucine aminopeptidase, and 5-nucleotidase were demonstrable, but were less active than in normal intestine. They also observed that in the columnar esophageal epithelium, the lysosomal β-galactosidase activity was less than in the intestine, whereas the β-glucuronidase activity was greater than in the stomach. Such an enzymatic pattern is at variance with that of the normal pattern in which the activity of both of these enzymes is greater in the intestinal absorptive mucosa than in the gastric secretory epithelium.[10] Not much attention has been paid thus far to the mucin secretion by this epithelium. Most of our specimens showed a capricious admixture of neutral (gastric) and acid (intestinal) mucins, some of which were sulfated, although one type generally predominated over the others. This makes us wonder whether the type of mucin produced is independent of or secondary to local stimuli, and what influence, if any, it might have on the course of the disease.

Therefore, this distal esophageal secretory mucosa is characterized by gastric, intestinal, and unclassifiable features. For this reason, we feel that it is pathologic and sui generis in that it has no equivalent in the normal and abnormal gastrointestinal tract. As mentioned previously, a similar opinion has been expressed by Trier.[63] Thus, we think that it cannot be considered as a gastric mucosa with intestinal metaplasia;[1, 3, 20] in fact, when the latter occurs in the stomach, it is characterized by a full complement of mature and immature intestinal cells,[18, 52] which is not the case in the esophagus.

The genesis of this epithelium has been a matter of controversy ever since it was described. Some authors favored a congenital malformation,[6, 34, 41] especially for those cases discovered early in life.[1] Indeed, the possibility cannot be excluded that occasionally islands of congenital heterotopic gastric mucosa present in the distal esophagus of some patients with gastroesophageal reflux might be the starting point of the alterations in the esophageal mucosa. Such cases, however, if they exist, would be the exception rather than the rule, as shown by esophagoscopic observations. Further, congenital gastric heterotopia in the esophagus differs from the secretory epithelium associated with reflux esophagitis in that it is generally in the form of islands and is located more frequently in the upper than in the distal part of the esophagus.[48, 56] Others, while favoring a congenital process, suggested that some examples of "gastric mucosa" in the esophagus might be acquired through healing of an ulceration caused by gastric reflux.[4] More evidence favoring an acquired pathogenesis has accumulated during the last few years. The association of columnar esophageal epithelium and gastric reflux with or without hiatal hernia has been repeatedly stressed.[3, 13, 55] This association is striking even in small children and infants. In addition, while many patients with gastroesophageal reflux display only minor or no inflammatory changes of the squamous mucosa,[7, 27, 57] columnar esophageal lining of the type described here is found almost exclusively in association with gastroesophageal reflux.

Progressive phases in the evolution of peptic esophagitis going from minimal nonspecific inflammatory changes to extensive replacement of the squamous lining by columnar epithelium have been depicted on the basis of esophagoscopic observations.[55] Furthermore, 3 cases have been reported in whom such progressive replacement could be histologically documented.[19, 21, 40] In another case, a subtotal esophagectomy and gastroesophageal anastomosis for a lye stricture were followed by reflux esophagitis and replacement of the preoperatively documented squamous esophageal mucosa by columnar epithelium over a period of 13 years.[42] Finally, experimental evidence was provided by Bremner et al[12] who showed that re-epithelization of stripped distal esophageal mucosa in the dog was by columnar cells in the presence of gastroesophageal reflux and predominantly by squamous epithelium if the cardiac sphincter was intact and competent. This is in keeping with the experimental studies of Thal[61] indicating that in an acid environment, the esophageal squamous epithelium is replaced by an ingrowth of columnar cells, as well as with the observations on the regeneration of the gastric mucosa of rats by Wong and Finckh.[66]

In our opinion, the clinical, esophagoscopic, structural, and experimental findings overwhelmingly support the theory that in a significant proportion of patients, the peptic injury produced by the gastroesophageal reflux is repaired by a meta-plastic columnar and secretory epithelium.

The progenitor cell that gives rise to such metaplastic and peculiar epithelium remains unknown. Some authors [12, 19, 23] have suggested a derivation from cardiac (gastric, junctional) cells, but Hamilton and Yardley [21] have pointed out that the columnar lining in the esophagus can develop even in absence of cardiac mucosa. In fact, they observed the development of columnar lining in the esophagus of a patient who underwent partial esophagogastrectomy for squamous carcinoma of the esophagus six years previously. Other suggestions include the esophageal glands,[3, 21] the squamous epithelium itself,[21] and a primordial esophageal or gastric stem cell.[9] Transition from squamous epithelium or from esophageal glands to columnar esophageal lining was not found in our material. We did find undifferen-tiated cells in some cases, but their nature was unclear, and we could not come to a satisfactory conclusion. We could only hypothesize that such cells might be undifferentiated foregut cells capable of mimicking in the course of their evolution various types of gastrointestinal cells without necessarily reaching full maturity. It is pertinent to point out that the foregut gives origin to the gastrointestinal tract including as far down as the upper half of the second part of the duodenum, which could explain in part the intestinal features of this esophageal lining.

The clinical importance of this lesion is apparent, especially when one con-siders its complications, and is underscored by its precancerous nature. Several cases of adenocarcinomas associated with esophageal columnar epithelium have been reported and have been the object of recent reviews.[8, 22, 42] These were all infiltrating tumors with the exception of one multifocal adenocarcinoma in situ.[8] It is difficult to establish from the literature the exact incidence of this carcinoma, because most authors report single cases and frequently do not specify whether the tumor involved the cardia as well. In a series of 140 cases of reflux esophagitis with metaplastic columnar changes previously reported from here, there were 3 adenocarcinomas (in 2 men and 1 woman) confined to the esophageal wall and separated from the cardia by a segment of columnar esophageal mucosa.[42] At the Mayo Clinic, 2 of 85 cases of "Barrett esophagus" subsequently developed an adenocarcinoma limited to the esophagus, and in 5 additional cases the 2 diseases were diagnosed simultaneously.[22] These figures represent a very high incidence when they are compared with the rarity of primary esophageal adenocarcinoma in the general population. In fact, in a series reported from the Memorial Sloan-Kettering Cancer Center, adenocarcinomas were 2.4 percent of all esophageal carcinomas,[65] the overall incidence of which has been reported as 8.3 and 1.9 per 100,000 population for white males and females in the United States [2] and as 9.5 and 2.6 respectively by the Tumor Registry of Geneva (Switzerland).

In the local series, there were 9 additional cases, all in men, in whom the carcinoma involved the distal esophagus lined by columnar epithelium and the cardia at the same time.[42] It is not possible to determine in such cases whether the carcinoma arose in the esophagus or in the cardia, but the concomitance of the two conditions is striking all the same.

Once the metaplastic lesion has set in, it is irreversible as judged by its persistence after surgical correction of the reflux. Its histologic appearance also remains essentially unchanged. Corrective surgery thus appears to be useful in limiting the onset and consequences of such complications as stenosis and peptic ulceration, but probably has only a limited influence on the precancerous potential of this lesion. For instance, one patient developed an adenocarcinoma in the distal esophagus lined by columnar epithelium nearly three years after his gastroesophageal reflux had been successfully corrected surgically.[42] This is of great practical significance and indicates that all patients with columnar esophageal lining should be frequently and carefully checked even after their gastroesophageal reflux is no longer a factor.

Acknowledgments

The authors are indebted to Miss Jacqueline Bräutigam and to Miss Hazel Holden for their able technical assistance.

References

1. Abrams L, Heath D: Lower esophagus lined with intestinal and gastric epithelia. Thorax 20:66, 1965
2. Ackerman LV, del Regato JA: Cancer. Diagnosis, treatment and prognosis, 4th ed. St Louis, Mosby, 1970, pp 408–9
3. Adler RH: The esophagus with columnar epithelium, its clinical significance. Geriatrics 25:109, 1965
4. Allison PR, Johnstone AS: The oesophagus lined with gastric mucous membrane. Thorax 8:87, 1953
5. Barrett NR: Chronic peptic ulcer of the oesophagus and "oesophagitis." Br J Surg 38:175, 1950
6. Barrett NR: The lower esophagus lined by columnar epithelium. Surgery 41:881, 1957
7. Behar J, Sheahan DC: Histologic abnormalities in reflux esophagitis. Arch Pathol 99:387, 1975
8. Belladonna JA, Hajdu SI, Bains MS, Winawer SJ: Adenocarcinoma in situ of Barrett's esophagus diagnosed by endoscopic cytology. N Engl J Med 291:895, 1974
9. Berenson MM, Herbst JJ, Freston JW: Enzyme and ultrastructural characteristics of esophageal columnar epithelium. Am J Dig Dis 19:895, 1974
10. Berenson MM, Herbst JJ, Freston JW: Esophageal columnar epithelial β-galactosidase and β-glucuronidase. Gastroenterology 68:1417, 1975
11. Bosher LH, Taylor FH: Heterotopic gastric mucosa in the esophagus with ulceration and stricture formation. J Thorac Cardiovasc Surg 21:306, 1951
12. Bremner CG, Lynch VP, Ellis FH: Barrett's esophagus: congenital or acquired? An experimental study of esophageal mucosal regeneration in the dog. Surgery 68:209, 1970
13. Burgess JN, Payne WS, Andersen HA, Weiland LH, Carlson HC: Barrett esophagus. The columnar-epithelial-lined lower esophagus. Mayo Clin Proc 46:728, 1971
14. Currie AR, Wheatley DN: Cilia of a distinctive structure $(9 + 0)$ in endocrine and other tissues. Postgrad Med J 42:403, 1966
15. Donnellan WL: The structure of the colonic mucosa. The epithelium and subepithelial reticulohistiocytic complex. Gastroenterology 49:496, 1965

16. Fawcett DW, Porter KR: A study of the fine structure of ciliated epithelia. J Morphol 94:221, 1954
17. Goldman H, Ming SC: Mucin in normal and neoplastic gastrointestinal epithelium. Histochemical distribution. Arch Pathol 85:580, 1968
18. Goldman H, Ming SC: Fine structure of intestinal metaplasia and adenocarcinoma of the human stomach. Lab Invest 18:203, 1968
19. Goldman MC, Beckman RC: Barrett syndrome. Case report with discussion about concepts of pathogenesis. Gastroenterology 39:104, 1960
20. Hage E, Pedersen SA: Morphological characteristics of the columnar epithelium lining the lower esophagus in patients with Barrett's syndrome. Virchows Arch (Pathol Anat) 357:219, 1972
21. Hamilton SR, Yardley JJ: Acquisition of columnar (Barrett type) epithelium in the distal esophagus after partial esophagogastrectomy. Lab Invest 32:425, 1975
22. Hawe A, Payne WS, Weiland LH, Fontana RS: Adenocarcinoma in the columnar epithelial lined lower (Barrett) oesophagus. Thorax 28:511, 1973
23. Hayward J: The lower end of the oesophagus. Thorax 16:36, 1961
24. Heitmann P, Strauszer T, Sapunar J, Larrain A: Lower esophagus lined with columnar epithelium: morphological and physiological correlation. Gastroenterology 53:611, 1967
25. Hershfield NB, Lind JF, Hildes JA, McMorris LS: Secretory function of Barrett's epithelium. Gut 6:535, 1965
26. Hill LD, Gelfand M, Bauermeister D: Simplified management of reflux esophagitis with stricture. Ann Surg 172:638, 1970
27. Ismail-Beigi F, Horton PF, Pope CE: II Histological consequences of gastro-esophageal reflux in man. Gastroenterology 58:163, 1970
28. Ito S: Anatomic structure of the gastric mucosa. In Code FC, Heidel W (eds): Handbook of Physiology, sect 6, Alimentary Canal, vol 2, Secretion. Washington, DC, American Physiological Society, 1967, pp 705–41
29. Jackson C: Peptic ulcer of the esophagus. JAMA 92:369, 1929
30. Johns BAE: Developmental changes in the oesophageal epithelium in man. J Anat 86:431, 1952
31. Johnston JH: Gastric lined esophagus associated with rings and stenosis. Ann Surg 173:641, 1971
32. Kaye GI, Lane N, Pascal R: Colonic pericryptal fibroblast sheath: replication, migration, and cytodifferentiation of a mesenchymal cell system in adult tissue. II. Fine structural aspects of normal rabbit and human colon. Gastroenterology 54:852, 1968
33. Kaye GI, Fenoglio CM, Pascal RR, Lane N: Comparative electron microscopic features of normal, hyperplastic, and adenomatous human colonic epithelium. Variations in cellular structure relative to the process of epithelial differentiation. Gastroenterology 64:926, 1973
34. Kleinsasser O, Friedmann G: Magenschleimhaut in Ösophagus. Ein Beitrag zur Frage der Genese der Hiatushernien. Z Laryng Rhinol Otol 51:751, 1972
35. Lillibridge CB: The fine structure of normal human gastric mucosa. Gastroenterology 47:269, 1964
36. Lortat-Jacob JL: L'endobrachy-oesophage. Ann Chir 11:1247, 1957
37. Mangla JC, Kim Y, Guarasci G, Schenk EA: Pepsinogens in epithelium of Barrett's esophagus. Gastroenterology 65:949, 1973
38. Millington PF, Finean JB: Electron microscope studies of the structure of the microvilli on principal epithelial cells of rat jejunum after treatment in hypo- and hypertonic saline. J Cell Biol 14:125, 1962
39. Monti MM, Fasel J, Savary M: Le problème histologique des hétérotopies épithéliales étendues du bas oesophage. Ann Oto-Laryng 86:380, 1969
40. Mossberg SM: The columnar-lined esophagus (Barrett syndrome)—An acquired condition? Gastroenterology 50:671, 1966
41. Mounier-Kuhn P, Gaillard J, Lafon H, Morgon A, Haguenauer JP: Oesophagites et architecture muqueuse. J Fr Otorhinolaryngol 17:721, 1968

42. Naef AP, Savary M, Ozzello L: Columnar-lined lower esophagus: an acquired lesion with malignant predisposition. Report on 140 cases of Barrett's esophagus with 12 adenocarcinomas. J Thorac Cardiovasc Surg 70:826, 1975

43. Nagle GJ, Kurtz SM: Electron microscopy of the human rectal mucosa. A comparison of idiopathic ulcerative colitis with inflammation of known etiologies. Am J Dig Dis (New Series) 12:541, 1967

44. Parker FG, Barnes EN, Kaye GI: The pericryptal fibroblast sheath. IV. Replication, migration, and differentiation of the subepithelial fibroblasts of the crypt and villus of the rabbit jejunum. Gastroenterology 67:607, 1974

45. Pearse AGE, Coulling I, Weavers B, Friesen S: The endocrine polypeptide cells of the human stomach, duodenum, and jejunum. Gut 11:649, 1970

46. Pittman FE, Pittman JC: Electron microscopy of intestinal mucosa. Arch Pathol 81:398, 1966

47. Raeburn C: Columnar ciliated epithelium in adult oesophagus. J Path Bact 63:157, 1951

48. Rector LE, Connerley ML: Aberrant mucosa in the esophagus in infants and in children. Arch Pathol 31:285, 1941

49. Rifaat MK, Iseri OA, Gottlieb LS: An ultrastructural study of the "extraneous coat" of human colonic mucosa. Gastroenterology 48:593, 1965

50. Rubin W: An unusual intimate relationship between endocrine cells and other types of epithelial cells in the human stomach. J Cell Biol 52:219, 1972

51. Rubin W: Endocrine cells in the normal human stomach. A fine structural study. Gastroenterology 63:784, 1972

52. Rubin W, Ross LL, Jeffries GH, Sleisenger MH: Intestinal heterotopia. A fine structural study. Lab Invest 15:1024, 1966

53. Rubin W, Ross LL, Sleisenger MH, Jeffries GH: The normal human gastric epithelia. A fine structural study. Lab Invest 19:598, 1968

54. Savary M: L'apport de la photographie en endoscopie oesophagienne basse. Ann Otolaryngol Chir Cervicofac 87:684, 1970

55. Savary M: L'expression endoscopique de l'oesophagite par reflux. Proc 13th Congress Internat Broncho-oesophagol Soc, Lyon, 1971. Villeurbane (France), Simep, 1972, pp 101–18

56. Savary M, Naef AP, Ozzello L, Roethlisberger B: Endobrachyôesophage et adénocarcinome. Schweiz Med Wochenschr 105:575, 1975

57. Seefeld von U, Krejs GJ, Brändli HH, Siebenmann RE, Blum AL: Reflux und Sodbrennen. Morphologische Aspekte Z Gastroenterol 12:36, 1974

58. Sevier AC, Munger BL: A silver method for paraffin sections of neural tissue. J Neuropathol Exp Neurol 24:130, 1965

59. Tahara E, Haizuka S, Kodama T, Yamada A: The relationship of gastrointestinal endocrine cells to gastric epithelial changes with special reference to gastric cancer. Acta Pathol Jap 25:161, 1975

60. Tateishi R, Tanuguchi H, Wada A, Horai T, Taniguchi K: Argyrophil cells and melanocytes in esophageal mucosa. Arch Pathol 98:87, 1974

61. Thal AP: Discussion of Hill LD, et al [26]

62. Trier JS: Studies on small intestinal crypt epithelium. I. The fine structure of the crypt epithelium of the proximal small intestine of fasting humans. J Cell Biol 18:599, 1963

63. Trier JS: Morphology of the epithelium of the distal esophagus in patients with mid-esophageal peptic strictures. Gastroenterology 58:444, 1970

64. Trier JS, Rubin CE: Electron microscopy of the small intestine: a review. Gastroenterology 49:574, 1965

65. Turnbull ADM, Goodner JT: Primary adenocarcinoma of the esophagus. Cancer 22:915, 1968

66. Wong J, Finckh ES: Heterotopia and ectopia of gastric epithelium produced by mucosal wounding in the rat. Gastroenterology 60:279, 1971

DEFINING THE PRECURSOR TISSUE OF ORDINARY LARGE BOWEL CARCINOMA:
Implications for Cancer Prevention

CECILIA M. FENOGLIO, GORDON I. KAYE,
ROBERT R. PASCAL, AND NATHAN LANE

The observations that atypism, carcinoma in situ, or intramucosal carcinoma is rarely seen except in adenomatous polyps and papillary adenomas and that invasive foci less than 5 millimeters in diameter are rarely seen except in these lesions, constitute evidence to support the belief that the vast majority of cancers arise in adenomatous polyps and papillary adenomas.[1] (1958)

Apart from the separate problem of cancer in ulcerative colitis we need to know whether there is an alternative to the concept that all large bowel cancers arise from pre-existing benign adenomatous polyps or villous adenomas. So far, no scientific evidence in support of an alternative theory of histogenesis has been described. In particular, the concept of cancer "de novo," whatever this means in morphological terms, remains hypothetical.[2] (1975)

In order to define the precursor tissue of ordinary large bowel carcinoma, particular attention will be given to the terminology. We have attempted to use simple accurate terms, with the help of diagrams and illustrations, so that internists, surgeons, radiologists, and pathologists will have the same mental image of what we are dealing with, in order to facilitate the communication that is so necessary for proper diagnosis and treatment in this field.

The term precursor tissue is synonymous with precancerous or preneoplastic tissues. This term not only implies that cancer *may* develop in such a lesion or abnormal tissue, but also that cancer *will* develop in such an abnormal focus with far greater frequency than in the seemingly morphologically normal adjacent tissue.

A further implication of the term precursor tissue is that, in the case of the large bowel, the detection and removal of this precursor tissue will reduce the incidence of colorectal carcinoma.

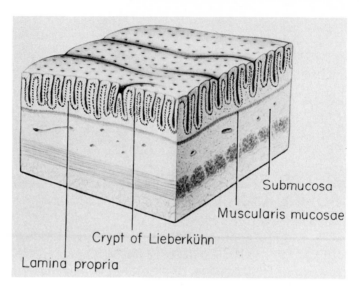

Fig. 1. Diagram of normal colon to emphasize the muscularis mucosae. It is of prime importance to remember that in neoplasia the muscularis mucosae is used to distinguish between an intramucosal and an invasive neoplasm.

This chapter will deal only with those benign lesions known as adenomas and hyperplastic polyps and only the ordinary moderately and well-differentiated adenocarcinomas.

The rare cases of undifferentiated carcinoma and carcinoma arising in ulcerative colitis will not be considered. Neither will we consider a variety of unrelated polypoid masses such as juvenile polyps, the polypoid hamartomas of Peutz-Jeghers syndrome, inflammatory pseudopolyps, polypoid leiomyomas, lymphoid masses, lipomas, etc. However, we will discuss those studies of familial polyposis cases in which we have gained some insights into colorectal neoplasia.

Basic Concepts

The evolution of ordinary large bowel carcinoma from its precursor tissue is best understood if one recalls a few features of normal colonic histology and cell kinetics.

The flat nonvillous colonic mucosa has simple test tube shaped glands known as the crypts of Lieberkuhn. The intervening mucosal tissue is called the lamina propria. A thin layer of smooth muscle, the muscularis mucosae, is the boundary line between the mucosa and submucosa, and it is this structure which is used to distinguish between an intramucosal and an invasive process (Fig. 1). The importance of this is discussed at length later in this chapter.

Normally, cell division is very active, but it is restricted to the deepest one-half or one-third of the crypts (Fig. 2). Cells produced by this active division migrate toward the surface and differentiate into two principal cell types, goblet cells and absorptive cells (Fig. 3).

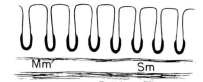

Fig. 2. Normal controlled replication is restricted to the deep portion of the crypts, as indicated by the heavy shading. (From Fenoglio and Lane: Cancer 34:819, 1974)

In three to four days, this dynamic process of division and migration is perfectly balanced by exfoliation from the free surface.

Benign Proliferations

If in one or several crypts there is an imbalance between the rates of cell division and cellular exfoliation, there will occur a net gain in the number of cells, and a protrusion or "polyp" will result. In older adults, such benign proliferations are very common. Therefore, in order to define a precursor relationship of some of these proliferations to carcinoma, it is essential to classify them. This classification is as follows:

1. These proliferations (polyps) are divided into two basic biologic types, hyperplastic polyps and adenomas.
2. Furthermore, the adenomas must be divided according to size, and it is desirable to specify their shape and histologic pattern as well.

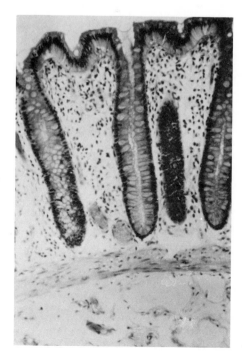

Fig. 3. Normally, cells migrate upwards and differentiate into two main cell types; the goblet cells are prominent in the crypts and the absorptive cells are more evident on the free surface. × 100.

3. Finally, it is essential to appreciate not only the absolute frequency of these proliferations, but especially the relative frequency of hyperplastic polyps to adenomas and the relative frequency of small and large adenomas.

Two Basic Types

The two biologic types of benign proliferations occurring in adults may be discussed in terms of hyperplasia and benign neoplasia. It is because of the different characteristics of hyperplasia versus neoplasia that these two kinds of proliferations have such a different meaning in terms of the subsequent development of large bowel cancer. Fortunately, these two types are easily distinguished histologically.[3-6]

Hyperplasia (Hyperplastic Polyps)

Grossly, these appear as sessile, discrete, smooth-surfaced and rounded "dewdrop" elevations usually less than 5 mm (Fig. 4). Microscopically, the excessive number of cells results in papillary infoldings of the epithelium within the crypts, producing a typical serrated or corkscrew appearance of the glands (Fig. 5). In support of the idea that this is merely a hyperplastic process, one observes that differentiation into goblet and absorptive cells is indistinguishable from normal. This correlates with the fact that in this hyperplastic lesion, cell division remains restricted to the lower portions of the crypts, as in the normal colon (Fig. 6).

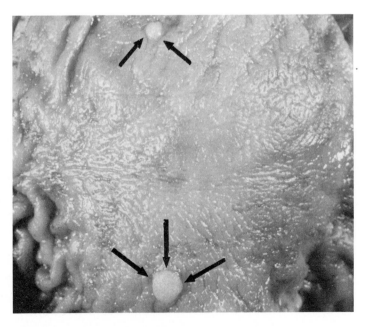

Fig. 4. Hyperplastic polyps usually measure a few millimeters in diameter and have a discrete "dewdrop" appearance.

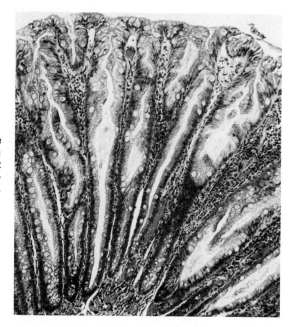

Fig. 5. In hyperplastic polyps, the papillary infolding of the epithelium is typical. The important point is that differentiation into goblet and absorptive cells is similar to normal. × 88.

Restriction of cell division that is similar to normal is an important characteristic of nonneoplastic tissues.

An additional histologic feature concerns an associated hyperplastic connective tissue change. Excess collagen production results in a thickening of the basement membrane beneath the surface epithelium. The dynamics of this phenomenon and how it contrasts with the situation in adenomas is discussed later.

Benign Neoplasia (Adenomas)

Grossly, these lesions are most commonly pedunculated with a raspberry-like surface, in contrast to the smooth surface of hyperplastic polyps (Fig. 7A). Less frequently, they may be bulky and sessile, or, rarely, flat and plaquelike (Fig. 7B and C). Unlike the hyperplastic polyps, their size may vary from only 1 or 2 mm to many centimeters. Several histologic patterns occur; either a tubular or a villous (papillary) appearance may be present, or these patterns may be combined (Fig. 8).

Fig. 6. The heavy lines show that in hyperplastic polyps, as in normal mucosa, the zone of replication remains restricted to the lower portion of the crypts. (From Fenoglio and Lane: Cancer 34:819, 1974)

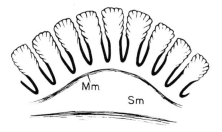

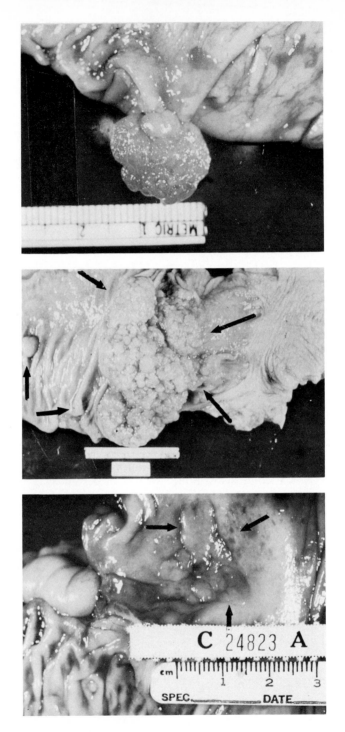

Fig. 7. The three typical gross appearances of adenomas. Top. Pedunculated adenoma. Center. Sessile adenomas. A bulky sessile adenoma, also known as papillary or villous adenoma, is in the center. A small rounded sessile adenoma is seen at the extreme right. Bottom. Flat, plaquelike adenoma.

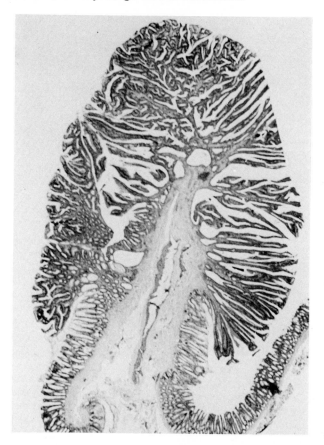

Fig. 8. Pedunculated adenoma with both papillary fronds and tubular areas. × 7. (From Grinnell and Lane: Surg Gynecol Obstet (Int Abstr Surg) 106:519, 1958)

The basic characteristics of the cells composing the adenomas are the same regardless of the variety of gross and microscopic patterns. In general, adenomatous epithelium is tall and very crowded, producing a "picket-fence" pattern with a marked increase in the nuclear cytoplasmic ratio (Fig. 9). Correlated with this nuclear change is a failure of orderly differentiation into goblet and absorptive cells. This, in turn, reflects the fact that the control mechanisms governing cell division are largely lost in adenomas, so that thymidine uptake, DNA synthesis, and mitosis occur at all levels in adenomatous epithelium (Fig. 10 and 11). This last is perhaps the key feature indicating the neoplastic nature of adenomatous tissue.

Morphologically and dynamically, these cells are indistinguishable from the partially differentiated cells that constitute the replicating population of the normal colonic crypt (Fig. 11).[5]

Associated Connective Tissue Features

Some years ago, our group became interested in certain specific connective tissue changes that occur in hyperplastic polyps and adenomas.[7-9] The normal

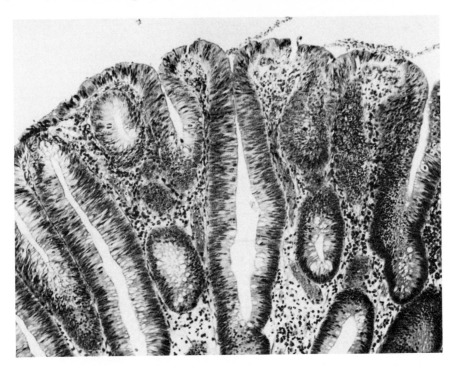

Fig. 9. In adenomas, there tends to be uniformity of the epithelium. The crowding of elongated nuclei produces the typical "picket-fence" appearance. Orderly differentiation into goblet and absorptive cells is largely lost. × 150. (From Lane et al: Gastroenterology 60:537, 1971)

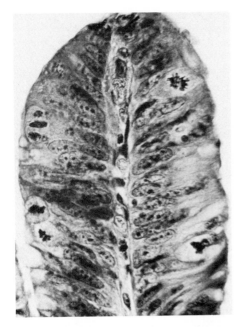

Fig. 10. In an adenoma, mitotic activity may be seen at all levels—even at the free surface. × 600. (From Lane et al: Gastroenterology 60:537, 1971)

Fig. 11. The heavy line indicates that in adenomas the zone of cell replication is *not* restricted. In contrast to normal mucosa and hyperplastic polyps, cell replication occurs in all regions of adenomatous epithelium. The loss of control of replication confirms the neoplastic nature of adenomas. (From Fenoglio and Lane: Cancer 34:819, 1974)

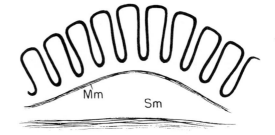

crypt is tightly invested by a sheath of fibroblasts, which appears to be directly apposed to the epithelium, with minimal intervening collagen (Fig. 12A and B). However, at the mouth of the crypt, and especially under the free surface epithelium, one normally observes a uniform band of collagen (Fig. 13). Because it appears as though it is supporting the surface epithelium, we have called this the *collagen table*. It was noted on autoradiographic and electron microscopic studies that the nuclei of the fibroblasts around the bottom of the crypt picked up tritiated thymidine, indicating replication at the same level in the crypt at which the epithelial cells were replicating. Furthermore, autoradiography and electron microscopy showed that these fibroblasts migrated toward the luminal surface and differentiated synchronously with the epithelium. In the normal mucosa, as in the epithelium, the fibroblasts lost the ability to pick up thymidine and replicate at the surface. These features are summarized in Figure 14.

In adenomas, the fibroblasts beneath the surface epithelium remain immature and show thymidine uptake, as does the adenomatous epithelium (Fig. 15). Collagen is minimally produced by these immature subepithelial fibroblasts, resulting in a collagen table that is thinner than that under the normal adjacent epithelium of that individual (Fig. 16). By contrast, in hyperplastic polyps, the mature fibroblasts underneath the fully differentiated and hyperplastic surface epithelium, produce a collagen table that is also hyperplastic and thicker than the adjacent normal collagen table of that particular person (Fig. 17). This epithelial-fibroblast partnership is further shown by the fact that the point of thickening or thinning of the collagen table corresponds precisely with the point of epithelial junction between normal and hyperplastic or normal and adenomatous epithelium.

These contrasting connective tissue changes further emphasize the fundamentally different nature of hyperplastic polyps and adenomas.

Carcinoembryonic Antigen

Carcinoembryonic antigen (CEA), as originally described by Gold and Friedman,[10] was defined as a tumor-associated antigen that is found in cancers of the colon as well as in fetal gastrointestinal tissues. When a radioimmunoassay was developed for the detection of this material in the blood, a 97 percent incidence of positivity was reported in patients with cancers of the colon.[11] This incidence decreased to 72 percent when a larger series of patients was studied.[12] It then became clear that this drop in the incidence of positive blood levels was due to the

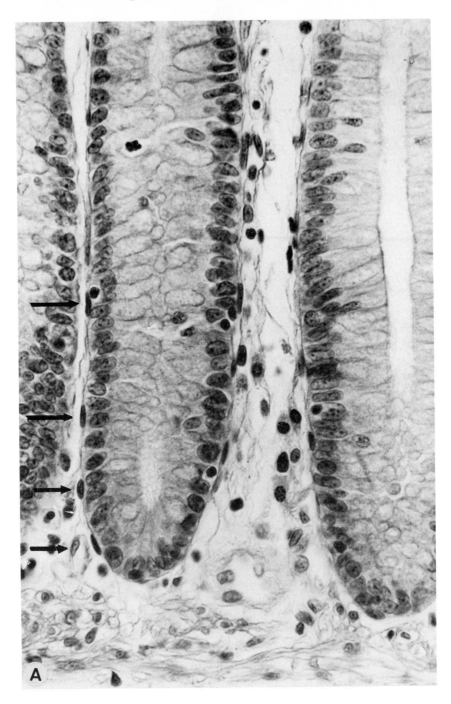

Fig. 12. Sagittal section A, and cross section B of normal colonic crypts. Note the sheath of flattened fibroblast nuclei closely investing the epithelium. These appear as a chain of elongated nuclei in A and as a complete ring in B. Other cells of the lamina propria appear to be randomly distributed. A: × 550; B: × 550. (From Pascal et al: Gastroenterology 54:835, 1968)

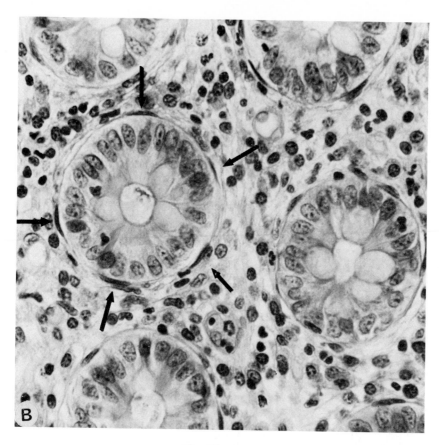

Fig. 12. (*cont.*)

inclusion of patients with early stages of disease and that the incidence of positivity for CEA in the blood correlates with the extent of the disease.[13]

CEA may be detected in tissue sections by using a monospecific antiserum in the three-layer bridge immunoperoxidase procedure for antigen detection as described by Hsu et al.[14]

Early studies in this laboratory using this technique indicate that CEA *may* be present in benign adenomatous epithelium,[15] as well as in the invasive cancers occurring in adenomas.[16] However, just as in the case with invasive cancer, CEA is present in some adenomas. CEA is not found in the cells lining the normal crypts of Lieberkuhn at any level. (The only exception to this is in the epithelium adjacent to a cancer or adenoma where CEA may be demonstrated on the cells at the luminal surface. This appears to represent a local spillover from the neighboring lesion.) CEA has not been demonstrated in the hyperplastic polyps examined to date. This, then, is further evidence that the adenomatous cells are truly neoplastic, since they may express a specific oncofetal antigen.

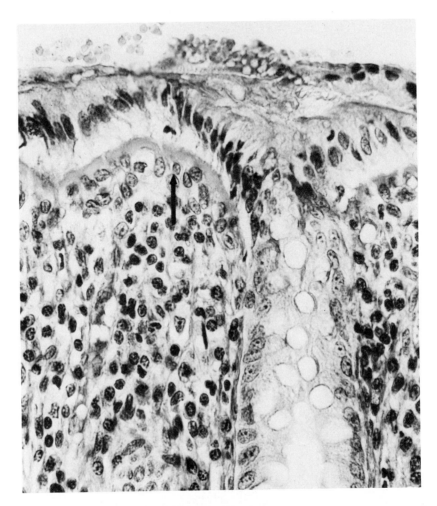

Fig. 13. At the surface of normal colonic mucosa, functional differentiation of the pericryptal fibroblast sheath is manifested by the production of a well-defined collagen table (arrow). Fewer fibroblast nuclei are seen under the absorptive epithelium of the surface. × 650. (From Pascal et al: Gastroenterology 54:835, 1968)

The Anatomic Origin of Adenomas

Bussey [17] has been able to detect adenomatous transformation of single crypts in grossly normal mucosal areas in familial polyposis specimens by using serial sections. He has, in effect, demonstrated "unicryptal" adenomas. In studies of colonic epithelium of patients with familial polyposis, Deschner and Lipkin [18] have found occasional crypts which, although histologically normal, show thymidine uptake continuing at or near the surface. These observations suggest a failure of those control mechanisms that normally restrict replication to the deep portion of

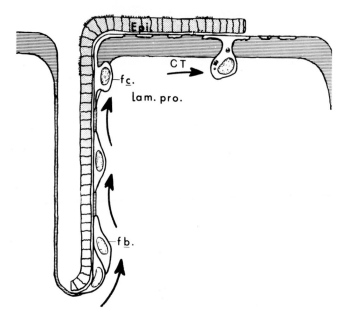

Fig. 14. Diagram showing the migration and maturation of the pericryptal fibroblast sheath in normal colonic mucosa. Like the epithelium, replication of fibroblasts (fb) is restricted to the deep zone of the crypt. As the fibroblasts migrate in synchrony with the epithelium, they too stop dividing and differentiate into functioning fibrocytes (fc), producing the normal collagen table (CT, hatched area).

Fig. 15. Autoradiography of adenomatous mucosa shows uptake of tritiated thymidine by nuclei of both the surface adenomatous epithelial cells and subjacent immature fibroblasts (arrow). × 800. (From Kaye et al: Gastroenterology 60:515, 1971)

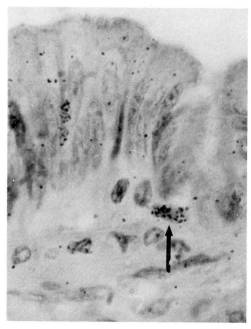

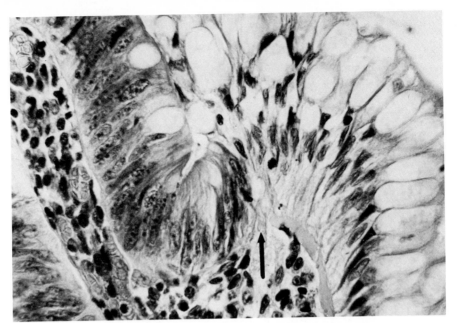

Fig. 16. Junction (arrow) of adenomatous (left) and normal (right) epithelium. There is so little collagen production under the adenomatous epithelium that the collagen table is thin and indistinct. A well-developed collagen table is seen under the normal epithelium. × 600. (From Lane et al: Gastroenterology 60:537, 1971)

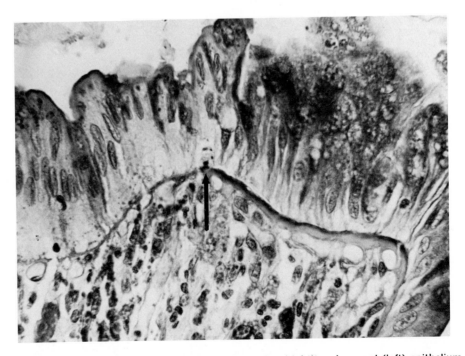

Fig. 17. Junction (arrow) of edge of hyperplastic polyp (right) and normal (left) epithelium. There is an overproduction of collagen resulting in a greatly thickened collagen table under the surface epithelium of hyperplastic polyps. × 600. (From Lane et al: Gastroenterology 60:537, 1971)

the crypt. This may be the earliest demonstration of an abnormality reflecting the transformation of normal to adenomatous epithelium.

Although adenomas ultimately may assume a wide variety of sizes, shapes, and histologic patterns, it seems that all of them have the same morphology at their inception. In studying minute adenomas, one observes a small number of crypts which are completely adenomatous.[3] Furthermore, the surface of these minute adenomas remains smooth (Fig. 18A). This indicates that at the outset, adenomatous tubules or papillary fronds do not grow preferentially from the free surface with preservation of normal colonic crypts below. When these minute adenomas (1 to 2 mm) are systematically studied using serial sections, one always observes that at the central point of origin of the lesion, the *full depth* of a few crypts is adenomatous. It is only in random tangential sections away from the center of the lesion that one may gain the misleading impression that the adenomatous epithelium has arisen in the upper portions of the crypts (Fig. 18B, C). This superficial position of the adenomatous epithelium toward the periphery of the adenoma is simply the result of spread of the adenomatous epithelium from the central nidus of origin (Fig. 19).

These observations support the following hypothesis concerning the precise site of origin of adenomatous epithelium in a crypt. It is known that normal cell division, which occurs deep in the crypt, is a controlled process giving rise to daughter cells that have been programmed to migrate upward and *stop* synthesizing DNA. If, in this replicating zone, the normal control mechanisms fail, an abnormal daughter cell population will result. Such cells will *continue* to synthesize DNA even after migrating upward. However, since it is in the deep third of the crypt that the original loss of control has taken place, this is the primary site of origin of the abnormally replicating adenomatous cell population. It is only subsequent to this that the on-going cell division in the entire crypt results in a sufficient number of adenomatous cells so that we are able to recognize that an adenoma has developed.

Size, Shape, and Histologic Pattern Relationships

Almost all hyperplastic polyps are minute and sessile. Greater structural variation is seen among adenomas, and there are several statistical correlations to be noted between size, shape, and histologic patterns.[19]

The average small adenomas, ie, in the size range of approximately 1 to 1.5 cm, tends to be pedunculated and to have a tubular pattern. Among larger adenomas, a greater proportion tend to be sessile and have a papillary (villous) pattern microscopically. The relationship between size and development of carcinoma in adenomas is discussed in the next section.

Absolute and Relative Frequencies

"Polyps" may be found in as many as 25 percent [20] of older adults who are repeatedly examined sigmoidoscopically over many years. Complete colon examination at autopsy has disclosed "polyps" in 50 percent of these specimens.[21]

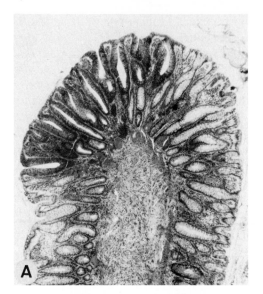

Fig. 18. Three sections through a small adenoma. A. This is a sagittal section through the center of a minute adenoma. It is evident that the neoplastic cells extend from the bases of the crypts to the smooth surface. In B, from the edge of the lesion, it would appear as if the adenomatous epithelium were arising in the superficial portion of a single crypt. In C, closer to, but not yet at the center of the lesion, the adenomatous crypts still appear to arise superficially. A: × 25; B: × 25; C: × 25. (From Lane and Lev: Cancer 16:751, 1963)

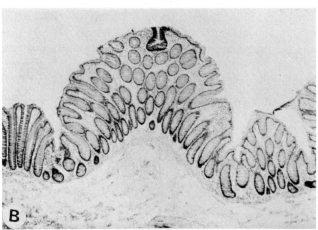

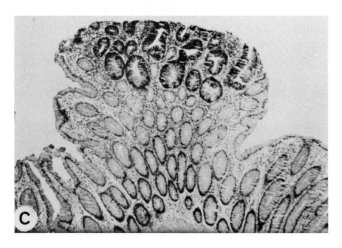

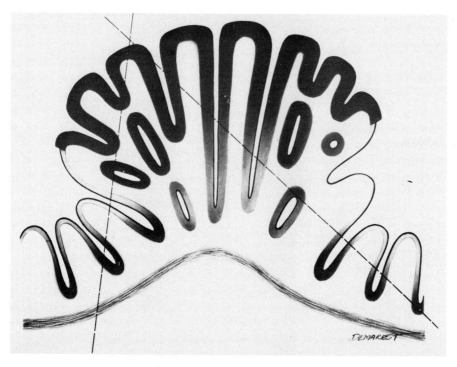

Fig. 19. Diagram of the adenoma shown in Figure 18. The neoplastic cells, which probably arise in the base of one central crypt, spread centrifugally to replace other crypts. Histologic sections not from the center of the lesion—such as indicated by the broken lines—can produce the appearances of Figures 18B and C. Such off-center sections would give the misleading impression that adenomatous epithelium arises superficially. (From Lane and Lev: Cancer 16:751, 1963)

An understanding of *relative* frequency is of greater importance than absolute figures such as these. Hyperplastic polyps are at least 10 times as frequent as all adenomas.[22] Adenomas smaller than 1.5 cm are about 10 times as common as larger adenomas.[6] Thus, the large adenomas represent only about 1 percent of all large bowel "polyps."

Unfortunately, the term "polyp" is often used indiscriminately. The frequency of all benign proliferations is so great that unless they are classified, as described in the preceding pages, according to type, size, and relative frequency no relationship to carcinoma is statistically discernible. With an understanding of proper classification, one can critically evaluate questions such as the overall frequency of "polyps," their distribution relative to carcinoma in the colon, and, most important, the incidence with which carcinoma may be found in various types of polyps.

Focal Carcinoma in Benign Proliferations

There are several practical anatomic features that clinicians and pathologists should understand when considering the frequency with which focal carcinoma may be found in benign proliferations.

Foci of carcinomatous or adenomatous tissue are not found, to our knowledge,

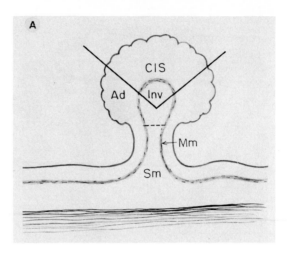

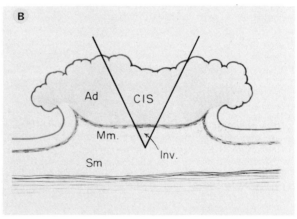

Fig. 20. A. Diagram of intramucosal (CIS) with focal invasive carcinoma (Inv) arising in a pedunculated adenoma (Ad). The wedge of invasive cancer is confined to the submucosa of the head of the adenoma. At this stage, metastases can occur, but are very rare. B. Focal invasive carcinoma arising in a sessile adenoma involves the submucosa of the bowel wall as soon as it crosses the muscularis mucosae. There is a greater frequency of metastasis from focal carcinoma in sessile (villous) adenomas than in pedunculated (polypoid) adenomas. (From Fenoglio and Lane: Cancer 34:819, 1974)

in hyperplastic polyps. It is generally agreed that they have no statistically significant relationship as a precursor tissue to either carcinoma or adenoma; nonetheless, it seems to be correct that they are frequently found in colons bearing adenomas or carcinomas as anatomically separate lesions.

The question of focal carcinoma in adenomas is more complex. Clinically significant focal carcinoma is found with sufficient frequency in the larger adenomas (larger than 1.5 cm) so that these may be considered as precancerous lesions. However, to evaluate critically any statement of the frequency with which carcinoma may be found in adenomas, it is mandatory to distinguish between intramucosal and invasive carcinoma.

Clear-cut examples of intramucosal carcinoma *do* exist and are individually important because they are the most minimal form and stage in which colon cancer can be recognized. However, statistics that include intramucosal carcinoma in the calculation of the frequency of carcinoma in adenomas are without practical value for two reasons. First of all, the distinction between atypia and intramucosal carcinoma is imprecise. Secondly, intramucosal carcinoma by itself, ie, without invasion across the muscularis mucosae, does not metastasize.[23] It is not *clinically* significant at the time it is observed in a specimen. Therefore, for the practical purpose of conservatively evaluating the frequency with which carcinoma may be found in adenomas, only lesions showing invasion through the muscularis mucosae should be counted as being clinically significant. Figures 20A through 22B show that in both pedunculated and sessile adenomas, it is the muscularis mucosae that is the dividing line between an intramucosal and an invasive neoplasm.

As noted, small adenomas (smaller than 1.5 cm) are approximately 10 times as common as large adenomas (larger than 1.5 cm). Focal invasive carcinoma occurs but is very rare in small adenomas. However, it may be found in 10 percent or more of larger adenomas. The likelihood of finding carcinoma increases with the size of the adenomas and is influenced further by the tendency of larger adenomas to be sessile and have villous (papillary) features.[6, 19] Thus, the subgroup "larger adenomas" may be considered a statistically significant precursor tissue for large bowel carcinoma.[1]

These findings indicate that the chance of encountering focal invasive cancer among all the benign proliferations, including the hyperplastic polyps, is incon-

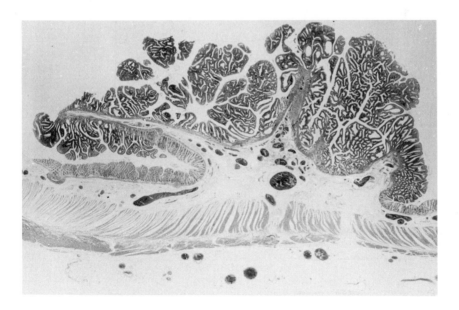

Fig. 21. A sessile adenoma of the papillary-villous type. (Note the proximity of the lesion to the richly vascularized submucosa.) This shows that with properly prepared sections one can precisely trace the muscularis mucosae, even when it follows a complex pathway, as in this specimen. × 6.

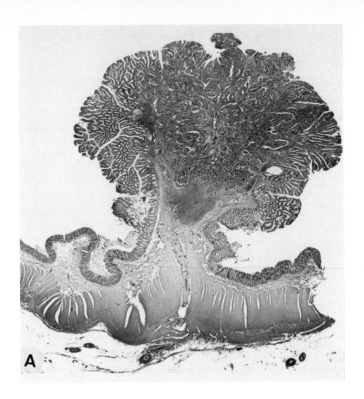

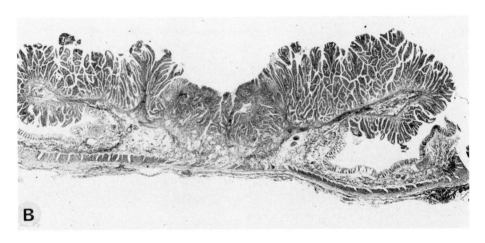

Fig. 22. A. Invasive carcinoma arising in a pedunculated adenoma. As diagrammatically illustrated in Figure 20A, it is clear that the cancer has crossed the muscularis mucosae, but has invaded only the submucosa of the head of the adenoma. × 7. (From Grinnell et al: Surg Gynecol Obstet (Int Abstr Surg) 106:519, 1958) B. Again using the muscularis mucosae as a boundary, it is evident in this sessile adenoma that an invasive focus of cancer has invaded the colonic submucosa. This corresponds to the diagram in Figure 20B. × 7.

sequential—perhaps a tenth of 1 percent or 1 in 1000. The risk is substantially greater in certain adenomas. Hence, we see the necessity of subclassifying polyps as to histologic type, frequency, and size. These relationships are summarized as follows:

Of 1000 "polyps," there will be 900 hyperplastic polyps; 90 small adenomas (focal carcinoma is rare); 10 large adenomas, of which 1 will have invasive carcinoma.

Thus, incidence of invasive carcinoma is 0.1 percent in all "polyps," *but* equals 10 percent in the large adenomas.

The Origin of Large Bowel Carcinoma

Has de novo carcinoma of the colon—as defined in modern terms of cellular dimensions—really been observed? Thus far in this chapter, we have documented that certain adenomas, ie, the larger ones (larger than 1.5 cm) are a significant precursor for ordinary large bowel carcinoma. The question remains whether all or almost all ordinary carcinoma evolves from adenomatous tissue or whether it arises de novo as well. In terms of modern cell biology, the expression de novo carcinoma can only mean that there is a direct one-step transformation into microscopically recognizable cancerous epithelium and glands from the epithelium of a normal crypt(s).

Some years ago, the de novo concept was given impetus by a study of 20 small cancers in which thorough study disclosed no associated adenomatous tissue.[24] Small carcinomas that were accepted as de novo were defined as any lesion up to 2 cm. At that time, this was considered small enough to reflect the morphology of the neoplastic process at its origin. The majority of the carcinomas were between 1 and 2 cm, and only 2 were 5 mm or less. All the lesions were invasive. We now believe that when carcinomas have reached such a size and stage, they may no longer be accepted as an accurate reflection of the morphology of the neoplasm at

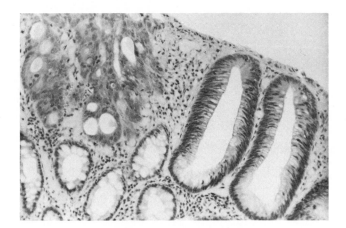

Fig. 23. A small focus of purely intramucosal carcinoma (upper left) arising in a flat adenoma under 0.5 cm in diameter. Further growth of the carcinoma would probably have obliterated the adenomatous epithelium on the right. × 80.

the time of its inception. One cannot exclude the possibility that antecedent adenomatous tissue was destroyed by the growth of the carcinoma.

At present, attitudes on this subject are more in keeping with the minute, even microscopic dimensions that are involved in the cellular origins of cancer. Therefore, for a small lesion to be acceptable as representing the morphology of a neoplasm at its inception, it should not be more than a few millimeters, or even a fraction of a millimeter in size.

Our experience is the same as Morson's,[25] ie, persisting adenomatous tissue is found in inverse proportion to the size of the carcinoma. Like Morson, we too have observed residual adenomatous tissue most commonly in small cancers, and we believe that as the invasive cancer progresses, adenomatous tissue is destroyed.

Occasionally, one encounters a minute or microcancer in a small adenoma. Such foci probably represent the most minimal stage or "degree" of cancer recognizable by present techniques. Figures 23 and 24A, B, and C illustrate two examples of this phenomenon. These adenomas did not exceed 5 mm. One contained a zone of

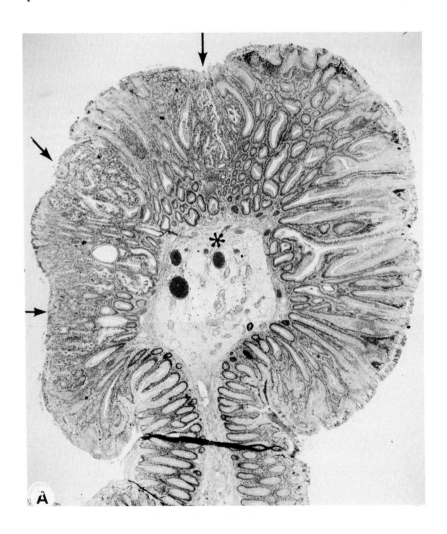

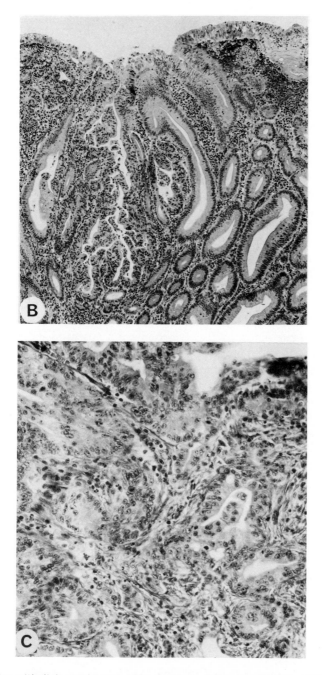

Fig. 24. Intraepithelial carcinoma *plus* focal invasive carcinoma, arising in a 5-mm adenoma, A. (facing page) The intraepithelial carcinoma (arrows) has already replaced much of the adenomatous epithelium. At higher magnification B, the disorganized, noninvasive carcinoma contrasts with the adenomatous glands. At one point in this adenoma (asterisk in A), but at a deeper level of sectioning, there was a focus of invasive carcinoma C that did not exceed 2 mm. Such foci of minute cancer (microcancer) have not been observed in normal, nonadenomatous mucosa. A: × 7; B: × 50; C: × 120.

only intramucosal carcinoma (Fig. 23), while the other also showed an invasive focus, which did not exceed 2 mm (Fig. 24). Since neither adenoma exceeded 5 mm, it is evident that only minimal additional growth of the carcinoma would have obliterated the evidence of the precursor adenomatous tissue.

With these very small dimensions in mind, it seems that such foci of minute or microcancer are found only in adenomatous tissue. In this minute size range, colorectal cancers have not been observed to date as a de novo process in normal nonadenomatous mucosa.

Relationship of Mucosal Lymphatics and Metastasis

Because the colonic mucosa is so richly vascularized, the absence of metastasis from intramucosal carcinoma in an adenoma is of some interest. A partial explanation emerged from a study of the distribution of colonic mucosal lymphatics, particularly in adenomatous tissue.[23] Initially, specimens of colonic carcinoma showing extensive intramural lymphatic spread were studied. Even with extensive intramural lymphatic permeation by cancer cells, the lamina propria of the normal mucosa never showed lymphatic involvement. This enigma prompted a light and electron microscopic study of the lamina propria of more than 20 specimens each, of normal mucosa, hyperplastic polyps, and adenomas. The ultrastructural criteria for distinguishing lymphatics from capillaries are well established.[23] The findings in each tissue indicated that lymphatics are absent in the mucosal lamina propria superficial to the muscularis mucosae. Although electron microscopic observation proves this with the greatest precision, the results are best visualized in the dimensions of conventional histology (Figs. 25 and 26). Thus, intramucosal carcinoma in adenomas does not gain access to lymphatics until it reaches the level of the muscularis mucosae.

In most adenomas, the distance from the adenomatous surface to its muscularis mucosae is many times the distance from the surface of normal mucosa to its muscularis mucosae (Figs. 20A, B, and 21). Therefore, should a focus of carcinoma arise near the surface of a large adenoma, it may grow to considerable size before reaching the muscularis mucosae and the lymphatics at this level. The lamina propria of adenomas is richly endowed with blood capillaries, and why intramucosal carcinoma does not metastasize via these channels is completely unknown.

Relevance of Familial Polyposis

Familial polyposis is the natural human model for the study of ordinary bowel carcinomas, since there is no known difference as far as morphogenesis is concerned between the adenomas and carcinomas in familial polyposis and in ordinary large bowel neoplasia.

The pathologic evidence provided by familial polyposis specimens supports the idea that most carcinomas evolve from adenomatous tissue.[17] In such specimens, minute and microscopic foci of carcinoma can be found, but they have been observed only in adenomatous epithelium. On the other hand, foci of neoplasia as small as a single crypt have been observed and proved to be adenomatous, but

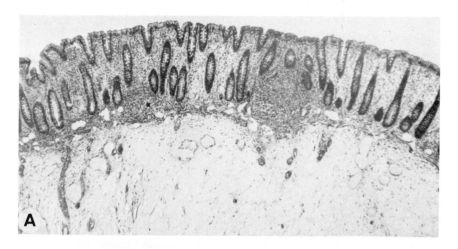

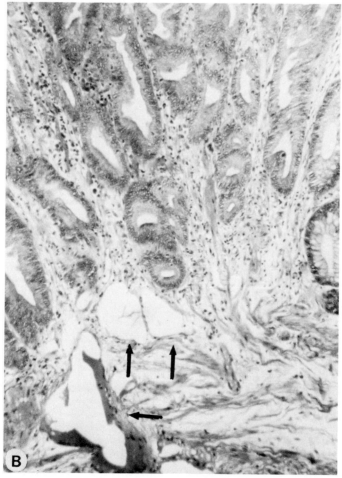

Fig. 25. A. In normal mucosa, the most superficial lymphatics form a plexus at the level of the muscularis mucosae ($\times$ 45). At the base of the hyperplastic polyps (B), superficial fibers of the muscularis mucosae with their associated lymphatics may be ''pulled up'' a short distance toward the intercryptal lamina propria (cont.).

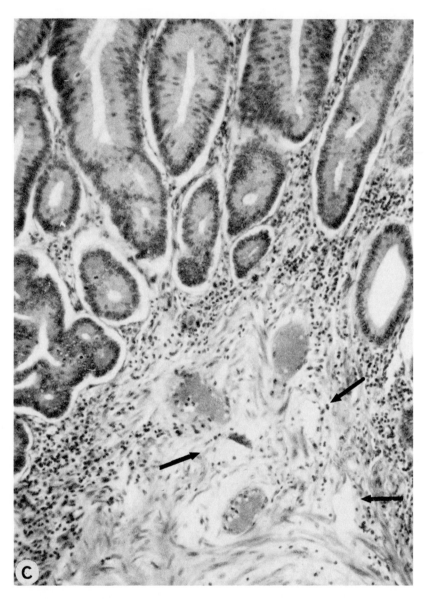

Fig. 25. (cont.) In adenomas C, elevation of the neoplastic crypts and "pulling up" of fibers of the muscularis mucosae may be quite marked and lymphatics may accompany them (arrows). B: × 79; C: × 88. (From Fenoglio et al: Gastroenterology 64:51, 1973)

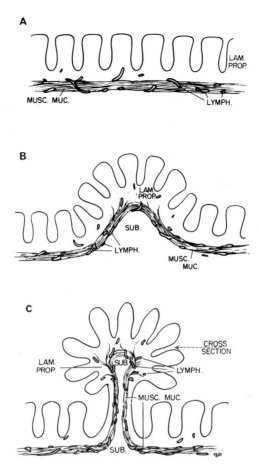

Fig. 26. Diagrammatic representation of the distribution of mucosal lymphatics in normal colon (A), hyperplastic polyps (B), and adenomas (C). The normal colonic mucosa shows a lymphatic plexus around the muscularis mucosae. From this, some blind loops extend upward for a short distance into the lamina propria, but no lymphatics are seen above the level of the base of the crypts. B. In hyperplastic polyps, the basic anatomic relationships are preserved. The major change is an architectural one in which the fibers of the muscularis are elevated. C. In the adenomas, there is a disorganization of the fibers of the muscularis mucosae, but the relationship of the lymphatics to the muscularis mucosae is preserved. (From Fenoglio et al: Gastroenterology 64:51, 1973.)

not carcinomatous. These observations are based on extensive microscopic study in polyposis cases of areas of grossly normal mucosa.[17] De novo carcinoma does not seem to occur in familial polyposis despite the remarkable predilection for carcinoma in this condition.

While much valuable information will be gained by the study of animal models, there is no evidence to suggest that large bowel neoplasms produced by carcinogen administration more accurately reflect the morphogenesis of ordinary large bowel cancer than what has been observed in familial polyposis. Indeed, unless new evidence causes us to downgrade familial polyposis as a model, it should be the yardstick against which experimental results should be measured.

Evidence from Periodic Sigmoidoscopy and Polypectomy in Relation to the Adenoma-Carcinoma Sequence

The 25-year study done at the University of Minnesota Cancer Detection Center appears to provide empiric proof for the contention that most ordinary adenocarcinomas arise from adenomatous tissue.[26] This study involved periodic sigmoidoscopic examination of thousands of individuals and the removal of mucosal protrusions. The statistically anticipated incidence of rectosigmoid carcinoma was reduced by 85 percent. It is not our purpose to discuss the pros and cons of the feasibility of such studies on a truly massive scale, but the experience from that clinic provides valuable empiric documentation for all the other evidence that suggests that the adenoma-carcinoma sequence is the usual pathway in the development of large bowel carcinoma.

Summary

The cardinal points of this chapter are concerned with ordinary moderately and well-differentiated adenocarcinoma, and those benign proliferations of adults known as hyperplastic polyps and adenomas. These two benign lesions are separate and distinct, and their classification by type, size, and relative frequency is necessary to understand the precursor tissue concept. Hyperplastic polyps, which are unrelated to neoplasia, are 10 times more common than adenomas. In turn, small adenomas (smaller than 1.5 cm) are 10 times more frequent than large adenomas (larger than 1.5 cm), so that these large adenomas constitute only about 1 percent of the benign proliferations we have considered. Cancer, intramucosal and invasive, *can* occur in small adenomas, but only the large adenomas will harbor invasive cancer with significant frequency, ie, 10 percent or more.

The cellular origin of cancer involves minute or microscopic dimensions. Hence, a lesion that is likely to reflect the morphology of a neoplasm at its inception must measure only a few millimeters—or perhaps a fraction of a millimeter. *It is essential to accept the discipline of these minute dimensions,* and in doing so, we note that minute or microcancer is observed only in adenomatous tissue and has not been reported as a de novo process in normal mucosa. The same observation applies to familial polyposis—even though there is a tremendous predilection for carcinoma in this condition. The University of Minnesota clinical study suggests that until dietary, immunologic, and other possible factors that might lead to the prevention of adenomas are clarified, the detection and removal of adenomatous tissue is the most reliable way of reducing the incidence of large bowel cancer at the present time.

References

1. Grinnell RS, Lane N: Benign and malignant adenomatous polyps and papillary

adenomas of the colon and rectum. An analysis of 1,856 tumors in 1,335 patients. Surg Gynecol Obstet (Int Abstr Surg) 106:519, 1958

2. Muto T, Bussey HJR, Morson BC: The evolution of cancer of the colon and rectum. Cancer 36:2251, 1975

3. Lane N, Lev R: Observations on the origin of adenomatous epithelium of the colon. Cancer 16:751, 1963

4. Lane N, Kaplan H, Pascal RR: Minute adenomatous and hyperplastic polyps of the colon: divergent patterns of epithelial growth with specific associated mesenchymal changes. Gastroenterology 60:537, 1971

5. Kaye GI, Fenoglio CM, Pascal RR, Lane N: Comparative electron microscopic features of normal, hyperplastic, and adenomatous human colonic epithelium. Gastroenterology 64:926, 1973

6. Fenoglio CM, Lane N: The anatomical precursor of colorectal carcinoma. Cancer 34:819, 1974

7. Pascal RR, Kaye GI, Lane N: Colonic pericryptal fibroblast sheath: replication, migration, and cytodifferentiation of a mesenchymal cell system in adult tissue I. Gastroenterology 54:835, 1968

8. Kaye GI, Lane N, Pascal RR: Colonic pericryptal fibroblast sheath: replication, migration, and cytodifferentiation of a mesenchymal cell system in adult tissue II. Gastroenterology 54:852, 1968

9. Kaye GI, Pascal RR, Lane N: The colonic pericryptal fibroblast sheath: replication, migration, and cytodifferentiation of a mesenchymal cell system in adult tissue III. Gastroenterology 60:515, 1971

10. Gold P, Freedman SO: Specific carcinoembryonic antigens of the human digestive system. J Exp Med 121:439, 1965

11. Thompson DMP, Krupey J, Freedman SO, Gold P: The radioimmunoassay of circulating carcinoembryonic antigen of the human digestive system. Proc Natl Acad Sci USA 64:161, 1969

12. Zamcheck N: The present status of CEA in diagnosis, prognosis and evaluation of therapy. Cancer 36:2460, 1975

13. Dahr P, Moore TL, Zamcheck N, et al: Carcinoembryonic antigen (CEA) in colon cancer. JAMA 221:31, 1972

14. Hsu KC, Zimmerman EA, Rudin L, et al: Application of immunoperoxidase bridge technique in studies of tumor tissues with antibody to tumor associated antigen (TAA). In: Proceedings of the Second Conference—Workshop on Embryonic and Fetal Antigens in Cancer. US Atomic Energy Commission, Division of Technical Information, Oak Ridge, Tenn, 1972, p 147

15. Marchand A, Fenoglio CM, Pascal R, Richart RM, Bennett S: Carcinoembryonic antigen in human ovarian neoplasms. Cancer Res 35:3807, 1975

16. Strauss RA, Pascal RR: Invasive and metastasizing carcinoma in a small adenomatous polyp of the colon: Report of a case with demonstration of a tumor associated antigen. Hum Pathol 6:256, 1975

17. Bussey HJR: Familial Polyposis Coli. Baltimore, Johns Hopkins Univ Press, 1975

18. Deschner EE, Lipkin M: Proliferative patterns in colonic mucosa in familial polyposis. Cancer 35:413, 1975

19. Morson BC: The polyp-cancer sequence in the large bowel. Proc R Soc Med 67:451, 1974

20. Gilbertsen VA, Knatterud GL, Lober PH, Wangensteen OH: Invasive carcinoma of the large intestine: A preventable disease? Surgery 57:363, 1965

21. Chapman I: Adenomatous polypi of large intestine: incidence and distribution. Ann Surg 157:223, 1963

22. Arthur JF: Structure and significance of metaplastic nodules in the rectal mucosa. J Clin Pathol 21:735, 1968

23. Fenoglio CM, Kaye GI, Lane N: Distribution of human colonic lymphatics in normal, hyperplastic and adenomatous tissue. Gastroenterology 64:51, 1973

24. Spratt JS, Jr, Ackerman LV: Small primary adenocarcinomas of the colon and rectum. JAMA 179:337, 1962
25. Morson BC: Factors influencing the prognosis of early cancer of the rectum. Proc R Soc Med 59:707, 1966
26. Gilbertsen VA: Proctosigmoidoscopy and polypectomy in reducing the incidence of rectal cancer. Cancer 34:936, 1974

SUDDEN UNEXPLAINED INFANT DEATH, 1970 THROUGH 1975
An Evolution in Understanding

MARIE VALDES-DAPENA

Is The Victim Normal?

The last six years have witnessed a remarkable change in our understanding of sudden unexpected and unexplained infant death; the change pertains to several aspects of our comprehension. Almost a decade ago, it was generally agreed that the usual victim of such a tragedy was a well-nourished and well-developed baby, usually 2 to 4 months of age whose sudden and unexpected death remained inexplicable after the performance of an adequate autopsy. It was granted by most that many of the affected infants had either a history of recent minor illness, especially an upper respiratory infection or histologic evidence of the same. But, no satisfactory cause of death could be ascertained at postmortem examination, and it was assumed that the babies had been basically well prior to their sudden demise.

Research conducted in recent years, however, has demonstrated that—*as a group*—these infants are different from normal anatomically, histologically, chemically, and even physiologically. Peterson et al,[75] in a study of 362 autopsied victims, showed that their crown-to-heel length, head circumference, and weight gain, by history, were significantly less than those of 270 living infants reared under optimal growth conditions. Naeye and Drage [66] encountered almost the same sort of revelation in a "prospective" study, a comparison of 124 victims with 372 matched controls. The mean body weight of the subjects had *fallen* from the fortieth to the twentieth percentile between birth and 4 months of age. Their body length and head circumference likewise exhibited similar retardation. Their postneonatal growth delay was shown to involve bones, brain, and other organs, all to about the same degree.

In 1976, evidence of another singular anatomic difference between normal infants and those who die suddenly, unexpectedly, and inexplicably was demonstrated at autopsy by Naeye et al.[68] In a study of 118 infants, they showed that many who die of the sudden infant death syndrome have abnormally heavy cardiac right ventricles.

All of the now known histologic differences between affected and normal infants have been brought to light by Naeye. In 1973, spurred by a desire to find supportive evidence that affected infants had indeed been subjected to chronic hypoxemia, he began to explore the possibility that they might exhibit abnormalities of the walls of their small pulmonary arteries. What he discovered was an increase in mean pulmonary arterial medial muscle mass produced by the combined effects of hyperplasia and hypertrophy.[64] This observation was later supported by Mason et al [59] and is being investigated further in our own laboratory.

The following year, in the course of the same quest, Naeye showed that again, *as a group,* infants who die of "crib death" exhibit significantly more retention of periadrenal brown fat during the first year of life than normal controls.[65] This observation, too, has since been confirmed by others.[113]

Along those same lines, Naeye also showed that affected infants exhibit undue retention of hepatic extramedullary hematopoiesis,[65] a finding later confirmed in our laboratory.[112]

Still in the realm of histologic differences, Naeye recently discovered that the victims also exhibit an increased volume of adrenal chromaffin cells;[68] this, too, he considers to be a consequence of chronic hypoxemia.

In a separate study of the brain stem, Naeye found that half of the victims had more astroglial fibers in those portions of the brain stem which regulate respiration than did matched controls.[66] Regarding this observation, however, he believes that the alteration is more likely secondary to chronic hypoxemia than its cause.

Naeye and Drage [67] have correlated all of these major anatomic and histologic observations as follows: The increase in weight of the cardiac right ventricle proves to be directly proportional to (a) the increase in muscle mass in the walls of small pulmonary arteries, (b) the degree of retention of periadrenal brown fat, and (c) the presence of hepatic erythropoiesis. He concludes that the pulmonary arterial abnormality is "probably the result of chronic alveolar hypoventilation while brown fat retention and hepatic erythropoiesis are likely consequences of chronic hypoxemia."

Dr. Henry Lardy and his co-workers at the University of Wisconsin have identified yet another aspect of the differences between infants who die of crib death and those of like age who appear to be normal.[56] They used hepatic tissue obtained at autopsy from 122 infants to determine the activity of certain gluconeogenic enzymes. Hepatic phosphoenolpyruvate carboxykinase activity proved to be considerably lower in the victims than in normal infants and, in many, the enzyme was defective "in its response to divalent transition metals such as Mn^{2+}," which they consider to be of special significance. They feel that this diminished enzyme activity could conceivably be responsible for fatal hypoglycemia but that, as is more likely, it may be nothing more than another secondary expression of adverse tissue reaction to some generalized phenomenon such as hypoxemia.

A number of investigators have recently explored the possibility that affected infants are or have been different from controls in regard to certain physiologic functions. Perhaps the most comprehensive of these studies was a review of the data collected from the Collaborative Perinatal Project of the National Institute of

Neurological and Communicative Disorders and Stroke. The initial intent had been to observe and document every aspect of the course of each of 59,379 conceptions and the ensuing pregnancies, including gestation, labor, and delivery, the neonatal period of each infant, and the development of every child up to 8 years of age. Of all these conceptions, 125 terminated as instances of sudden death in infancy. These 125 infants were compared with living matched controls from the same group by Naeye and Drage.[66] The victims of sudden death were noted, in retrospect, to have had more low Apgar scores than controls, all components of the scoring system except skin color contributing to that abnormality. About twice as many of the study subjects as controls had required neonatal resuscitation, positive respiratory pressure, and the administration of oxygen. Future victims had experienced a greater rate of the respiratory distress syndrome and more had received antibiotics. Feeding problems were common among them, their bottle feeding had been delayed and feeding by gavage was more often required.

A variety of neurologic abnormalities were observed more frequently among future victims of crib death than in the matched controls; they included jitteriness or tremulousness, an abnormal Moro reflex, generalized muscular hypotonia, abnormal reflexes, and spontaneous hypo- or hyperthermia. The data for all of these differences prove to be statistically significant.

Naeye and his co-workers [69] approached the issue of functional or physiologic differences between affected infants and controls, during life, in still another manner. They conducted a separate retrospective study of the behavioral patterns of 46 infants who had died of crib death and compared them with those of their own siblings using an open-ended interview with the parents. The parents, whose infants had died within the preceding 3 years, were asked to describe the behavior, growth, and development of the affected babies and to make their own comparisons with those of siblings at comparable ages. Following the free interview, each set of parents completed a 70-item, self-administered Carey questionnaire.

By comparison, those infants who had later died of crib death, appeared to have been less active during life than their sibling controls. They exhibited less intense responses to a variety of stimuli. They were more often breathless and easily exhausted during feeding and had cries of different pitch. All of these differences were statistically significant and correlated well with postmortem morphologic evidences of hypoxemia.

Data on postnatal growth were obtained from baby books and physicians' records. Two-thirds of the victims had experienced a decrease in body weight percentile after birth in comparison to only one-third of the controls (P less than 0.05 Chi square). The mean decrease for victims was 7.6 ± 4.4 percentile points, whereas the sibling controls exhibited a mean *increase* of 2.8 ± 5.3 points.

In at least three separate instances, detailed physiologic studies were carried out on individual infants who later died inexplicably. In the first of these,[50] the intranatal fetal heart rate patterns of an infant who subsequently died suddenly and inexplicably showed variable decelerations indicative of umbilical cord compression. These patterns were unusual, closely resembling those of more immature fetuses in whom the mechanisms for the control of heart rate are not fully developed or have been blunted by the administration of atropine. Recordings of this same infant's heart rate immediately after birth showed more persistent tachycardia and less beat-to-beat variability than is usually found in clinically normal infants at equivalent gestational age.

In another such instance, the crying of an apparently healthy infant, who later died of crib death, was recorded on the fourth day of life in the department of Otolaryngology at the Johns Hopkins University School of Medicine.[86] The crying was perceived as unusual at the time; it was later analyzed and compared with that of four normal controls. The sounds produced by the subject were weaker and of shorter duration. Extremely high-pitched cries were more often exhibited by the victim. The cries were frequently weak and breathy. Abrupt changes in pitch and the presence of more than one pitch in the same segment of crying were also noted. These features suggested to the investigators abnormal function of the larynx and the vocal tract above the larynx.

Dr. Lee Salk and his team at Cornell [81] encountered yet another infant who subsequently succumbed to crib death in the course of a study of normal neonatal learning ability using cardiac habituation to an auditory stimulus. In retrospective review of the records, they discovered that the infant in question had showed greater lability and poorer stabilization of cardiac rate than 24 healthy neonatal controls. This observation suggested to Dr. Salk dysfunction of the central mechanism for stabilizing the autonomic response.

In view of all of these morphologic, chemical, and functional differences between groups of infants and individual infants who die suddenly, unexpectedly, and inexplicably and normal controls, it would now seem apparent that babies who die of crib death are not normal at the time of death and probably are never entirely normal. To put it another way, *as a group,* infants who ultimately die of crib death exhibit structural and functional abnormalities during life and at postmortem examination, which serve to indicate that in some way, not as yet defined, they are physiologically defective. This is, of course, a revelation inasmuch as just a few years ago virtually everyone assumed that they were in no way abnormal.

In this regard, however, a word of caution is in order. Despite the fact that anatomic, histologic, and physiologic differences between groups of infants have been described in detail, there is not as yet a single one of these differences that can be employed, before or after the death, as a predictive or diagnostic criterion. The fact of the matter is that there is not yet one positive criterion that can be employed by the clinician to identify the future victim, nor is there as yet one positive criterion that the pathologist can use to identify the subject at autopsy.

This is of the utmost importance to recognize, because some general pathologists, having heard that babies who die of crib death, for example, exhibit relatively more periadrenal brown fat than normal controls, have assumed that this feature represents a means of establishing the diagnosis at the time of postmortem examination—it does not. Nor do any of the other features mentioned; they are only characteristics of the group as a whole.

Observations at Autopsy

Morphologic observations at autopsy in the "typical" instance of sudden, unexpected, unexplained infant death have been described repeatedly in the literature both in the past,[2] and more recently.[7, 109, 110]

Characteristic observations include the following:

1. The body usually appears to be well developed and well nourished.
2. Frothy and even blood-tinged mucus may be present in and about the external nares.
3. Petechiae are often prominent over the pleural surfaces, especially the visceral surfaces, under the capsule and within the substance of the thymus, and in the epicardium.
4. The thymus is usually quite large, within limits of normal.
5. Blood in the heart is usually liquid rather than clotted.
6. The lungs fill their respective pleural cavities completely and often exhibit moderate edema and congestion.
7. The larynx or trachea often contain a little frothy, thin mucoid fluid and, at times, aspirated gastric content usually in the form of milk curd.
8. Lymphoid structures throughout the body, such as the mesenteric lymph nodes, are almost too well preserved.
9. The adrenals tend to be small, within limits of normal.
10. The urinary bladder is usually empty.
11. The stomach often contains abundant curd.

Other organs and tissues as examined grossly are usually not remarkable. Characteristic microscopic observations include:

1. Histologic features corresponding to numbers 3, 4, 6, 7, 8, and 9.
2. In the lungs, interalveolar walls are normally thick and cellular.
3. There may be foci of fibrinoid necrosis in the larynx or diffuse "subacute" inflammation involving the mucosa.
4. In the tracheal mucosa, the same sort of infiltrates including plasma cells may be seen.

Bacterial cultures of heart's blood with concomitant cultures of the spleen for confirmation reveal the presence of isolated significant pathogenic organisms in not more than 5 percent of these autopsies. Cultures of the lungs and upper airway characteristically yield a variety of organisms. Interpretation of their significance, especially in the absence of morphologic evidence of disease, is difficult if not impossible.

The Causes of Sudden, Unexpected, *Explained* Infant Deaths

Every once in a while, the postmortem examination of an apparently healthy infant of appropriate age reveals a recognizable, incontrovertible cause of death. There are the rare discoveries of extensive involvement of the heart and brain in the pathologic lesions characteristic of tuberous sclerosis, for example. But these occurrences are so infrequent as to be unworthy of inclusion in a working list of disease entities that might be expected to become evident under such circumstances.

At a recent conference for forensic pathologists in Santa Fe,[70] a group of those assembled compiled the following catalogue of disease processes they felt might reasonably be expected to become evident during the course of an autopsy on the body of an infant who had died suddenly and unexpectedly.

1. General:
    Sepsis (including meningococcemia)
2. Heart:
    Endocardial sclerosis (subendocardial fibroelastosis):
    Congenital aortic stenosis
    Myocarditis (especially Coxsackie)
3. Lungs:
    Pneumonia
    Bronchiolitis
4. Kidneys:
    Evidence of poisoning (eg, salt poisoning)
5. Gastrointestinal tract:
    Enterocolitis (eg, Shigella, Salmonella)
    Evidence of cystic fibrosis of the pancreas (particularly in hot weather)
6. Liver:
    Hepatitis (especially Coxsackie)
    Evidence of poisoning
7. Pancreas:
    Pancreatitis (especially Coxsackie)
    Evidence of poisoning (especially boric acid)
    Cystic fibrosis (particularly in hot weather)
8. Adrenal:
    Congenital adrenal hyperplasia
9. Brain:
    Meningitis
    Encephalitis
    Evidence of trauma (especially subdural hemorrhage)
    Arteriovenous malformation
10. Skeleton:
    Skull fracture
    Other evidences of "child battering"

This list was compiled by the group of working forensic pathologists assembled there, not by any means as an exhaustive treatise on the subject, but rather as a practical guide or reminder as to what sorts of identifiable disease processes may eventuate in the sudden and unexpected death of an apparently well infant.

Minimal Pathologic Changes and the Dilemma They Pose for the Pathologist

Virtually all pathologists who have performed substantial numbers of infant autopsies, have encountered the insoluble problem of what to do about the case in which there are identifiable lesions of minimal to moderate intensity which, of themselves, would not appear adequate to have caused death. One of the most common of these is inflammation of the larynx or trachea, observed in at least 50 percent of the sudden deaths of seemingly well infants. Another is the presence of neutrophiles, in relatively small numbers, scattered about pulmonary alveoli. Still another is bronchiolitis, observed in just a few of the sections of lung examined in any one case. Not uncommonly, careful microscopic study of the heart will reveal an occasional cluster of inflammatory cells within the myocardium.

As mentioned elsewhere in this chapter a few such autopsies will reveal the histologic changes characteristic of cytomegaloviral infection. However, in those instances in which attempts at viral isolation have been conducted in conjunction with the microscopic study of tissues, the sites of recovery of the viruses unfortunately have not corresponded to those in which morphologic lesions have been demonstrated and vice versa.

In the situations described here, most pathologists with an appreciable body of experience in the area have elected arbitrarily to group such cases into a subset of the so-called sudden infant death syndrome with minimal to moderate pathologic alterations probably insufficient, of themselves, to have been responsible for death.

Recent Developments Regarding Epidemiologic and Clinical Factors

Incidence

A review of recently published reports on the epidemiology of sudden, unexpected, unexplained infant deaths reveals considerable variation from place to place. The rate of occurrence varies from 0.06 per 1000 livebirths in Sweden [35] to 3.00 per 1000 livebirths in Ontario, Canada [93] (Table 1).

One of the most interesting aspects of this particular issue concerns the apparent decrease which has been observed lately, not only in the numbers of

TABLE 1. Recent Data on Comparative Rates of Occurrence of the Sudden Infant Death Syndrome

Author	Year	Location	Rate/1000 Livebirths
Fohlin [35]	1974	Stockholm, Sweden	0.06
Block [15]	1973	Ashkelon Dist., Israel	0.31
Baak [4]	1974	Netherlands	0.42
Houstek [51]	1970	Czechoslovakia	0.8
Kraus [54]	1972	California	1.55
Borhani [18]	1973	Sacramento Co., California	1.7
Beal [5]	1972	South Australia	1.7
Tonkin [100]	1974	Auckland, New Zealand	1.9
Valdes-Dapena [114]	1974	Philadelphia	1.92 (in 1972)
Camps [22, 23]	1970	Great Britain	2.0
Adelson [1]	1975	Cuyahoga Co., Ohio	2.08 (in 1974)
Bergman [14a]	1972	King Co., Washington	2.32
Turner [102]	1975	Western Australia	2.5
Fedrick [33]	1973	Oxford Linkage Area, Great Britain	2.78
Froggatt [40a]	1971	Northern Ireland	2.8
Steele [93]	1970	Ontario, Canada	3.0

**TABLE 2. Documented Diminution in Rate of Occurrence of the
Sudden Infant Death Syndrome**

Author	*Years*	*Location*	*Rates/1000 Livebirths*
Houstek [51]	1952–67	Czechoslovakia	3.0 –0.8
Valdes-Dapena [114]	1960–74	Philadelphia	2.5 –1.9
Borhani [18]	1964–70	California	2.0 –0.9
Adelson [1]	1965–70	Cuyahoga Co., Ohio	3.45–2.07
Mason [60]	1965–74	Memphis	3.10–0.9

infants dying of crib death but also in the relative rate of occurrence per 1000 live-births. Comparison of the figures in Table 1, for example, with those that appear in a similar chart prepared in 1969 [108] reveals the fact that, in general, relative rates are lower now than they were as little as seven years ago. However, the fact that the rate had really diminished to a statistically significant degree in specific populations under continued and relatively sophisticated surveillance for the occurrence of the phenomenon did not become apparent until 1974.[109] Retrospective review of the available reliable data shows that in at least five circumscribed populations there has been a similar substantial documented decrease (Table 2).

We have observed, however, as have others,[51] that this decrease parallels that for all infant deaths during the same period of time. One can only speculate as to the significance of both trends. At least in Philadelphia, the drop is not paralleled by any reduction in the rate of prematurity, but it does prove to be quite similar to a steady decrease in inadequate delivery of prenatal care.

Socioeconomic Factors

For many years, investigators have been aware that, in general terms, the socially and economically underprivileged are more susceptible to crib death than the well-to-do. In the last eight years, however, a number of interested workers have concentrated on attempts to analyze pertinent data in some systematic fashion.

Bergman et al [14a] examined the incidence of crib death from the standpoint of family income, and determined that in King County, Washington, 38 percent of affected families earned less than $5000 a year and 89 percent, less than $10,000. Borhani et al [18] also approached the problem along those lines determining rates in each of 5 groups of census tracts according to average income. Where the median family income exceeded $13,500, the rate of crib death was 1.3 per 1000 live-births, but where income was less than $6500 the rate was 2.9. Kraus and Borhani [53] studied the occupational status of the father and discovered that the risk for the infant of fathers without a job or occupied as nonfarm laborers was higher than for the infants of fathers with professional, technical, or managerial positions.

In the late 1960s, the work of Strimer and his colleagues,[98] as well as our own,[111] was directed toward a clearer understanding of the relationship of social and economic factors to sudden infant death. We concluded that (a) the rate was higher among the poor than among the well-to-do, no matter the race or minority status and (b) the rate was higher among minority nonwhites (predominantly black) than among whites, despite income.

Factors Related to the Infant

AGE OF THE INFANT AT DEATH.   A number of workers in the past, as well as in recent years, have examined the incidence of sudden, unexplained infant deaths by age at death. Froggatt [39] in his careful study of 162 cases observed the mean age to be 18.1 weeks and the median 13.8. Kraus and Borhani's study [53] is particularly interesting inasmuch as they compared an observed mean age of 2.9 months and a median of 2.4 with comparable peaks for infant deaths due to all other causes in the same geographic area (4.6 and 3.3 months respectively). The differences prove to be statistically significant.

Kraus and others comment on the rather surprising fact that infants are relatively immune to sudden, unexplained death during the first 3 weeks of life.

BIRTH WEIGHT OF THE INFANT AND PREMATURITY.   Kraus and Borhani [53] noted a direct and inverse gradient between the weight of the affected baby at birth and the rate of postneonatal, sudden unexplained death ranging from 0.87 per 1000 livebirths among those who had weighed 4501 gm and more at birth, up to 6.55 per 1000 livebirths in those whose birth weight had been between 1501 and 2000 gm. Bergman et al [14a] similarly observed that the incidence of death among infants whose birth weight had been between 3.5 and 4.0 pounds was 10 times greater than that for infants who had weighed between 7.5 and 8.5 pounds at birth.

Froggatt et al [40a, b] on the other hand, using multiple regression analysis determined that birth weight may correlate with, but is not per se an important determinant of sudden, unexplained infant death. In addition, according to the analytic study of Kraus et al,[54] however, prematurity itself is not a strong determining factor.

SEX OF THE INFANT.   In their survey, Kraus and Borhani [53] reported the rate of occurrence of sudden death among male infants to be 1.82 per 1000 livebirths as compared with a rate of only 1.26 for females.

In five other series published in the 1970s, the sex ratio is strikingly consistent (Table 3). However, it is important to point out that in the Kraus series the ratio is not significantly different from the ratio of males to females among livebirths, and in Froggatt's, the ratio is similar to that for all infant mortality.

RACE OF THE INFANT.   The most detailed information available presently on

TABLE 3. Percent Males in 5 Recently Published Series of Sudden Unexplained Infant Deaths

Author	Year	Location	Percent Male
Houstek [51]	1970	Czechoslovakia	58
Fedrick [33]	1973	Oxford Linkage Area, Great Britain	58
Froggatt [40a]	1971	Belfast, Northern Ireland	58.6
Borhani [18]	1973	California	58.6
Bergman [14a]	1972	King County, Washington	59

racial differences in the sudden infant death event are those derived from Kraus' series of 525 autopsied infants.[53] The distribution of deaths by race was found to be significantly different from that expected on the basis of proportionate distribution of livebirths (Table 4).

TABLE 4. Race of the Infant in Series of 525 Sudden
Unexplained Infant Deaths *

Race	Rate/1000 Livebirths
Oriental (Chinese and Japanese American)	0.51
White (other than Mexican American)	1.32
Mexican American	1.74
Black	2.92
American Indian	5.93

* From Kraus and Borhani.[53]

As an amplification of this, Bergman et al [14a] showed a marked excess in death rates for males if they were white but not for nonwhites. Similarly Kraus and his co-workers [53, 54] observed the male excess among whites and Orientals, but not among blacks and American Indians. In fact, the death rate he observed among American Indian female infants (7.13 per 1000 livebirths) is the highest rate thus far reported for any sex-race group.

MULTIPLE BIRTHS.   The risk of sudden death for the infant born of a multiple birth is undoubtedly greater than that of the singleton birth. Kraus and Borhani [53] presented risk figures of 8.33 per 1000 livebirths for triplets, 3.87 for twins, and 1.46 for singletons. It is likely, however, from these and other data that the increased risk is fundamentally related to birth weight.

In a recently published study of twin deaths, it was noted that like-sexed and unliked-sexed pairs are equally affected, suggesting that environmental rather than genetic factors are more influential.[92]

GENETIC FACTORS AND RECURRENCES WITHIN FAMILIES.   Judging from currently available data, it would seem that sudden, unexplained infant death is not genetically controlled. Beckwith [7] has reviewed the reported cases of recurrence among subsequent siblings in 11 published series and declared the somewhat enhanced risk subsequent siblings experience to be less than would be expected were it a mendelian trait.

In Froggatt's series [40a, b] the recurrence rate among siblings was 4 to 7 times the random risk, or between 11.1 and 22.1 per 1000 siblings at risk. The previously mentioned twin study provides further evidence that the event is not inherited— even as a recessive trait. There is no report in the literature to date of this event occurring in an instance of parental consanguinity.

HEALTH OF THE AFFECTED INFANT.   As recently as a decade ago, all concerned would have attested to the fact that usually the infant who dies suddenly and inexplicably has been, in general, a healthy baby—not often ill—and well developed. Now there is a growing body of evidence to the contrary.

Borhani's report [18] noted that 64 percent of the 128 infants considered had had an episode of sickness, mostly a cold or "the sniffles," some time before death. More than 50 percent of the illnesses occurred during the two weeks preceding death.

Froggatt's assessment [40a, b] of the affected infants' postnatal health, in his study of 162 cases, led him to the conclusion they had experienced an increased incidence of minor illness during the week, and especially the last 24 hours, before death.

FEEDING OF THE INFANT.   Froggatt's detailed analysis [40a, b] of the feeding histories of affected infants revealed almost identical feeding patterns for those affected and matched controls. Of the infants in Houstek's series,[51] 32 were fully breast fed, and 7 of Bergman's [14a] had never received any cow's milk but had been given instead soy and goat's milk formulas. We are aware of 5 instances in which infants have died of crib death often having been exclusively breast fed, and Froggatt has reported 2 such cases.[40a]

This information leads us to believe that sensitivity to the proteins of cow's milk is probably not related to unexplained infant death and that breast feeding, even when exclusive of any supplemental feeding, does not protect against the event.

SLEEP STATE AT THE TIME OF DEATH.   Inasmuch as the great majority of unexplained infant deaths occur between midnight and 9 A.M., are not observed, and are apparently silent and without struggle, it is assumed that they happen while the infant is asleep. This is, of course, undocumented since no such death has yet been recorded while the subject was being monitored for sleep state.

POSITION OF THE INFANT AT DEATH.   In the series of 170 sudden infant deaths analyzed by Bergman et al,[14a] specific data are given with regard to the position of the infant's body in death. In 50 percent, the infant lay on the abdomen, half of these face down and half, to the side. Four percent lay on their backs and 46 percent on their sides. Froggatt [39] reported that 76 percent were lying on their sides; and in Houstek's experience,[51] 7 percent died in their mothers' arms, 61 percent lying flat on their backs, 10 percent on the abdomen, and 8 percent on the side. Thus, there seems to be no consistent pattern as to position, much would appear to depend upon local custom and the matter is probably of no consequence.

Factors Related to the Mother

MATERNAL AGE AND BIRTH ORDER.   Even in the last 5 years, several authors have reported what has been repeatedly observed in the past: The highest rate of sudden, unexplained infant death is seen among mothers less than 20 years old, with a gradient indicating clearly that the older the mother, the lower the risk of sudden death for her baby.[14a, 53, 54] Using multifactorial analysis, Froggatt [40a] determined a significantly increased risk under the circumstances of combined young maternal age and increased parity.

LEGITIMACY OF BIRTH.   In Kraus' report,[54] it is noted that the rate of death among illegitimate infants was almost twice as high as that for babies considered to have been legitimate.

PRENATAL CARE AND HEALTH OF THE MOTHER.   The risk for crib death among infants whose mothers have received no prenatal care at all appears to be more than four times as great as that for those infants whose mothers have received such care consistently, beginning in the early months of pregnancy.[53, 95]

Apparently, infants born to mothers maintained on methadone for opium addiction are at special risk in this regard.[77] Protestos,[78] Bergman,[10] Schrauzer et al,[84] and Steele [94, 95] have all observed a higher rate of occurrence among the infants of mothers who smoke than among those of mothers who do not.

Environmental Factors

SEASONAL VARIATION AND WEATHER AS A FACTOR.   As in the past, most investigators who have reported recently on this phenomenon record a preponderance of deaths during the winter months.[14a, 18, 33, 40a, 51, 53] This curve is independent of monthly fluctuation in the number of livebirths, and the temporal distribution is different from that of other postneonatal deaths.[40a, 53]

WEATHER AS A FACTOR.   Probably the single most definitive analysis of the weather as a potential factor in the cause of sudden, unexplained infant death is that of Fedrick.[33] She has documented the mean measurements for each of 8 meteorologic measurements by month over a 5-year period and correlated those data with the rate of occurrence of crib death in each 30-day period; as might have been predicted, she has demonstrated a striking negative association with temperature as well as with hours of sunshine and positive correlations with wind speed, relative humidity, and snowfall.

DAY OF THE WEEK.   In our own experience [111] and that of Borhani et al,[18] no one day of the week showed any striking correlation with increased numbers of crib deaths. Froggatt [40a, b] reported more deaths on Sundays, Peterson et al [75] an excess on Saturdays, Richards and McIntosh [80c] on Tuesdays, and Fedrick [33] on Thursdays.

TIME OF DAY.   Inasmuch as the great majority of unexplained infant deaths are not actually observed, most investigators arbitrarily calculate the time of death as the midpoint between the moment the infant was last seen alive and the moment he was discovered dead. Using 3 consecutive 8-hour periods beginning with midnight, Froggatt et al [40a] found the following percentage distribution: 50.0, 36.4, and 13.6.

PLACE OF DEATH.   According to the data of Fedrick,[33] 70 percent of the crib deaths in her series occurred at home or at some other noninstitutional address, 6.8 percent died en route to the hospital, and 22.3 percent in the hospital. This distribution is probably representative of the experience of most investigators. However, many series include the occasional sudden death in a baby carriage or car bed.

SPACE-TIME CLUSTERING.   Bergman et al [14a] reported a suggestion of "epidemicity" in the form of scattered small clusters in time. However, employing two different methods of statistical approach to the issue, Froggatt and his coworkers [40a, b] concluded that, on the basis of their experience, "if clustering (or 'contagion') exists, there is no evidence of it from these tests at least one of which would readily demonstrate clustering of such infective diseases as measles and poliomyelitis, as well as some which may have only an infective component, eg, Burkitt's tumor."

Results of Recent Research

Morphologic Observations at Autopsy

In addition to the recent morphologic observations published by Naeye and others, there are two new reports from Dr. J. L. Emery and his co-workers in Sheffield, England. In the first,[32] they relate their search for the site of origin of free neutral fat-laden macrophages in the cerebrospinal fluid of infants with subacute brain damage. The largest concentrations were found in the region of the fornix, the corpus callosum and its radiations, and around small blood vessels. Striking increases in the number of such cells were noted in two groups of children, those dying in the postperinatal period following episodes of respiratory distress and in a large proportion of older children presenting as unexpected deaths in infancy. The authors suggest that these changes are not specific and probably represent the result of cerebral hypoxia.

In their second paper,[26] they described in great detail lesions of the vocal cords in 91 infants dying as "cot deaths." Pathologic changes of this type have been documented before;[2, 76, 107, 116] however, this is a far more comprehensive treatment of the subject than has been published to date. Cullity and Emery [26] noted, as have others, that these lesions are not unique to infants who die in this manner, but are seen in others.

The Upper Airway: Its Morphology and Function

In a recent publication,[101] Dr. S. Tonkin of Auckland, New Zealand, presented a new hypothesis suggesting that obstruction of the airway at the level of the posterior pharynx is responsible for crib death. She proposed that this oropharyngeal occlusion results from several unique anatomic features of the upper airway of the human infant and may involve pharyngeal relaxation during sleep, a hypermobile mandible, and perhaps an enlarged tongue.

Years ago, Beckwith [6] and Bergman et al [12] proposed the hypothesis that this sort of death was caused by a sudden spasm of the larynx; however, they found it impossible to relate that phenomenon to the state of sleep, so intimately a part of the usual history. Furthermore, their attempts to re-create the event in an experimental model were not entirely successful. In addition, shortly thereafter, French et al [36] demonstrated the absence of any postmortem radiographic evidence of nasopharyngeal obstruction in these infants.

Of particular interest with regard to the upper airway and its possible relationship to the phenomenon of sudden death in infants is the recent work of Downing and Lee [31] of Yale using the piglet as an experimental model and Sessle et al,[87] of Toronto using kittens and cats. The animal was anesthetized, and the investigators cannulated both the distal and the proximal segments of the trachea separately. While pressure changes were being recorded in the distal portion, a number of different test fluids were introduced into the larynx. Whereas normal saline produced little or no change in the animals' respiratory pattern or arterial pressure, the instillation of distilled water or cow's milk triggered an inhibitory chemoreflex with apnea in the majority, which was fatal in many. Topical application of procaine or transection of the superior laryngeal nerve abolished the response, but electrical stimulation of the superior laryngeal nerve mimicked the original experiment.

Additional studies demonstrated that the apneic response to chemical laryngeal stimulation is enhanced when the animal's central respiratory drive is depressed by the administration of chloralose or by severe anemia.

As an extension of these experiments, Sessle's group recorded the activity of hundreds of single cells in the solitary tract nucleus of cats and kittens during peripheral stimulation to nasal mucosa, recurrent laryngeal nerves, etc. The rhythmic discharge of these cells was suppressed, particularly in kittens, by a variety of stimuli, suggesting that the effect on respiration of neurologic feedback from the upper respiratory tract may be great in young animals and may be relevant to their sudden death.

Years ago, Shaw,[89] a prominent pediatrician, proposed that occlusion of the upper airway by nasal mucosal swelling during upper respiratory infection was responsible for the majority of crib deaths. This author contended that infants of the appropriate age are obligate nose breathers and cannot respond to obstruction of their nasal passages by breathing orally. This interesting hypothesis is accepted by many clinicians but has not yet been substantiated in the human, although it has in the infant monkey.[37] The principal difficulty with this hypothesis, however, is that obligate nose breathing is normally present from birth on, whereas the peak incidence of crib death occurs from 2 to 4 months of age, largely sparing the first months of life.

Currently, investigators are engaged in exploring a variety of aspects of the upper airway and the possibility of its participation in a mechanism or mechanisms for sudden infant death. These explorations include studies of the gross anatomy,[99a] detailed morphometry in x-rays,[34] the changing histologic features during this critical period of life,[34, 99a] functional aspects by way of motion pictures taken through a fiberoptic endoscope,[34] physiologic and reflex responses,[83, 99a] and biomechanical studies.[34]

The Role of Viral Infection

In three independent research projects [19, 80a, 105] reported in the early 1970s, a variety of viruses were isolated from a variety of anatomic sites in sizable series of autopsies that included at least 341 instances of crib death. Virtually every virus that could have been recovered and identified at the time was. These included parainfluenza 3 and 1, respiratory syncytial virus, adenovirus types 1, 2, 3, and untyped, rhinovirus, herpes simplex, enterovirus (nonpolio and untyped as well as polio), echovirus, Coxsackie virus B, and others. No one virus predominated in any series, and the sites of recovery included bowel, trachea, nasal passages, lung, myocardium, thymic extract, brain, suprarenal fat, blood cells, and serum. The rate of isolation among these infants as compared with that from control subjects did not suggest that viral infection was, in itself, an important cause for sudden infant death. The accumulated data rather pointed away from disseminated viral infection as a major factor in any ultimate mechanism. The possibility remains, however, that these ordinary viruses may participate in some mechanism, not yet understood, which eventuates in this type of death.

Recently, the role of epidemics of viral disease was systematically investigated [71] over a 42-month period in Chicago, during which time 778 such deaths occurred in the community, and there were seven independent identifiable outbreaks of specific viral infections. Influenza A was the only infection found to have a statistically significant association with sudden infant death, but the association was not highly significant statistically. Four epidemics of respiratory syncytial virus infection were not statistically associated with the sudden deaths.

We have observed individual instances of generalized cytomegalovirus infection in infants who appeared to die suddenly and unexpectedly, and such cases have been reported in recent literature [79, 91] as well. However, it would not seem that this particular infection can, of itself, play an important role in any ultimate mechanism among the majority of crib deaths.

Results of Recent Biochemical Research

For many years, some authors contended that altered electrolyte levels might be responsible for the sudden infant death syndrome. Because of technical limitations, however, the theory could neither be proved nor disproved. Recently, using postmortem analysis of vitreous humor, it has been possible to determine the concentrations of certain chemicals, inasmuch it has been established that their concentration in vitreous humor does indeed reflect antemortem serum concentration. In a study of 27 infants who died of crib death and 9 controls, Blumenfeld and Catherman [16] found no significant differences in the concentrations of sodium, potassium, chloride, calcium, or magnesium and on that basis declared that crib death is probably not attributable to chronic imbalance of any of these electrolytes nor to any condition that might produce such an imbalance.

In a similar study conducted in Sheffield, England, Dr. John L. Emery and his associates [32, 41] found hypernatremia, either with or without uremia, in half of a series of 25 "cot deaths." However, a special powder provided by the government there for the preparation of infant formulas is apparently frequently incorrectly dissolved by mothers, resulting in the relatively common administration of high solute feedings and water deficiency. This, it would seem, must be the explanation for the discrepancy between their results and those of Blumenfeld and Catherman.[16]

Preliminary data are currently accumulating in the laboratory of Dr. Harold Mars [58] of Case Western Reserve suggesting that biogenic amine metabolism may be intimately involved in the genesis of neonatal apneic episodes and also of the sudden infant death syndrome. The biogenic amines are potent biologic substances either possessing neurotransmitter functions or acting as modulators of neurophysiologic activity. Dr. Mars' attention was drawn to the matter by the chance observation of an altered urinary excretion pattern of dopa, dopamine, serotonin, and other amines in a "near-miss" infant. Later, he examined concentrations of those substances in the caudate nuclei and brain stems of 13 infants who had died of sudden death and three controls. Although no specific conclusions could be drawn from the data because of variability in content, it did appear that the concentrations of dopa, dopamine, noradrenalin, and decarboxylase were different in the two groups. He is continuing with this investigation at the present time.

The Role of Infection, Immunologic Mechanisms, and Immunologic Capability

In early life, the infant is suddenly exposed to a wide variety of antigens including microorganisms, pharmacologic agents, and a wide range of environmental substances. His immune reaction to any of these may differ markedly from that of the adult and may serve to jeopardize rather than protect him.[27] It is conceivable that two specific aspects of that encounter may set the stage for the sudden infant death syndrome: primary encounters with a multitude of antigens including infectious agents and a rapidly developing immune response.

There are, unfortunately, many aspects of immune mechanisms at this particular age which are not yet fully understood. These include the various components of the complement system and the ways in which they can be activated, the ontogeny and function of interferon, the serum and cellular aspects of phagocytosis, the role of the autonomic nervous system and hormonal factors as they influence the allergic response, and cell-mediated immune reactions.[27]

The innumerable facets, the complexity, and the interplay of host responses to antigenic challenge would appear at this time to constitute an almost insurmountable task for the investigator who seeks to clarify them and the role or roles they may play with regard to crib death.

In recent years, isolated specific studies have been conducted elucidating just a few of the countless aspects of these systems. In 1971, Urquhart and his co-workers [104] published their observation that antiglobulin antibody had been found in half of 39 instances of sudden infant death and half of 8 deaths due to lower respiratory or gastrointestinal infection. On the other hand, the antibody was found in only 5 percent of 21 living controls with a variety of inflammatory processes. The authors' assumption was that this antibody might produce fatal anaphylaxis.[104] However, these observations were not confirmed in the work of Clausen and others [25] who in 1973, reported *no* elevation of antiglobulin antibodies in the 7 samples of sera they examined.

In 1969, Khan [52] demonstrated elevated IgM in the sera of 18 of 24 (75 percent) crib deaths and 11 of 14 explained infant deaths, which led him to believe that infection may have been a factor in the ultimate mechanism of death. Similarly, Urquhart [106] in 1972, found elevation of IgM in 67 percent (26 of 39). By contrast, Clausen et al [25] in 1973 and Turner et al [103] in 1975 both observed that IgM levels in the sera of victims closely resembled those of noninfected control groups.

Beckwith,[7] in a separate study of 8400 cord bloods found no elevation of IgM in any of 15 infants who, on follow-up, had been discovered to have succumbed to the syndrome of sudden infant death.

Serum levels of IgE at autopsy have been investigated by at least two groups. Clausen et al [25] found them to be similar to those for controls in 17 cases of sudden death, whereas Turner and his co-workers [103] observed the prevalence of specific IgE antibodies to house-dust mite, Aspergillus fumigatus, and bovine beta-lactoglobulin to be significantly greater among crib deaths than among controls.

Titers for specific antibodies to 14 common viral agents were determined in serum obtained at autopsy and proved to be similar among both sudden deaths and control patients.[25] The third component of complement has been reported as not depressed [25] and serum interferon not increased.[80a]

Studies in Progress

Apnea as a Hypothetical Mechanism for Sudden Unexplained Infant Death

Undoubtedly, the single most exciting current hypothesis as to the ultimate mechanism of at least some crib deaths is that of sudden spontaneous protracted apnea, probably related to sleep. This thesis was popularized in 1972 by Steinschneider [96] with his observation that two infants he had been monitoring because of repeated episodes of apnea died suddenly, unexpectedly, and inexplicably. There are unquestionably features of this proposal that are compatible with facts already established concerning crib death. The unrevealing nature of the postmortem examination is one. The tendency for such deaths to occur late at night seems to correspond with the suggested relationship of these apneic spells to sleep.

Recently, Steinschneider [97] and Guilleminault et al [43] have shown that infants subject to repeated apneic spells will experience them more frequently during episodes of nasopharyngitis; in accordance with that observation is the oft-noted presence of inflammatory change in the upper airway in 50 to 60 percent of autopsies on infants who die of crib death.

Of fundamental importance in this regard is the definition of the term *apnea*. Apparently, all infants normally experience many little episodes or short periods of not breathing, or the cessation of breathing. These are said to be a physiologic component of sleep in all infants, and thus it becomes rather arbitrary to decide upon the physiologic limits of such episodes. For purposes of research, Dement and Anders [29] chose to define apnea as those periods of the cessation of respiration exceeding 10 seconds. Episodes from 3 to 9 seconds they refer to as "respiratory pauses." Steinschneider [96] has used 15 seconds as the dividing line, defining anything exceeding that as apnea.

Guilleminault et al,[43] and Dement and Anders [29] of Stanford's Neonatal Sleep Research Unit have described three different kinds of sleep-apnea: central or diaphragmatic, in which chest movements cease; upper airway or obstructive apnea, in which chest and diaphragm move but no air moves in or out of the nose; and mixed central and obstructive. These investigators feel that the distinction between the three different types of apnea is important because (a) the most severe episodes of bradycardia are associated with upper airway or mixed types, (b) the associated bradycardia lasts longer with upper airway and mixed types than it does with central apnea, and (c) there is greater oxygen desaturation during upper airway apnea.

Using long-term (from 12 to 24 hours) polygraphic recordings, they monitored 40 infants of appropriate age in three categories: 25 children of parents suffering from sleep apnea; 15 premature babies; and 8 so-called near-misses.

On every infant they monitored the following:

1. Electroencephalogram
2. Electro-oculogram
3. Chin electromyogram
4. Respiration by means of 2 strain gauges, 1 thoracic and 1 abdominal
5. Respiration by means of 2 thermistors, in front of the mouth and in front of the nostril
6. Electrocardiogram
7. Behavioral criteria (checked by observers)

In some near-miss infants, an endoesophageal pressure transducer was employed to monitor endothoracic pressure, and in all of them, the oxygen saturation curve was followed continuously by means of an ear oximeter.

From these studies, they have learned that none of the offspring of adults with sleep apnea appeared to be abnormal with regard to any of the factors examined. Furthermore, they noted that normal premature infants often experience apneic episodes. Those weighing less than 2000 gm experience predominantly central apnea without accompanying bradycardia, whereas those weighing more than 2000 gm have obstructive or a mixed type of apnea often associated with bradycardia.

All of their eight near-misses were encountered during the winter, and two had positive family histories (one child had two near-misses among siblings and the other, a sibling who had succumbed to crib death). All three types of apnea were observed in near-miss infants; however one of them exhibited no apnea at all but only short spontaneous runs of bradycardia.

In this regard, it should be mentioned that in the study of 15 near-miss infants conducted by Friedman et al [38] at the Los Angeles LAC-USC Medical Center polygraphic recordings of seven variable factors were obtained (eight for 12 hours and seven for 2 hours). The near-miss infants as a group showed less apnea than age-matched controls. They exhibited less beat-to-beat cardiac variability, and no one single variable separated the near-miss infants from controls.

A number of investigators have hypothesized that rapid eye movement (REM) or active sleep would be the "at risk" period. The recordings of Guilleminault et al [43] and Kraus et al,[55] however, indicated that the worst apneic episodes (longest duration and greatest oxygen desaturation during upper airway apnea associated with bradycardia) occurred *not* during REM sleep but always in quiet or indeterminate sleep.

In summary then, the role of apnea with regard to sudden unexplained infant death is not yet clearly defined, although there are some suggestions that it may represent the ultimate mechanism of death for some, or even many, of these deaths.

For that reason, the National Institute of Child Health and Human Development is supporting a number of careful investigations of the matter. In the laboratory of Elliott Weitzman in Montefiore Hospital and Medical Center in New York City near-misses and appropriate controls are being monitored for selected respiratory, cardiac, and neurophysiologic factors.[115] In Los Angeles, the group of Hodgman et al [49] is deeply involved in 12-hour continuous polygraphic recordings on subsequent siblings of infants who have died inexplicably or of near-misses together with low-risk control groups. The data accumulated are being correlated with prenatal recordings of fetal activity and fetal electrocardiograms. They intend to describe the development of sleep and cardiopulmonary regulation in infants at high and low risk in an attempt to identify normal and abnormal patterns that might provide clues to the mechanism of sudden unexplained death.

Other related current investigations include sleep studies in twins,[42] a survey of biogenic amine metabolism as a reflection of immaturity or instability of the autonomic nervous system,[58] apnea resulting from nasal occlusion in infant pigs,[17] and the development of sleep state patterns and the characteristics of apneic episodes in kittens.[61]

One important aspect of this hypothesis is its practical clinical application. If spontaneous protracted apnea is indeed responsible for a significant number of crib deaths, then apnea monitoring, and even home monitoring, would appear to be indicated and, in fact, this is being employed or recommended by some physicians in certain instances. There are, however, three significant difficulties in this regard: The infant at risk cannot yet be definitively identified. Secondly, as Guilleminault et al [43] pointed out, apnea monitors, such as are used in the home, detect only the presence or absence of thoracic or abdominal movements and will be ineffective in cases of upper airway obstruction in which respiratory movements actually *increase*. Finally, at least one infant has been reported to have died of crib death while on an apnea monitor in a hospital intensive care nursery.[57]

Some prominent pediatricians oppose the use of home monitors simply because the mechanical device is fraught with technical difficulties and is therefore apt to alarm parents unnecessarily and all too frequently. They are convinced that the mechanism is a distinct obstacle to normal, natural, easy mother-infant relationships, interfering physically, psychologically, and emotionally.[13] Furthermore, they contend that the entire atmosphere of the home "burdened" with such a monitor is altered in a deleterious fashion and that parents, ever aware of the device, are necessarily tense and anxious all the time. Even the American Academy of Pediatrics [3] has taken an official stand on this side of the disagreement.

However, there are many parents, in addition to professionals, who favor home monitors, especially those parents who have already lost one infant to this tragedy and fear more than anything else the loss of another. They are willing to make any sacrifice and suffer any inconvenience for the sake of the assurance that, should their living infant stop breathing for an undue period of time, they will be alerted by a monitor in time to save the child's life.

And so today, the controversy still smoulders with supporters on both sides. Systematic investigation of the feasibility and psychological effects of apnea monitoring at home are underway in at least two medical centers.[45, 48]

Identification of the Infant at Risk

Ideally, physicians should be able to identify the infant at risk for the sudden infant death syndrome before the fact. However, despite recent developments in our knowledge concerning the potential victim and his various characteristics, no one can yet single him out. We do know that he is more likely than not to be a male from a minority group, of low socioeconomic origin, and to have been born of a young mother either prematurely or of low birth weight. There are apt to have been problems with establishment of his respiration initially. He was probably rather quiet with a relatively poor or peculiar cry or poor capacity to suck. There will be a history that he did not develop or gain weight adequately, etc. Yet even these features are so nonspecific and so common that they are actually insufficient to yield a high-risk population for purposes of investigation.

There are two approaches that could conceivably be used to identify a group of infants as being at special risk for this event, whether for purposes of investigation or even prevention. The first it to assume that the criteria are known (eg, frequent protracted episodes of apnea) and to select accordingly, and the second approach is to establish criteria on the basis of retrospective analysis of historical characteristics.

An interesting example of the former was published by Friedman and her co-workers [38] from the University of Southern California. They selected 15 infants characterized as near-misses on the basis of unexplained apneic episodes occurring after the neonatal period, the assumption being that spontaneous protracted apnea is the essential criterion. Their 12-hour polygraphic records were compared with those for age-matched controls. Although there were individual exceptions, the near-miss infants, as a group, showed less apnea, less beat-to-beat cardiac variability, and longer episodes of wakefulness than the controls. No one single variable separated the near-misses from control infants; however, one infant being studied exhibited bradycardia; one, fixed heart rate; and one, apnea. None died subsequently (to the time of publication).

An example of the latter approach, by contrast, is that of Carpenter and Emery.[24a, b] The investigators first analyzed retrospectively the detailed obstetric and perinatal histories of 119 sudden unexpected infant deaths (explained and unexplained), an obviously high-risk group, and 135 live controls born in the same hospitals. Eight variable factors that could be ascertained at or soon after birth were selected out of 40 as having the most prognostic value. These were:

1. Mother's age. Infants of young mothers are most susceptible.
2. Birth order. The risk for the infant increases as his order increases.
3. Maternal blood group. A is the most vulnerable, O next, and B or AB least.
4. Intention to breast feed. A bottle-fed baby is more at risk.
5. Duration of second stage of labor. The shorter this stage the greater the risk.
6. Urinary tract infection. Maternal urinary tract infections during gestation increases the risk.
7. Polyhydramnios.
8. Prematurity. Prematurity increases the risk if the infant is less than 2500 gm or 37 weeks gestation.

The investigators calculated that this high-risk group had had a relative probability of dying 8.6 times greater than that of the controls. Their ensuing prospective or second-stage study was based upon this set of 8 criteria.

There were 4 second or prospective study groups: Group 1 included all of the infants born the following year predicted to be at low risk (5077); Group 2 included roughly half of those thought to be at high risk who were then supplied with regular nursing-care visits to the home (354); Group 3 included the other half of the high-risk group for whom no such visits were supplied (477); and Group 4 included 80 families who although at high risk elected not to participate in the project at all.

Of the 6003 livebirths that occurred in 1973 in Sheffield, there were 12 sudden infant deaths. The observed relative risk among infants of Group 3, or those high-risk infants deliberately *not* followed at home, was 6.1 times greater than that for the low-risk infants (Group 1). None of the high-risk infants followed at home (Group 2) died. And the risk for those who were thought to be at high risk and who had not elected to participate in any way in the study (Group 4), was greatest of all, 9.1 times greater than that for the low-risk group. The numbers of admissions to hospital among the 3 high-risk groups paralleled these data. The authors concluded that this broad-based mode of selection would appear to be the most feasible.

Since statistics show that subsequent siblings of infants who have died of crib death are at greater risk (4 to 7 times) than children of the same age in the population in general,[40b] some investigators have elected to employ them as subjects for their research endeavors. Their probability of dying suddenly and inexplicably, however, is still only 8 to 14 out of every 1000 livebirths.

Along the same lines, other scientists have selected the twins of affected infants as logical study subjects. It has been determined [92] that surviving twins are indeed at greater risk than others; of 17 pairs of twins who died suddenly at home, 14 co-twins died within 30 days of the first deaths.

Nevertheless, in both of these relationships, it has been ascertained that the increased vulnerability of the survivor is not based on inheritance but rather upon a common "environmental" experience.

The exception to this may be the occasional set of sibs or twins, both with recurrent apneic or cyanotic spells, each of whom eventually succumbs to the syndrome.[96] Families of that type may be manifesting a familial disease which at the moment lurks unrecognized within the great body of sudden, unexplained infant deaths.

The Experimental Animal as a Model

Despite expectations to the contrary, no naturally occurring animal equivalent to the human sudden infant death syndrome has yet been identified and definitively documented. However, since the human infant cannot be used in the conduct of many experiments that appear to be indicated in light of new knowledge in the area, a number of investigators have begun to employ animals in their systematic approach to these explorations.

Apes and monkeys have been and are being used in research into the developmental aspects of the anatomy, histology, physiologic responses, and dynamics of the upper airway.[28, 34, 37, 99] At least two laboratories are engaged in examination of the relationship of fatal apnea to the laryngeal chemoreceptor system and naso-laryngeal-cardiopulmonary reflexes in infant pigs.[17, 31]

Kittens and cats are the subjects of at least five projects now in progress in the exploration of the role of viral infection, immunoglobulins, the physiologic responses of the upper airway, respiratory behavior in its relationship to sleep state, and the long QT syndrome.[28, 61, 72, 85, 87] Three current studies of relevant cardiovascular physiology and protective laryngeal closure reflexes involve the use of fetal, newborn, and infant dogs of different breeds.[28, 83, 88] Other animals being utilized as experimental models are rats, rabbits, calves, guinea pigs, and lambs.[20, 28, 30, 88]

Current Issues of Interest

Welfare of Families

In the summer of 1972, Bergman [9] conducted a nationwide survey to determine how the families of infants who died suddenly and inexplicably were being treated in various cities and counties throughout this country. He and his co-workers discovered that although affected parents were being dealt with in a humane manner in a number of areas, the situation was deplorable in many others. Ignorance and apathy were largely to blame for inadequate support and counseling. But in some instances, the attitudes of those in authority were inexcusably suspicious and even accusatory.

With those data at hand, he and other members of the National Foundation for Sudden Infant Death, Inc., launched an independent program in an attempt to influence local authorities to improve their systems of case management. Simultaneously they, together with members of The Guild for Infant Survival, another parent group, sought to persuade Congress to pass a law to improve the management of such situations. The law was passed, and as a consequence, in the summer of 1975, 24 management centers were established in different cities and states across the country. The objectives of these centers are (a) to provide autopsies for infants who die suddenly and unexpectedly; (b) to provide information about sudden and unexplained infant death in general and about the specific relevant autopsy observations in particular to affected families, as soon as possible; (c) to provide follow-up counseling for families as long as indicated; and (d) to establish educational programs on the subject for all concerned and especially doctors, nurses, police, and firemen.

In the fall of 1975, Bergman [14b] reported on the early results of his campaign —both through the independent program of the Foundation and the 24 management centers. In general, there had been appreciable improvement, at least in most of the sites revisited for evaluation.

Certainly, all physicians involved in these tragic situations have a responsibility to aid the afflicted families in any way or ways they can.[11, 62] In some instances, the pathologists performing the autopsies have assisted to the extent that they themselves talk with the parents, after completion of the necropsy, informing them directly and promptly of their findings and assuring them that as parents and guardians of the child they had not overlooked any recognizable disease process. This in itself removes some element of guilt and provides a measure of assurance.

Breast Feeding

Some have suggested that bottle feeding may predispose infants to sudden death either by means of a hypersensitivity reaction to the foreign proteins contained in the formula [73] or by means of an acquired immune deficit.[44] Although sudden, unexplained infant death does occur more frequently among artificially fed than breast-fed infants, in any civilized population at the present time, there are far more bottle-fed than breast-fed babies. However, Schrauzer et al [84] did perform a statistical analysis in San Diego County and found no difference between suddenly dead infants and controls with regard to breast feeding. As a matter of fact, crib-death babies who had been either totally or partially breast fed died at an earlier age than those who had been fed by formula.

The issue of allergy to the proteins of cow's milk has been dealt with at some length elsewhere.[108] It would seem now an untenable hypothesis.

We have observed at least five instances of crib death occurring in infants who had never received any feeding except breast milk. Other investigators have also reported sudden, unexplained death in infants exclusively breast fed.[8] This at least suggests that the immunologic components of mother's milk do not necessarily protect against the event.

Other Current Hypotheses

In 1972, Dr. Joan Caddell [20] proposed the hypothesis that sudden, unexpected death in infancy is a preventable condition resulting from the magnesium deprivation syndrome of growth. This syndrome is most striking in young, rapidly developing infants and animals receiving magnesium-poor breast milk or on an artificial diet poor in magnesium in relation to its content of calcium, phosphorus, and protein, nutrients that increase the metabolic requirement for magnesium. Premature and low–birth weight infants with poor magnesium stores and rapid growth rates are most vulnerable. She suggested that the pathogenesis of the syndrome of sudden infant death was based on magnesium deficiency leading to the liberation of histamine and histamine shock with bronchospasm, apnea, emphysema, and increased vascular permeability resulting in pulmonary edema and circulatory collapse.

Swift and Emery,[99b] later in 1972 [99a] published their observation that magnesium levels in the vitreous humor in four cases of "cot death" were completely within the range of normal. Later, others [16, 74] noted normal levels in a total of 32 victims.[7, 8, 16]

Despite these two sets of observations, Dr. Caddell is continuing her research in this area studying the magnesium status of postpartum women, neonates, and infants from one to six months of age employing a parenteral magnesium-loading test. She is also using very young rats fed magnesium deficient diets as animal models.[21]

In 1971, it was first proposed [63] that deficiency of selenium or vitamin E might be responsible for crib death. This thesis was later refuted by others in publications in 1973 [82] and 1975.[84] Vitamin E and plasma selenium levels among infants dying of the sudden infant death syndrome proved to be approximately the same as those of normal controls.

Progress in Research to Date

Dr. Eileen Hasselmeyer [46, 47] has described the path of investigation in the realm of crib death as being similar to that of other complex medical problems of the past. First came observation and documentation resulting in recognition of the problem by the scientific and lay communities in the late 1950s. Recognition served to stimulate epidemiologic research efforts of the early 1960s and descriptions of the pathologic features of the entity. Later, a host of hypotheses were formulated, a definition was agreed upon, and diagnostic criteria established. A considerable body of scientific literature began to accumulate in the late 1960s. And now, in the mid-1970s academic interest has peaked, and numerous worthwhile research endeavors are proceeding apace.

Research in the Future

Highly qualified investigators are currently exploring a wide variety of approaches to better understanding the ultimate mechanism of the sudden, unexpected, and unexplained infant death. Included are studies directed at better understanding the development of cardiopulmonary reflexes, chemosensitive systems, particularly in the upper airway, the results of "respiratory loading" in the infant, maturation of the larynx, immunologic aspects, the possibility of genetic susceptibility, and possible neurophysiologic factors. At least two academic centers are engaged in detailed follow-up studies of selected infants judged to be at special risk.

The National Institute of Child Health and Human Development is and has been for some years deeply committed to a program intended to stimulate and support solid productive research in this area. There can be no question that they have accomplished a great deal, and we look forward with optimism to the results of the work they have caused to be done.

Conclusion

In summary, the first half of this decade has witnessed almost revolutionary changes with regard to sudden, unexplained infant deaths. Perhaps the most significant of these is the concept—ever increasing in strength and support—that the victim of the tragedy is not fundamentally a normal or healthy infant and probably never was, even before birth.

Secondly, there has been a tremendous increase in awareness of and interest in the topic, not only among medical people and academicians (who now more than ever have begun to explore the phenomenon systematically), but also among the laity.

And lastly, government agencies have taken a more active role, not only in promoting research, which they were doing previously, but also in providing for the welfare of afflicted families. Now more than ever, it seems conceivable that we may one day understand the cause or causes of these many deaths that are presently inexplicable and thus may prevent their occurrence.

References

1. Adelson L: Personal communication, 1975
2. Adelson L, Kinney ER: Sudden and unexpected death in infancy and childhood. Pediatrics 17:663, 1956
3. American Academy of Pediatrics. Committee on Infant and Preschool Child. Home monitoring for sudden infant death. Pediatrics 55(1):144, 1975
4. SIDS—Proc Francis E. Camps Int Symp Sudden and Unexpected Death in Infancy, Toronto, Ontario, Canada, May 15–17, 1974
5. Beal S: Sudden infant death syndrome. Med J Aust 2:1223, 1972
6. Beckwith JB: Observations on the pathological anatomy of the sudden infant death syndrome, pp 83–107. See Bergman et al [12]
7. Beckwith JB: The sudden infant death syndrome. Curr Probl Pediatr 3(8):1, 1973
8. Beckwith JB: Personal communication, 1975
9. Bergman AB: The management of sudden infant death syndrome (SIDS) in the United States, 1972. New York, National Foundation for Sudden Infant Death, 1973
10. Bergman A: Relationship of passive cigarette smoking to sudden infant death syndrome. J Pediatr 58:665, 1976
11. Bergman AB: Psychological aspects of sudden unexpected death in infants and children. Review and commentary. Pediatr Clin North Am 21:115, 1974
12. Bergman AB, Beckwith JB, Ray CG (eds): Proceedings of the Second International Conference on Causes of Sudden Death in Infants. Seattle, Univ of Washington Press, 1970, p 248
13. Bergman AB, Beckwith JB, Ray CG: Commentaries re the apnea monitor business. Pediatrics 56:1, 1975
14a. Bergman AB, Ray CG, Pomeroy MA, Wahl PW, Beckwith JB: Studies of the sudden infant death syndrome in King County, Washington. III. Epidemiology. Pediatrics 49(6):860, 1972
14b. Bergman AB: Current classification of primary counties in each standard metropolitan statistical area (SMSA) with reference to changes in management of SIDS cases in 1972 and 1975. See Hasselmeyer [47]
15. Block A: SIDS in the Ashkelon district. A 10-year survey. Isr J Med Sci 9:452, 1973
16. Blumenfeld TA, Catherman RL: Postmortem vitreous concentration of Na, K, Cl, Ca and Mg in sudden infant death syndrome. Pediatr Res 9:344 (Abstract), 1975
17. Bonner A: Spontaneous apnea in infant pigs. See Hasselmeyer [47]
18. Borhani NL, Rooney PA, Kraus JF: Post-neonatal sudden unexplained death in a California county. Calif Med 118:12, 1973
19. Brandt CD: Infectious agents from cases of sudden infant death syndrome and from members of their community, pp 161–74. See Bergman et al [12]

20. Caddell JL: Magnesium deprivation in sudden unexpected infant death. Lancet 2:258, 1972
21. Caddell JL: Testing the hypothesis: Magnesium deprivation in SIDS. See Hasselmeyer [47]
22. Camps EF (ed): Confidential enquiry into post-neonatal deaths, 1964–1966. Rep Public Health Med Subj (Lond) 125:1, 1970
23. Camps EF: The cot or crib death. Br J Hosp Med 4:779, 1970
24a. Carpenter RB, Emery JL: Identification and follow-up of infants at risk for sudden death in infancy. Nature 250:729, 1974
24b. SIDS—Proc Francis E. Camps Int Symp Sudden and Unexpected Death in Infancy, Toronto, Ontario, Canada, May 15–17, 1974
25. Clausen CR, Ray CG, Hebestreit N: Studies of the sudden infant death syndrome in King County, Washington. IV. Immunologic studies. Pediatrics 52:45, 1973
26. Cullity GJ, Emery JL: Ulceration and necrosis of vocal cords in hospital and unexpected child deaths. J Pathol 115:27, 1975
27. Dancis J (ed): Research planning workshops on the sudden infant death syndrome: (2) Developmental aspects of infection and immunity. Bethesda, Maryland, May 26–27, 1972. Public Health Service Pub No NIH-74-578, GPO Washington, DC
28. Dawes GS, Harding R, Johnson P, McClelland M: An animal model for sudden infant death. See Hasselmeyer [47]
29. Dement WW, Anders T: Summary of research on the relationship between sleep apnea and the sudden infant death syndrome. See Hasselmeyer [47]
30. Dennenberg V: Consequences of infant risk factors in humans and animals. See Hasselmeyer [47]
31. Downing SE, Lee JC: Central respiratory drive and the laryngeal chemoreflex: Mechanisms for fatal apnea in the piglet model. See Hasselmeyer [47]
32. Emery JL, Gadson DR: Neutral fat in the brains of infants dying in the perinatal period and presenting as unexpected death in infancy. Scientific Program of the Pathological Society of Great Britain and Ireland, January 9–11, 1975. London, 1975
33. Fedrick J: Sudden unexpected death in infants in the Oxford Record Linkage Area. An analysis with respect to time and place. Br J Prev Med 27:217, 1973
34. Fink BR: Maturation of larynx in relation to infant death. See Hasselmeyer [47]
35. SIDS—Proc Francis E. Camps Int Symp Sudden and Unexpected Death in Infancy, Toronto, Ontario, Canada, May 15–17, 1974
36. French JW, Beckwith JB, Graham CB, Guntheroth WG: Lack of postmortem radiographic evidence of nasopharyngeal obstruction in the sudden infant death syndrome. J Pediatr 81:1145, 1972
37. French JW, Morgan BC, Guntheroth WG: Infant monkeys—a model for crib death. Am J Dis Child 123:480, 1972
38. Friedman ME, Geidel S, Havens B, Hoppenbrowers T, Hodgman JE: Near-miss for sudden infant death syndrome. Clin Res 23(2):142A, 1975
39. Froggatt P: Epidemiologic aspects of Northern Ireland Study, pp 32–46. See Bergman et al [12]
40a. Froggatt P, Lynas MA, Marshall TK: Sudden unexpected death in infants (cot death) report of a collaborative study in Northern Ireland. Ulster Med J 40:116, 1971
40b. Froggatt P, Lynas MA, MacKenzie G: Epidemiology of sudden unexpected death in infants (cot death) in Northern Ireland. Br J Prev Soc Med 25:119, 1971
41. Gadson DR, Emery JL: Fatty change in the brain in perinatal and unexpected death. Arch Dis Child 51(1):42, 1976
42. Gould JB: A study of monozygous and dizygous twins to ascertain possible neurophysiological factors for the sudden infant death syndrome. See Hasselmeyer [47]

43. Guilleminault C, Peraita R, Souquet M, Dement WC: Apneas during sleep in infants: Possible relationship with sudden infant death syndrome. Science 190: 677, 1975

44. Gunther M: The neonate's immunity gap, breast feeding and cot death. Lancet 1(7904):441, 1975

45. Hall CW: Cardiorespiratory responses of infants. See Hasselmeyer [47]

46. Hasselmeyer EG: An introductory overview. In Robinson RR (ed): SIDS. Toronto, Ontario, Canada, 1974, pp 15–20

47. Hasselmeyer EG: Research perspectives in the sudden infant death syndrome, 1975. DHEW Publication No. (NIH) 76- 1976. Washington, DC, DHEW Public Health Service, National Institutes of Health, 1976

48. Henning L: Psychological aspects of the use of an apnea monitor in the home. See Hasselmeyer [47]

49. Hodgman JE, Harper R, Hoppenbrouwers T, Sterman MB: Development of sleep and cardiopulmonary variables in infants at high and low risk for SIDS. See Hasselmeyer [47]

50. Hon EH: Some biophysical fetal data on a SIDS infant. See Hasselmeyer [47]

51. Houstek D: Sudden infant death syndrome in Czechoslovakia: Epidemiologic aspects, pp 55–63. See Bergman et al [12]

52. Khan WN, Ali RV, Werthmann M, Ross SJ: Immunoglobulin M determinations in neonates and infants as an adjunct to the diagnosis of infection. J Pediatr 75:1282, 1969

53. Kraus JF, Borhani NO: Post-neonatal sudden unexpected death in California: A cohort study. Am J Epidemiol 95:497, 1972

54. Kraus JF, Franti CE, Borhani NO: Discriminatory risk factors in post-neonatal sudden unexplained death. Am J Epidemiol 96:328, 1972

55. Kraus JF, Alfred N, Auld PAM: Apnea in premature infants. See Hasselmeyer [47]

56. Lardy HS, Bentle LA, Wagner MJ, et al: Defective phosphoenolpyruvate carboxykinase in victims of sudden infant death syndrome. See Hasselmeyer [47]

57. Lewak N: Sudden infant death syndrome in a hospitalized infant on an apnea monitor. Pediatrics 56(2):296, 1975

58. Mars H: Biogenic amine metabolism in apnea and crib death. See Hasselmeyer [47]

59. Mason JM, Mason LH, Jackson M, et al: Pulmonary vessels in SIDS. N Engl J Med 292:479, 1975

60. Mason JM: Personal communication, 1975

61. McGinty DJ: Animal studies of physiological mechanisms associated with cardiopulmonary instability during sleep. See Hasselmeyer [47]

62. McClelland CO, Fleming DG, Katona P: Letter: The physician's responsibility in the management of sudden infant death syndrome. Am J Dis Child 129(1): 138, 1975

63. Money DF: Cot deaths and deficiency of vitamin E and selenium. Br Med J 4:559, 1971

64. Naeye RL: Pulmonary arterial abnormalities in the sudden infant death syndrome. N Engl J Med 289:1167, 1973

65. Naeye RL: Hypoxemia and the sudden infant death syndrome. Science 186:837, 1974

66. Naeye RL, Drage J: Sudden infant death syndrome, a prospective study. Ped Res 9:298 (Abstract), 1975, and Soc Ped Res, Proc of the Meeting, Amer Ped Soc Denver, Col, April 16–19, 1975

67. Naeye RL, Drage J: Sudden infant death syndrome, a prospective study, and other reports. See Hasselmeyer [47]

68. Naeye RL, Whalen P, Ryser M, Fisher R: Cardiac and other abnormalities in the sudden infant death syndrome. Am J Pathol 82:1, 1976

69. Naeye RL, Messmer J, Specht T, Merritt TA: Sudden infant death syndrome, temperament before death. J Pediatr 88:511, 1976

70. National Conference of Pathologists on Sudden Infant Death Syndrome. Santa

Fe, New Mexico. Supported by Sudden Infant Death Syndrome Information and Counseling Grant MCH-000022, Office for Maternal and Child Health, BCHS, PHS, HEW, November, 1975

71. Nelson KE, Greenberg MA, Mufson MA, Moses VK: The sudden infant death syndrome and epidemic viral disease. Am J Epidemiol 101(5):423, 1975

72. Padgett GA, Hegreberg GA, Prieur DJ: Sudden death in cats: A spontaneously occurring model for SIDS of man. See Hasselmeyer [47]

73. Parish WE, Barrett AM, Coombs RRA, Gunther M, Camps FE: Hypersensitivity to milk and sudden death in infancy. Lancet 2:1106, 1960

74. Peterson DR, Beckwith JB: Magnesium deprivation in sudden unexpected infant death. Lancet 2:330, 1973

75. Peterson DR, Benson E, Fisher L, Chinn N, Beckwith JB: Postnatal growth and the sudden infant death syndrome. Am J Epidemiol 99(6):389, 1974

76. Pinkham JR, Beckwith JB: Vocal cord lesions in the sudden infant death syndrome, pp 104–7. See Bergman et al [12]

77. Pierson PS, Howard P, Kleber H: Sudden deaths in infants born to methadone-maintained addicts. JAMA 220(13):1733, 1972

78. Protestos CD, Carpenter RG, McWeeny PM, Emery JL: Obstetric and perinatal histories of children who died unexpectedly (cot death). Arch Dis Child 48(11):835, 1973

79. Raven C: Sudden infant death syndrome. JAMA 235:249 (Letter to the editors), 1976

80a. Ray CG, Beckwith JB, Hebestreit NM, Bergman AB: Studies of the sudden infant death syndrome in King County, Washington. I. The role of viruses. JAMA 211:619, 1970

80b. Ray CG, Hebestreit NM: Studies of the sudden infant death syndrome in King County, Washington. II. Attempts to demonstrate evidence of viremia. Pediatrics 48:79, 1971

80c. Richards ID, McIntosh HT: Confidential inquiry into 226 consecutive infant deaths. Arch Dis Child 47:697, 1972

81. Salk L, Grellong BA, Dietrich J: Sudden infant death: Normal cardiac habituation and poor autonomic control. N Engl J Med 241:219, 1974

82. Saltzstein SL, Schrauzer GN, Rhead WJ: Letter: Sudden infant deaths and deficiencies in diet. JAMA 226:466, 1973

83. Sasaki CT: Postnatal respiratory development as related to the sudden infant death syndrome. See Hasselmeyer [47]

84. Schrauzer GN, Rhead WJ, Saltzstein SL: Sudden infant death syndrome: Plasma vitamin E levels and dietary factors. Ann Clin Lab Sci 5(1):31, 1975

85. Schwartz PJ: Experimental reproduction of the long Q-T syndrome and SIDS. See Hasselmeyer [47]

86. Seitz RE, Nathanson SN: Abnormal cry in an infant dying suddenly and unexpectedly. See Hasselmeyer [47]

87. Sessle BJ, Storey AT, Lund JP, Greenwood LF: Neural mechanisms contributing to upper respiratory tract function in adult cat and kitten. See Hasselmeyer [47]

88. Sinha SN: Cardiovascular physiology in experimental models in relationship to the mechanisms for death in SIDS. See Hasselmeyer [47]

89. Shaw EB: Sudden unexpected death in infancy syndrome. Am J Dis Child 116:115, 1968

90. SIDS 1974 Proceedings of the Francis E. Camps International Symposium on Sudden and Unexpected Deaths in Infancy. Robinson RR (ed). Canadian Foundation for the Study of Infant Deaths. Toronto, Ontario, Canada, 1974, p 364

91. Smith SD, Cho CT: Letter: Cytomegalovirus pneumonia in sudden infant death syndrome. JAMA 233(8):861, 1975

92. Spiers PS: Estimated rates of concordancy for the sudden infant death syndrome in twins. Am J Epidemiol 100(1):1, 1974

93. Steele R: Sudden infant death syndrome in Ontario, Canada: Epidemiologic aspects, p 64. See Bergman et al [12]

94. SIDS—Proc Francis E. Camps Int Symp Sudden and Unexpected Death in Infancy, Toronto, Ontario, Canada, May 15–17, 1974

95. Steele R, Langworth JT: The relationship of ante-natal and post-natal factors to sudden unexpected death in infancy. Can Med Assoc J 94:1165, 1966

96. Steinschneider A: Prolonged apnea and the sudden infant death syndrome: Clinical and laboratory observations. Pediatrics 50:646, 1972

97. Steinschneider A: Nasopharyngitis and prolonged apnea. Pediatrics 56(1):967, 1975

98. Strimer R, Adelson L, Oseasohn R: Epidemiologic features of 1,134 sudden unexpected infant deaths. JAMA 209:1493, 1969

99a. Sutton D: Infant primate upper airway: Anatomy and physiology. See Hasselmeyer [47]

99b. Swift PG, Emery JL: Magnesium and sudden unexpected infant death. Lancet 2:871, 1972

100. SIDS—Proc Francis E. Camps Int Symp Sudden and Unexpected Death in Infancy, Toronto, Ontario, Canada, May 15–17, 1974

101. Tonkin S: Sudden infant death syndrome: Hypothesis of causation. Pediatrics 55(5):650, 1975

102. Turner KJ, Baldo BA, Hilton JM: RAST studies: IgE antibodies to Dermatophagoides pteronyssinus (house dust mite), Aspergillus fumigatus and beta-lactoglobulin in sudden death in infancy syndrome (SIDS). Dev Biol Stand 29:308, 1975

103. Turner KJ, Baldo BA, Hilton JM: IgE antibodies to Dermatophagoides pteronyssinus (house dust mite), Aspergillus fumigatus, and bovine beta-lactoglobulin in sudden infant death syndrome. Br Med J 1:357, 1975

104. Urquhart GE, Logan RW, Izatt MM: Sudden unexplained death in infancy and hyperimmunization. J Clin Pathol 24:736, 1971

105. Urquhart GE, Grist NR: Virological studies of sudden unexplained infant deaths in Glasgow, 1967–1970. J Clin Pathol 25:443, 1972

106. Urquhart GE, Izatt MM, Logan RW: Cot death: An immune complex disease. Lancet 1:210 (Letter to the editor), 1972

107. Valdes-Dapena MA: Crib deaths and focal fibrinoid necrosis of the infant larynx. J Forensic Sci 3:503, 1958

108. Valdes-Dapena MA: Progress in sudden infant death research, 1963–69, pp 3–13. See Bergman et al [12]

109. Valdes-Dapena MA: Sudden death in infancy: A report for pathologists. Perspect Pediatr Pathol 2:1, 1975

110. Valdes-Dapena MA: The sudden infant death syndrome—1975—an update for pathologists. Bull Int Acad Pathol 16:15, 1975

111. Valdes-Dapena MA, Birle LJ, McGovern JA, McGillen JF, Colwell FH: Sudden unexpected death in infancy: A statistical analysis of certain socio-economic factors. J Pediatr 73:387, 1968

112. Valdes-Dapena MA, Gillane MM, Catherman R: Abnormal extramedullary hematopoiesis in the sudden infant death syndrome. See Hasselmeyer [47]

113. Valdes-Dapena MA, Gillane MM, Catherman R: Brown fat retention in the sudden infant death syndrome. Arch Pathol Lab Med 100:547, 1976

114. Valdes-Dapena MA, McGovern JA, Birle LJ, Auerbach VH: Changes in annual incidence rates of sudden unexpected deaths among infants in Philadelphia, 1960–1972. J Pediatr 84(5):776 (Letter to the editor), 1974

115. Weitzmann E, Cornwell AC: Evaluation and follow-up of selected respiratory, cardiac and neurophysiologic parameters in infants. See Hasselmeyer [47]

116. Werne J, Garrow I: Sudden, apparently unexplained death during infancy. I. Pathological findings in infants observed to die suddenly. Am J Pathol 29:817, 1953

THE SIGNIFICANCE OF EPITHELIAL POLYPS OF THE LARGE BOWEL

HARLAN J. SPJUT AND ROLANDO G. ESTRADA

Since the paper published in 1958 by Spratt et al,[1] there have been considerable controversy and innumerable publications related to the certainty or uncertainty of epithelial polyps becoming adenocarcinomas of the large intestine. One of the significant conclusions of the paper was, "The theory of the origin of adenocarcinomas of the colon within adenomatous polyps had little to support it." Others [2] have supported the findings of Spratt and his associates, on the other hand, Lane and associates,[3] and Wychulis and associates [4] have advocated a strong relationship between the occurrence of adenomatous polyps and adenocarcinoma.

In part, at least, the problem of the significance of the epithelial polyp revolves around the rather broad definition of adenomatous polyp used by many pathologists. Most accept four major types of epithelial polyps: adematous, mixed, villous, and hyperplastic. Yet these are often ignored, as becomes apparent when papers report "adenomatous polyps" giving rise to carcinoma with metastases. We reviewed 13 recently published case reports [5-17] and found that none of the authors have illustrated an adenomatous polyp, but have shown mixed polyps or villous tumors with carcinoma. Then there are the papers that are poorly illustrated or not illustrated at all, which merely adds to the confusion. In other words, we have been unable to find a single illustrated case in which a pure adenomatous polyp contained an invasive carcinoma that metastasized.

Except for hyperplastic polyps and the characteristic villous tumors, perhaps a specific histologic definition of epithelial polyps of the large intestine is of no consequence. However, it has been pointed out by various observers [18, 19] that there apparently is significance to the villous component of epithelial polyps. With these points in mind, we reviewed a group of epithelial polyps from the large intestine with the view of segregating these into histomorphologic groups as a means of determining the significance of the pathologic features. Nonepithelial polypoid lesions, carcinoids, pseudopolyps, hamartomas, and inflammatory polyps were not considered in this review.

TABLE 1. Distribution of Polyps and Polyps with CIS* and Adenocarcinoma

Localization	Total Number of Polyps (%)	Polyps with CIS NO. (%)	% †	Carcinomas Arising in Polyps NO. (%)	% †
Cecum	26 (3.24)	0 (—)	0	0 (—)	0
Ascending	53 (6.61)	1 (5)	0.12	1 (5.88)	0.12
Transverse	49 (6.11)	2 (10)	0.24	2 (11.8)	0.24
Descending	69 (8.61)	0 (—)	0	1 (5.9)	0.12
Sigmoid	310 (38.7)	9 (45)	1.12	9 (52.9)	1.12
Rectum	294 (36.7)	8 (40)	0.99	4 (23.5)	0.49
Total	801	20	2.49	17	2.12

* Carcinoma in situ.
† This is percent of total number of polyps (801).

Materials and Methods

Eight hundred and one epithelial polyps from 611 patients were reviewed. These were consecutive patients and seen in the following hospitals in Houston: Ben Taub General Hospital, The Methodist Hospital, and St. Luke's Episcopal Hospital. The majority of the polyps were removed either by colonoscopic excision, proctoscopic excision, or open polypectomy. Another group included those polyps

TABLE 2.

Type of Polyp	Total No.	Av. Age (yr)	F	M	Localization CECUM	ASCEND.	TRANSV.
Adenomatous	250 (31.2)	60	85 (34)	165 (66)	15 (6)	20 (8)	23 (9.2)
Adenomatous (1–4% villous)	80 (10)	61	28 (35)	52 (65)	0 (—)	6 (7.5)	4 (5)
Adenomatous (5–20% villous)	110 (13.7)	61.4	42 (38.2)	68 (61.8)	3 (2.7)	4 (3.6)	6 (5.5)
Adenomatous (21–50% villous)	114 (14.2)	60	51 (44.7)	63 (55.3)	6 (5.2)	8 (7)	5 (4.3)
Villous tumors	123 (15.4)	61.7	64 (52.1)	59 (47.9)	0 (—)	2 (1.6)	7 (5.7)
Hyperplastic polyps	124 (15.5)	53	37 (29.8)	87 (70.2)	2 (1.6)	4 (3.2)	6 (4.8)

Percentages given in parentheses.

found in a segment of bowel associated with an infiltrative carcinoma that had been resected; 290 (47 percent) of the patients were women; 321 (53 percent) were men. The mean age of the patients was 59.8 years, with an age range of 23 to 90 years; 39 (13.4 percent) of the women were under 50, and 70 (24.1 percent) were over 70 years of age. Among the men, 64 (19.9 percent) were over 70, and 57 (14.6 percent) were under the age of 50 years. The distribution of the polyps can be seen in Table 1. In general, the distribution is similar to that which has been previously reported in the literature in that the majority of the polyps were located in the rectum and sigmoid with the remainder of the large intestine being rather uniformly involved. As can be seen in Table 2, there are some slight variations in the distribution of the major histologic types, namely adenomatous, mixed, hyperplastic, and villous tumors. There were 250 (31.2 percent) adenomatous polyps, 304 (36.7 percent) polyps with a varied percentage of villous component, 123 (15.4 percent) villous tumors, and 124 (15.5 percent) hyperplastic polyps. This histologic distribution was similar to that reported by Kurzon and associates.[19]

Results

For this study, an epithelial polyp is defined as a proliferation of mucosal epithelium, glandular and surface, to form a protrusion into the bowel lumen. The four major histologic types that we considered are: adenomatous, mixed (villoglandular polyps), villous tumors, and hyperplastic polyps. With some exceptions, it is difficult to differentiate the various epithelial polyps from the gross appearance (Figs. 1 and 2). It is true that certain characteristic villous tumors are identifiable (Fig. 3). These have recognizable villous patterns, are broad based, and often have a convoluted multilobate surface. An occasional villous tumor is pedunculated. In general, the lesions are larger than the other histologic types, but these range in size from 0.6 cm up to 8.5 cm in our study. Thus, the smallest lesion falls readily within the range of hyperplastic and adenomatous polyps.

Summary of Data

Localization			Size (cm)			Carcinomas	
DESC.	SIGM.	RECTUM	SMALL	LARGE	AVERAGE	CIS	CA
47 (18.8)	75 (30)	70 (28)	0.3	2.5	0.65	0 —	0 —
8 (10)	31 (38.7)	31 (38.7)	0.2	2.0	0.6	5 (6)	0 —
8 (7.3)	43 (39)	38 (34.5)	0.3	2.5	1.06	3 (2.7)	0 —
6 (5.2)	55 (48.2)	34 (29.8)	0.3	4.5	1.48	5 (4.4)	7 (6.14)
9 (7.3)	39 (31.7)	66 (53.6)	0.6	8.5	1.72	7 (5.7)	10 (8.13)
6 (4.8)	44 (35.5)	61 (49.2)	0.3	2.0	0.5	0 —	0 —

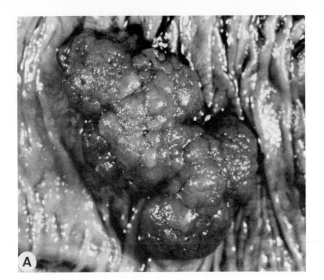

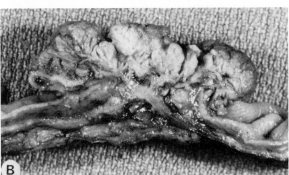

Fig. 1. A and B. An adenomatous polyp with an estimated 25 percent villous component. The lesion occurred in the sigmoid colon of a 65-year-old woman.

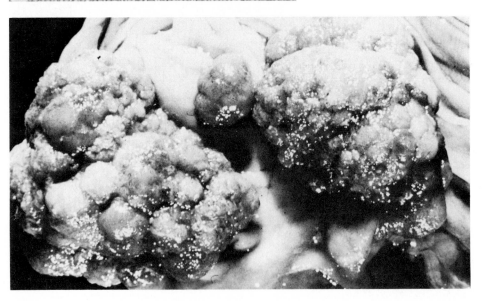

Fig. 2. Two villous tumors (large) and an adenomatous polyp (single, small) showing the similarity to Figures 1A and B. These were resected from the ascending colon of a 52-year-old woman. $\times$ 1.75.

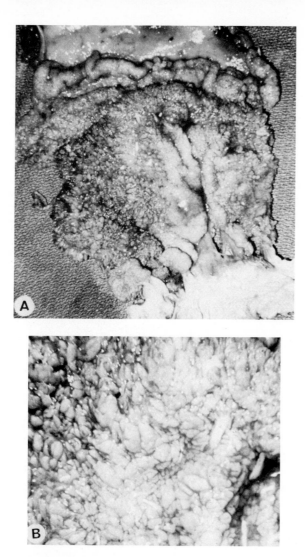

Fig. 3. A villous tumor of the rectum with characteristic villous pattern. This occurred in a 63-year-old female. B: × 3.

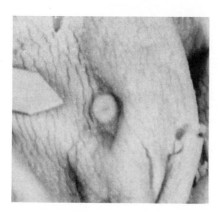

Fig. 4. A hyperplastic polyp of the large bowel. The patient was male, 62 years of age. × 2.

151

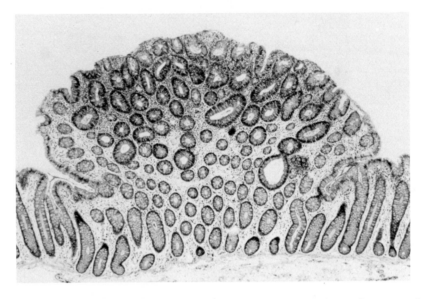

Fig. 5. This is a pure adenomatous polyp demonstrating the cytologic changes: reduced goblet cells and nuclear stratification. H&E. × 40.

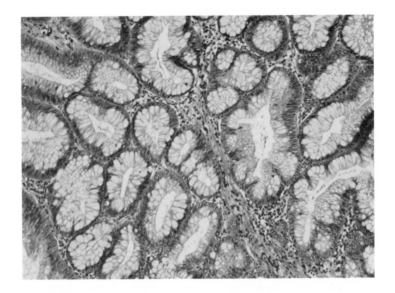

Fig. 6. A gland portraying characteristic adenomatous features. H&E. × 200.

Hyperplastic polyps are generally small mucosal protrusions without a stalk and for the most part are less than 5 mm in diameter (Fig. 4). These lesions have smooth, perhaps slightly roughened, pink-tan surfaces. Again, the size is not necessarily specific, as adenomatous polyps may have the same configuration and size. According to Lane and associates,[3] at least 90 percent of polyps less than 5 mm in diameter will turn out to be hyperplastic. The pedunculated mixed and adenomatous polyps are indistinguishable from each other on their uncut or cut surfaces.

We recognize that there are various names used for adenomatous polyps, such as adenoma or tubular polyp. We have chosen to retain the name adenomatous due to its widespread usage. Adenomatous polyps are composed of well-defined glands that add to the mass of the normal mucosa thus causing the polypoid protrusion. A central fibrovascular core sometimes containing muscularis mucosae is present. This is in continuity with the normal muscularis mucosae and submucosa.

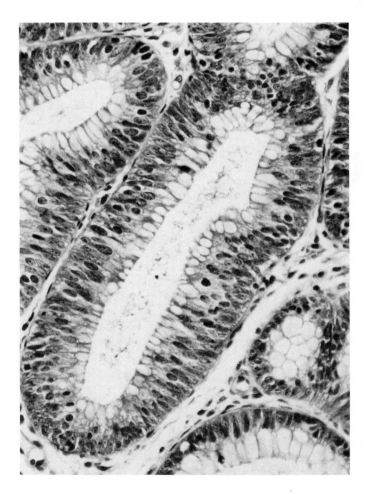

Fig. 7. Adenomatous polyp representing a variation in which goblet cells remain prominent. This pattern should not be confused with that of a hyperplastic polyp. H&E. × 85.

In the individual glands of the polyp, there is a tendency for the nuclei to become elongated and stratified when compared to the normal basally located ovoid nuclei (Figs. 5 and 6). In addition, goblet cells are generally less frequent than normal. The cytoplasm of the cells of the adenomatous polyp is denser and, at times, amphophilic and perhaps acidophilic. These alterations are noted throughout the body of the polyp. There are variations from this basic definition in that some adenomatous polyps are composed of glands that have rather abundant goblet cells (Fig. 7), and in others goblet cells are few and the nuclear component prominent, tending to atypical alterations. There may be some branching of the glands in the atypical foci. Ordinarily at the edges of the body of the polyp, there is an abrupt transition between the normal colonic mucosa and the adenomatous epithelium. At times, transition may be noted. Only occasionally have we noted adenomatous alterations of the mucosa of the stalk of a polyp away from the main lesion.

Mixed (villoglandular) polyps are not as clearly defined as are adenomatous polyps. There may be differences of opinion as to what represents a villus. Our definition of a villus is a narrow fibrovascular core covered by epithelium that has adenomatous alterations like those just described (Fig. 8). In other words, these fine, fingerlike structures are similar to those that would be expected in a characteristic villous tumor. We have more or less arbitrarily designated epithelial polyps as mixed if an estimated 20 percent of the polyp has a villous pattern and the remainder had an adenomatous pattern (Fig. 9). These patterns may be intermingled.

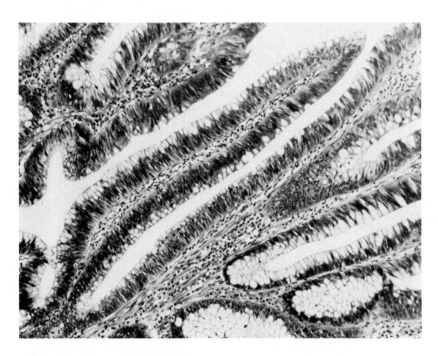

Fig. 8. A single villus. This corresponds to formations that we consider to be a villus in estimating the percent of such structures in an adenomatous polyp. H&E. $\times$ 100.

It is recognized that epithelial polyps have less than 20 percent villous components, with many having less than 5 percent by our estimates (Fig. 10). We wish to emphasize that the villous components represent only an estimate of the total surface of the polyps as studied on hematoxylin and eosin stained slides.

We have defined a villous tumor as an epithelial polyp which exhibits 50 percent or more villous pattern. In other words, lesions that we designate as villous tumors do have an adenomatous component. In fact, among the 123 villous tumors in this study, none were purely villous. The villi are defined as previously noted, ie, long, fingerlike, epithelial-covered structures with the narrow fibro-vascular core (Fig. 11). The epithelium has an adenomatous alteration, ie, nuclear stratification, decreased prominence of goblet cells, and increased density of the cytoplasm. In some of the flat lesions, the villous projections almost appear to spring directly from the mucosa.

Lane and his associates [3] have carefully defined the hyperplastic polyp. Our definition conforms with theirs from the histologic standpoint. For all practical purposes, these lesions are small, less than 5 mm, and sessile. The epithelium of the glands and the surface of the polyps show a somewhat serrated margin with only little nuclear stratification. Generally, the nuclei tend to lie at the bottom of

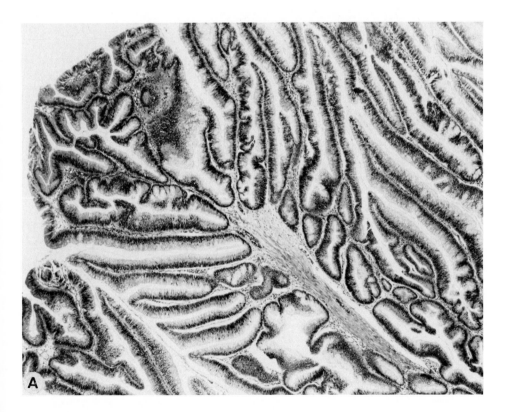

Fig. 9A and **B.** Adenomatous polyps with villous components. Definite glandular structures are present. H&E. × 69 (cont. on p. 156).

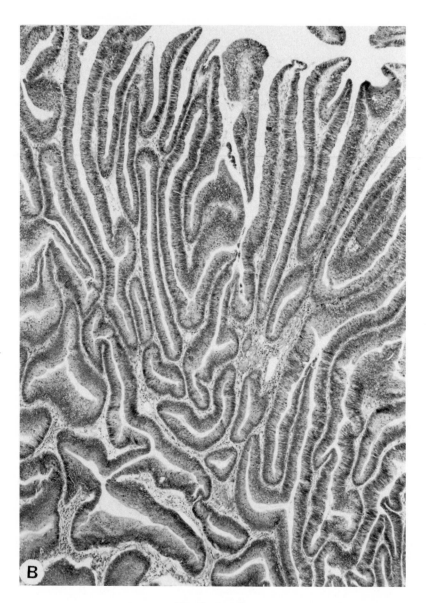

Fig. 9. (*cont.*)

the cells. The epithelium has an acidophilic coloration, and the goblet cells are usually prominent (Figs. 12 to 14). These polyps were the most homogenous group in the study.

Carcinoma in situ (CIS) was observed only in adenomatous polyps with a villous component and in villous tumors. The lesion was not observed in pure adenomatous or hyperplastic polyps. The polyps containing CIS ranged from 0.5 to 2 cm in greatest dimension and averaged 1.4 cm. Carcinoma in situ is defined histologically as a complex arrangement of the glandular components of a polyp, and we expect to see branching of the glandular structures, increased nuclear stratification, nuclear pleomorphism, and increased numbers of mitotic figures (Fig. 15A–D). The non–CIS portions of the polyp serve as baselines by which to judge these changes. Invasion is not seen, and step sections through a block or blocks may be necessary in order to verify this. Carcinomas in situ are generally focal and do not involve a major portion of any of the polyps in our study. We have not diagnosed CIS merely on the basis of intense nuclear stratification. We have insisted upon the presence of multibranching of the glandular structures and the nuclear alterations described above. The location of CIS bearing polyps and the histologic type of polyp are seen in Tables 1 and 3.

An invasive carcinoma is defined as glands having the characteristics of an adenocarcinoma with definite evidence of invasion of the body or stalk of the

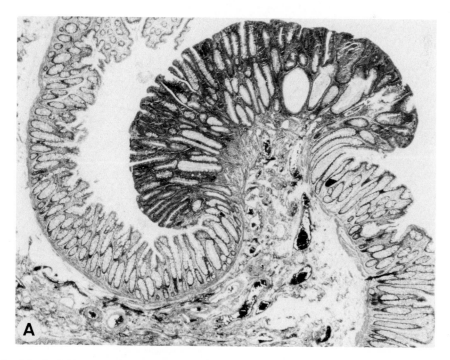

Fig. 10. A. Adenomatous polyp with an estimated less than 10 percent villous portion. H&E. A: × 25; B: × 50. (cont. on p. 158)

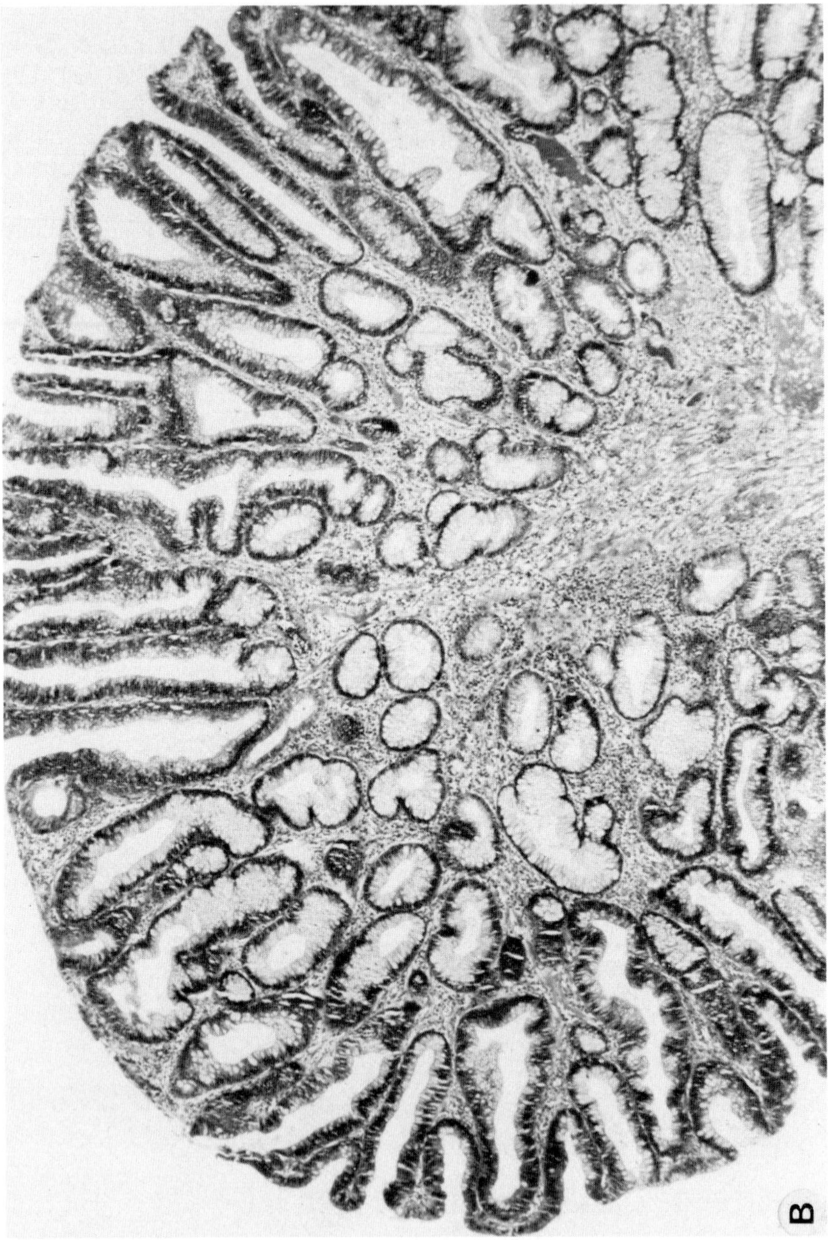

Fig. 10. B. See legend on previous page.

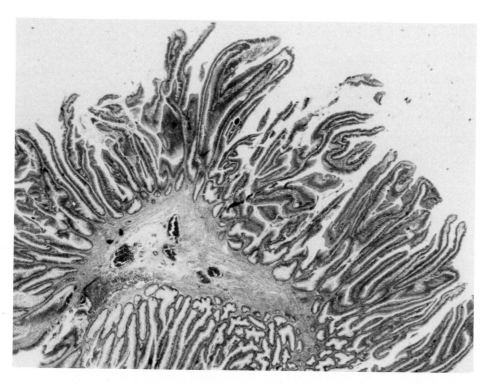

Fig. 11. Portion of a rectal villous tumor removed from a 71-year-old woman. This lesion had an estimated 80 percent villous component. A carcinoma with a nodal metastasis was present. H&E. × 29.5.

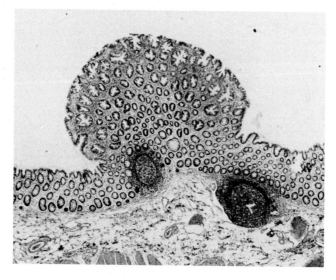

Fig. 12. A hyperplastic polyp with "sawtooth" epithelial pattern. H&E. × 25.

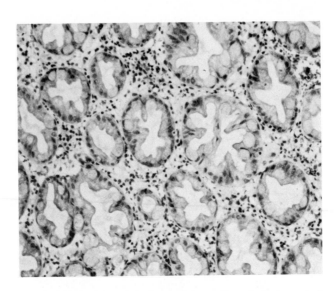

Fig. 13. At higher magnification, the typical glandular pattern is to be noted and compared with the adenomatous polyps in Figures 5, 6, and 7. H&E. × 80.

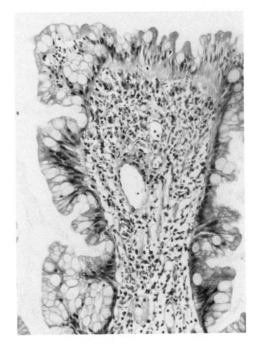

Fig. 14. Portion of a hyperplastic polyp illustrating the hyperplastic alterations at the surface of the lesion. H&E. × 170.

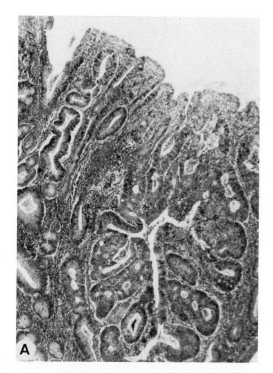

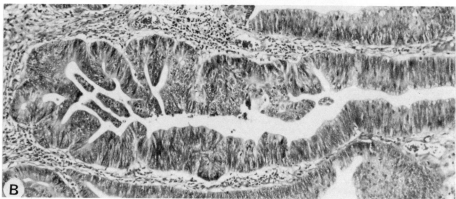

Fig. 15. A. Complex glandular structure of CIS in an adenomatous polyp (less than 5 percent villous). This occurred in a 15-mm polyp from a 70-year-old woman. H&E. × 34. B. Glandular budding and papillary formation in CIS in a villous tumor. H&E. × 85 (cont.).

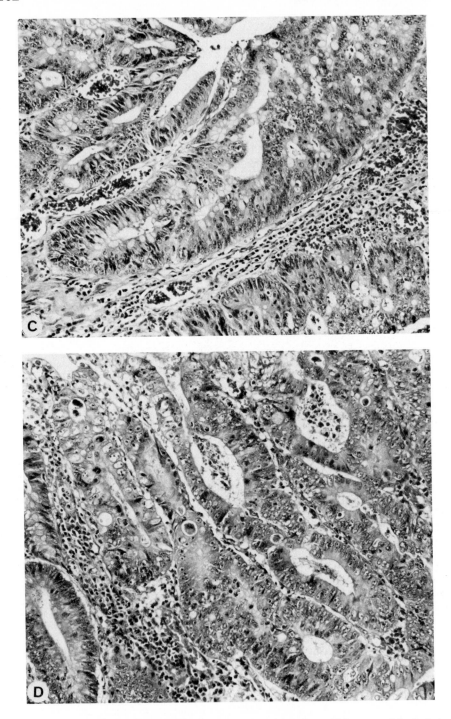

Fig. 15. (cont.). C. CIS with intricate glandular formation. This was detected in an adenomatous polyp with a 20 percent villous component. It was resected from a 65-year-old man. H&E. × 127.5. D. CIS displaying nuclear pleomorphism. H&E. × 127.5.

TABLE 3. Type and Location of Polyps Bearing CIS and Carcinomas *

Type of Polyp	Cecum		Ascend.		Transv.		Desc.		Sigmoid		Rectum	
	CIS	CA	CIS	CA	CIS	CA	CIS	CA	CIS	CA	CIS	CA
Adenomatous (pure)	—	—	—	—	—	—	—	—	—	—	—	—
Adenomatous (1–4% villous)	—	—	1	—	1	—	—	—	1	—	2	—
Adenomatous (5–20% villous)	—	—	—	—	—	—	—	—	1	—	2	—
Adenomatous (21–50% villous)	—	—	—	1	1	1	—	—	3	4	1	1
Villous tumors	—	—	—	—	—	1	—	1	4	5	3	3

* Number of polyps.

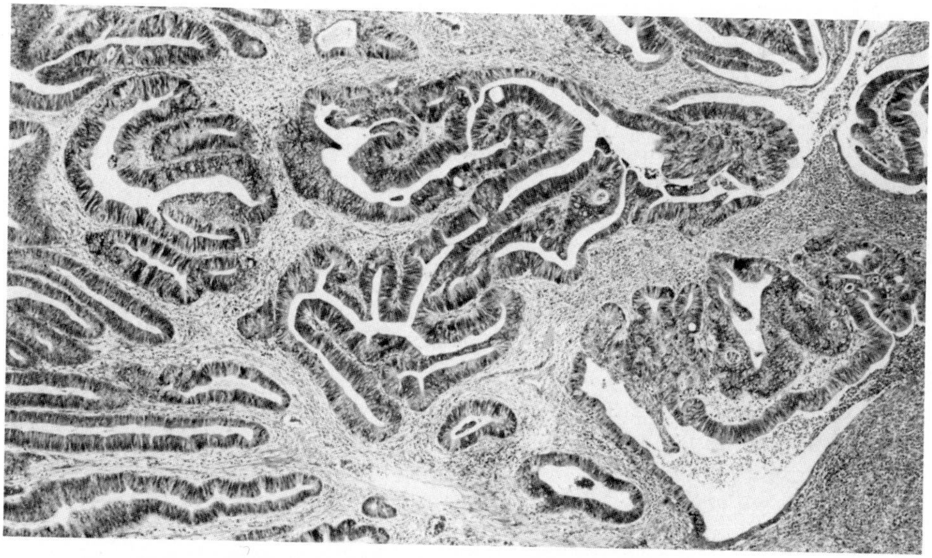

Fig. 16. An invasive adenocarcinoma in a villous tumor of the sigmoid colon. It was removed from a 48-year-old woman. There were no metastases. H&E. × 97.5.

polyp (Fig. 16). The invasiveness has to be verified by step sections through the suspected area so as to rule out the possibility of infoldings that give a false impression of infiltration. This has been pointed out by Castleman and Krickstein.[2] The type and location of polyps containing adenocarcinoma are seen in Tables 1 and 3. Adenomatous polyps with villi that contained a carcinoma ranged from 1.4 to 4 cm in size and averaged 2.4 cm; those arising in villous tumors varied from 1.0 to 8.5 cm and averaged 4.4 cm.

Correlative Studies

The 250 adenomatous polyps represent 31 percent of the total group. These were purely adenomatous without a villous component. An additional 80 polyps had less than 5 percent estimated villous pattern that, in some instances, was but a single villus. The average age of patients having adenomatous polyps was 60 years, with 66 percent of the patients male and 34 percent female. The adenomatous polyps ranged in size from 0.3 to 3.5 cm, with an average size of 0.65 cm. The distribution of adenomatous polyps was similar to that described in other papers, and was as follows: cecum, 6 percent; ascending colon, 8 percent; transverse colon, 9 percent; descending colon, 19 percent; sigmoid colon, 30 percent; and the rectum, 28 percent. This varies only slightly from the total number of polyps (Table 2). None of the pure adenomatous polyps exhibited CIS or carcinoma.

The adenomatous polyps with a villous component (5 to 20 percent) had an average size of 1.1 cm. In fact, 63 percent of the polyps measured more than 1 cm in greatest dimension. The patients had an average age of 61.4 years, with 38 percent female and 62 percent male. The distribution of the adenomatous polyps with a villous component in the large intestine was as follows: rectum, 38 percent; sigmoid, 43 percent; descending colon, 8 percent; transverse colon, 6 percent; ascending colon, 4 percent; and cecum, 3 percent. Compared to adenomatous polyps with less than a 5 percent villous component, it appears that those with greater than a 5 percent villous component tend to be slightly larger lesions, but the risk of harboring a carcinoma in situ does not appear to be greater. We found little difference in the distribution of these lesions (Table 2).

The mixed (villoglandular) polyps were arbitrarily defined as those that contained a 20 to 50 percent villous component. These polyps averaged 1.48 cm in size with a range of 0.3 to 4.5 cm. The average age of the patients was 60 years, with 45 percent of the patients female and 55 percent male. Thus, one can say that these polyps tended to be larger than adenomatous, or adenomatous with a lesser villous component, and the male/female ratio approached 1. The distribution of the mixed polyps was similar to that previously noted for the other histologic types and was as follows: rectum, 30 percent; sigmoid, 48 percent; descending colon, 5.5 percent; transverse colon, 4 percent; ascending colon, 7 percent; and cecum 5.5 percent. In 5 (4.4 percent) of these lesions, a CIS was detected. In addition, 6 (6.1 percent) had an invasive carcinoma (Table 2).

Villous tumors had an average size of 1.7 cm, with a size range of 0.6 to 8.5 cm. The localization of these tumors was as follows: rectum, 53.6 percent;

sigmoid, 31.7 percent; descending colon, 7.3 percent; transverse colon, 5.7 percent, and ascending colon, 1.6 percent (Table 2). Most villous tumors are located in the rectal and sigmoidal areas. This represents a difference compared with other types of polyps. The average age of the patients is 61.7 years with an age range of 55 to 65 years; 48 percent of the patients were male and 52 percent female. As in most other studies, this lesion represents the one in which the highest risk of a carcinoma or CIS occurs. In our group, 7 (5.7 percent) of the villous tumors contained a CIS and 10 (8.1 percent) an invasive carcinoma. This represents 14 percent of the 123 villous tumors. This figure is lower than many reported in the literature, with the range often being up to 50 percent and generally in the region of 25 to 35 percent.

Hyperplastic polyps are a common epithelial polypoid lesion of the large intestine. As has been previously stated, they are ordinarily small, less than 5 mm in diameter, and seldom pedunculated. In our group of epithelial polyps, hyperplastic polyps constituted 14.2 percent of the total. The age distribution of patients bearing these polyps is somewhat different than the total: 26 percent of the patients were less than 49 years of age and 40 percent were between 50 and 60 years of age (Table 2); 34 percent of the patients were older than 60 years of age, and there was a pronounced predominance of men. The distribution in large intestine is similar to the total number, that is 88 percent of the lesions were located in the rectum and sigmoid, 3.8 percent in the descending colon, 3.8 percent in the transverse colon, 3 percent in the ascending colon, and 1 percent in the cecum. The size is similar to what Lane and his associates [3] reported, ranging from 3 to 8 mm. We had one unusual lesion that measured 2 cm in greatest dimension; this occurred in a 53-year-old woman who had multiple hyperplastic polyps. It is also of interest that in the large lesion, there were adenomatous foci. In addition, we have encountered 1 hyperplastic polyp that was pedunculated. Nine patients had multiple hyperplastic polyps with the youngest patient, a 23-year-old woman, having multiple hyperplastic polyps and a carcinoma of the rectum. With the exception of the 1 large lesion that contained adenomatous foci, there were no atypical epithelial alterations or villous components in the hyperplastic polyps; none suggested carcinoma in situ.

In recent years, the colonoscopic examination has become popular, and 36 percent of the polyps studied in this group of patients were removed through the colonoscope. We had thought that there would be a somewhat different distribution of the polyps removed through the colonoscope, when compared to polyps that had been removed through the sigmoidoscope by polypectomy and in association with resection of a carcinoma. This did not prove to be so. The distribution of the polyps and the age of the patients having the polyps removed was quite similar. The localization was found to be as follows: 56 percent in the sigmoidal area, 16.4 percent in the descending colon, 11.2 percent transverse colon, 4.3 percent ascending colon, 5 percent in the cecum with only 7 being removed from the rectum. This distribution is similar to that reported for 196 polyps removed through the colonoscope at the Mayo Clinic.[20] The slight increase in percentage of lesions located in the cecum probably reflects the ability of the colonoscope to reach this area. The small number of rectal lesions would be a function of location and availability to the proctoscope. The lesions removed through the colonoscope varied in size from 4 mm to 3 cm, with 92 percent of the polyps 1.5 cm in diameter or less. The histologic types removed through the colonoscope were not different from what would be expected: 74.3 percent were classified as adenomatous, 12.5 percent as mixed, 11.6 percent as hyperplastic, and 1.6 percent as villous.

Included in the study were 80 polyps (10 percent) found in segmental resections of the colon due to infiltrating carcinoma. The histologic patterns as well as distribution of these polyps were not different from those just described, nor was there an increased incidence of CIS, as had been reported.[11, 21]

A major interest in this review was the significance of a villous component in an epithelial polyp of the large intestine. As has been suggested in the literature, a villous component increases the risk of a carcinoma arising within the polyp, and villous components are more likely to be seen as the polyp enlarges. In epithelial polyps containing 25 to 50 percent of a villous component, we could find little correlation between the presence of the villous component and the size. For example, there were five polyps that measured 3 mm in greatest dimensions. These five had 25, 40, 40, 40, and 50 percent villous components respectively. For those polyps measuring greater than 3 cm, the distribution of the villous component was similar, with the majority being in the range of 25 to 40 percent. One significant finding, however, is that carcinoma and carcinoma in situ were found in the larger lesions, often those exceeding 2 cm in greatest dimension. The two occurred in the largest lesions, which measured 4 and 4.5 cm in diameter. Carcinomas and CIS are seldom found in lesions smaller than 1.0 cm. Carcinoma in situ was demonstrated in adenomatous polyps containing a villous component varying from 1 to 20 percent. These lesions were smaller on the average than adenomatous polyps with a greater proportion of villous pattern (Table 2).

Discussion

It has been our contention that the epithelial polyp–carcinoma relationship is not an inevitability. There are those who disagree with this view, feeling that there is a reasonably strong or strong relationship between epithelial polyps and carcinoma of the large intestine.[3, 4] The answer to the polyp–carcinoma question is not easy to delineate. There are many variables in regard to histopathologic definitions and type of material included in various reviews that add to the problem.

For example, Hughes,[22] in a review of autopsy material, pointed out that from his figures adenomatous polyps of the large intestine may indeed be self-limited lesions. In discussing the age incidences, he noted that there were no increases in size of these lesions when one individual was compared to another in the same age group. If his observations are correct, then it would be unusual for a malignancy to develop in a lesion that reaches a certain size and then remains stable. Rather than jousting with the question of the epithelial polyp–carcinoma relationship, perhaps the size, the configuration, the histologic type, history of previous epithelial polyps, and the age of the patient should be taken into consideration in determining the risks for an individual of either having or developing a carcinoma of the large intestine or the risk that any given histologic type of epithelial polyp harbors a carcinoma.

It is accepted that there is a relationship between the size of the polyp and its chance of containing a carcinoma. This risk increases as the lesion exceeds the size of 10 mm.[1] Below this size, the chance of its being a carcinoma is said to be less than that of the risk of a surgical intervention to remove that polyp. In addition, the presence of a stalk as identified sigmoidoscopically or radiographically is a strong indication that the lesion is benign.[23] For those lesions that are followed radiographically, a change in the configuration from a smooth, rounded outline to one that has other shapes is an indication that a malignancy is present.

Age of a patient within the cancer age group does not apparently increase the risk of carcinoma in a polyp; at least in our groups, the average age and ranges were much the same. If Hughes' observations are valid, there is a negative correlation between age and size; in turn, size is related to risk of carcinoma and CIS in a polyp. The observation has been noted in follow-up studies that patients who had previous epithelial polyps removed have a higher risk of developing a carcinoma than do those patients who have not. Prager et al [25] found twice the number of carcinomas than expected in a 15-year follow-up study of 305 patients.

The histologic type is important in the sense that it has been noted that hyperplastic polyps for all practical purposes have no relationship with the presence or absence of a carcinoma. Although there are variations, at least from our observations, these lesions tend to remain small and rarely have an adenomatous alteration. Other histologic types may represent increased risks for epithelial abnormalities ranging from atypical hyperplasia to carcinoma in situ, to invasive carcinoma. As noted from our figures, there appears to be little or no risk of carcinoma in situ or of an invasive carcinoma with the lesions that we have defined as pure adenomatous polyps. With the presence of a villous constituent, this changes (Table 3). The largest number of carcinomas and CIS occur in the villous tumors. Thus, there seems to be validity in estimating the villous component of epithelial polyps. As noted previously, the observations of villi in adenomatous polyps have been made on several occasions, including those that are described as "diminutive." [24]

On this note, it is worth stating again that the "adenomatous polyps" that have been reported in the literature as containing invasive carcinomas and having metastases are not purely adenomatous but have a villous component, and some could readily be designated as villous tumors. This distinction may indeed be important in determining the risk of a particular lesion containing carcinoma or carcinoma in situ. From our review, two-thirds of epithelial polyps removed from the large intestine are not purely adenomatous. Discounting the hyperplastic polyps, the majority will have a villous component, be it small. The villous component varies from those having a single villus to those that are dominantly villous and designated as villous tumors.

The widely accepted classification of epithelial polyps has been mentioned previously in this chapter. Perhaps it would be of practical importance to designate the lesions with an estimated villous component. For example, adenomatous polyps with no villous component or adenomatous polyps with a given percentage, eg, an adenomatous polyp with 15 percent villous component or adenomatous polyp with a 40 percent villous component. There would be no need for the name mixed or villoglandular polyp. The designation of villous tumor would be retained for those lesions with an estimated 50 percent or more villous component. This line of reasoning suggests that there may be a continuum in the development of adenomatous polyps, particularly those that contain a villous component. It is conceivable that the lesions begin with villi, judging from the small size of many of ours, and then proceed to those lesions that are designated as villous tumors. This is speculative and obviously open to question and further study.

When all is said and done concerning the controversy related to the epithelial polyp and adenocarcinoma of the large intestine, the significance of all the discussion concerns the practical problems related to the treatment of a patient who is demonstrated to have a polypoid lesion. Does one prevent carcinoma of the large intestine by removing epithelial polyps, particularly those that are not designated as villous tumors? Perhaps in rare circumstances this may be so. It seems more likely that the identification of the adenomatous polyp, with or without the villous components, identifies patients who are at higher risk of developing carcinoma of the large intestine. This does not mean to say that there may not be an occasional situation in which there is conversion of one of the epithelial polyps other than the villous lesions to a carcinoma. If this is so, then the villous component becomes an important feature, a feature that should be indicated by the pathologists. If one accepts the cases reported in literature as "adenomatous polyps" that have become carcinomatous with metastases, then the villous component can be demonstrated to be important and indicating the risk of a carcinoma. Also, as has been previously mentioned, the size of the lesion in relationship to malignancy, the radiographic and gross configuration, the presence or absence of a stalk also tend to identify lesions that are significant, ie, significant from the standpoint of potential malignancy and those that should be removed.

With careful histologic definition, it would seem that it is not necessary to remove all polypoid lesions suspected of being epithelial polyps of the large intestine. But this is usually, if not always, retrospective information. Thus, if a patient is undergoing colonoscopic or sigmoidoscopic examination, it seems reasonable that any polypoid lesion encountered should be biopsied if not removed. However, if a patient has a lesion discovered radiographically and it has a smooth outline, measures 10 mm or less in diameter, and has a stalk, then there would be little reason to remove this lesion unless it is causing symptoms that need remedy. This would be particularly true in elderly persons and patients considered to be a high surgical risk. As has been shown by Marshak,[23] there seems to be little chance that these lesions will undergo a malignant alteration.

Even though there is an indication that a villous element increases the risk of CIS and carcinoma in adenomatous polyps, the long-term significance remains to be determined. With the use of careful radiographic studies of the large bowel [23] and employment of the colonoscope, prospective studies are possible—prospective in the sense of knowing precisely the type of epithelial polyp and the estimated percent of villi in a polyp removed from a patient followed at suitable intervals by reexamination.

Summary

We have reviewed 801 epithelial polyps removed from large intestines of 611 patients. Among these, there were 250 pure adenomatous, 304 adenomatous polyps with villi, 123 villous, and 124 hyperplastic polyps. Of the lesions classified as purely adenomatous, there were no observed carcinomas or carcinomas in situ. It would appear that a villous component may be an important indicator of the chance of the lesions harboring a carcinoma in situ or an invasive carcinoma. On the basis of our review, it would seem that it would be reasonable for a pathologist to indicate the estimated percentage of villous component in epithelial polyps of the large intestine.

References

1. Spratt JS, Jr, Ackerman LV, Moyer CA: Relationship of polyps of the colon to colonic cancer. Ann Surg 148:682, 1958
2. Castleman B, Krickstein HJ: Do adenomatous polyps of the colon become malignant? N Engl J Med 267:469, 1962
3. Lane N, Kaplan H, Pascal RP: Minute adenomatous and hyperplastic polyps of the colon: Divergent patterns of epithelial growth with specific associated mesenchymal changes. Gastroenterology 60:537, 1971
4. Wychulis AR, Dockerty MB, Jackman RJ, Beahrs OH: Histopathology of small polyps of the large intestine. Surg Gynecol Obstet 124:87, 1967
5. Kraus FT: Pedunculated adenomatous polyp with carcinoma on the tip and metastasis to lymph nodes. Dis Colon Rectum 8:283, 1965
6. Manheimer LH: Metastasis to the liver from a colonic polyp. Report of a case. N Engl J Med 272:144, 1965
7. Palacios RL, Wellman KF: Adenomatous polyp of colon with adenocarcinoma and pulmonary metastasis. Gastroenterology 51:82, 1966
8. Kaye GI, Lane N: Distribution of human colonic lymphatics in normal, hyperplastic and adenomatous tissue: Its relationship to metastasis from small carcinomas in pedunculated adenomas, with two case reports. Gastroenterology 64:51, 1973
9. Willox GL, MacGregor JW: Malignant polyp of the colon and rectum. Arch Surg 92:514, 1966
10. Lane N, Kaye GI: Pedunculated adenomatous polyp of the colon with carcinoma, lymph node metastasis and suture-line recurrence. Am J Clin Pathol 48:170, 1967
11. Silverberg SC: Focally malignant adenomatous polyps of the colon and rectum. Surg Gynecol Obstet 131:103, 1970
12. Bigelow B, Winkelman J: Polyps of colon and rectum. Cancer 17:1177, 1964
13. Kobayashi S: Early colonic carcinoma presenting as a pedunculated polyp. Gastrointest Endosc 20(3):118, 1974
14. Gunn LC: The treatment of pedunculated adenomatous colorectal polyps with focal cancer. Surg Gynecol Obstet 141(4):604, 1975
15. Strauss RS, Pascal RR: Invasive and metastasizing cancer in a small adenomatous polyp of the colon. Report of a case with demonstration of a tumor-associated antigen. Hum Pathol 6(2):256, 1975
16. Shatney CH, Lober PH, Sosin H: Metastasis from a pedunculated adenomatous polyp with focally invasive carcinoma. Dis Colon Rectum 18(1):67, 1975
17. Shatney CH: The treatment of pedunculated adenomatous colorectal polyp with focal cancer. Surg Gynecol Obstet 139(6):845, 1974

18. Fung CHK, Goldman H: The incidence and significance of villous change in adenomatous polyps. Am J Clin Pathol 53:21, 1970
19. Kurzon RM, Ortega R, Rywlin AM: The significance of papillary features in polyps of the large intestine. Am J Clin Pathol 62:447, 1974
20. Spencer RJ, Coates HL, Anderson MJ, Jr: Colonoscopic polypectomies. Mayo Clin Proc 49:40, 1974
21. Kalus M: Carcinoma and adenomatous polyps of the colon and rectum in biopsy and organ tissue culture. Cancer 30:972, 1972
22. Hughes LE: The incidence of benign and malignant neoplasms of the colon and rectum: A post-mortem study. Aust NZJ Surg 38:30, 1968
23. Marshak RH, Lindner AE, Maklansky D: Adenomatous polyps of the colon. A rational approach. JAMA 235:2856, 1976
24. Pagtalnan RJG, Dockerty MB, Jackman RJ, Anderson MJ, Jr: The histopathology of diminutive polyps of the large intestine. Surg Gynecol Obstet 120: 1259, 1965
25. Prager EM, Swinton NW, Young JL, Veidenheimer MC, Corman ML: Follow-up study of patients with benign mucosal polyps discovered by proctosigmoidoscopy. Dis Colon Rectum 17:322, 1974

PATHOGENETIC MECHANISMS IN HEPATIC CIRRHOSIS OF THALASSEMIA MAJOR: LIGHT AND ELECTRON MICROSCOPIC STUDIES

THEODORE C. IANCU, BENJAMIN H. LANDING, AND HARRY B. NEUSTEIN

With the clinical collaboration of Carol B. Hyman, Jorge A. Ortega, and Jordan J. Weitzman, Childrens Hospital of Los Angeles

Thalassemia major (TM) produces not only severe chronic anemia, but progressive dysfunction of many organs. Hemosiderosis and hepatic cirrhosis occur even in the absence of administration of iron or of repeated blood transfusions. To gain better understanding of the liver involvement in TM, patients in a longitudinal clinical study involving hypertransfusion therapy underwent serial liver biopsies during infancy, childhood, and adolescence, in addition to clinical, hematologic, and biochemical studies. The purpose of the biopsies was to establish whether the high transfusion regimen produced more severe or more rapid progression of hemosiderosis and liver damage than the less aggressive transfusion regimen conventional in 1969, when the high transfusion program was begun. Tissues were also examined from deceased patients, both from the study group and from those who expired before 1969. Electron microscopic study of liver specimens from infants with TM has provided an opportunity for insight into early organelle and cell changes in TM.

Material and Methods

The 11 patients included in the study group were diagnosed as having thalassemia, either before, or at the time of, their first presentation at Childrens Hospital of Los Angeles (CHLA). The group included 9 patients with homozygous beta-thalassemia, and 1 patient each with beta-delta thalassemia and thalassemia intermedia. Hematologic data and serum vitamin E levels were obtained prior to treatment by a high transfusion regimen with vitamin E and folate supplementation. A total of 35 percutaneous needle biopsies of liver were performed on these 11 patients from the study group. Additional information was obtained from autopsies of the 4 patients who died while under study, as well as from 8 autopsies of patients with TM who died during the years preceding the study. The livers from autopsies of 5 patients who had aplastic anemia were also examined, to compare their liver lesions with those of the thalassemic patients. Eight initial liver biopsies and 10 of skin had spectrographic determinations of iron, phosphorus, copper, zinc, manganese, and magnesium levels.

Light Microscopy

Formalin-fixed and paraffin-embedded liver biopsies were examined after staining with hematoxylin-eosin, Masson trichrome, periodic acid–Schiff, ferrocyanide, and indirect aldehyde fuchsin stains for enzyme activity were also done on some frozen tissue specimens, but not consistently enough for analysis. Thick (1 to 2 μm) sections of epon-embedded blocks stained with toluidine blue, or Paragon stain, were also examined and compared with paraffin-embedded sections.

Electron Microscopy

Sixteen liver biopsies from 10 patients were processed for electron microscopy. Small (1 mm $\times$ 1 mm) liver fragments were fixed in 2 percent chilled glutaraldehyde, postfixed in 1 percent phosphate-buffered osmium tetroxide, dehydrated in graded alcohols and embedded in Epon 812 resin. Thick (1 to 2 μm) sections were used for orientation. Ultrathin sections (600 to 800 Å) were mounted on formvar-carbon-coated one-hole copper grids, and stained with uranyl acetate and lead citrate. Unstained sections from all biopsies were also examined. Sections were viewed and photographed using a Siemens 1A electron microscope.

Results

The hematologic data, including serum iron, folate, and vitamin E levels, are shown in Table 1. Table 1 shows the severe degree of anemia found in all patients before HTP treatment, as well as the low levels of serum folate and vitamin E before supplements were given. Table 2 shows iron concentrations of skin and liver at the time of the first biopsy for eight of the patients, as well as phosphorus, copper, zinc, manganese, and magnesium concentrations of these specimens. The skin and liver iron concentrations (Table 2) were greatly increased, even in the early biopsies, and were found to increase with age of the patient. The youngest patient had the lowest increase in liver iron (4 times normal), whereas the oldest patient had the highest increase (37 times normal). Significant elevations of phosphorus, magnesium, and copper were noted in both skin and liver specimens; the magnitude of the increase was, however, variable and less than the increase in iron concentration, even in the older patients.

TABLE 1. Clinical Data—Patients with Thalassemia Major on High Transfusion Program (HTP)

| Pt. No. | Sex/Age at start of HTP (yr) | Lowest recorded Hgb (g/dl)/ Pre-HTP* Hgb (g/dl) | Hepatitis B serum test | Splenectomy performed before start of HTP | Prior to HTP | | | Vitamin E (Serum α-tocopherol) (μg/ml)† | Age when liver biopsies performed (yr) |
					GMS Fe RECEIVED FROM Tx	SERUM Fe/ TIBC (μg/ml)	SERUM FOLATE (μg/ml)		
1TC	F/19	5.2/7.4	Neg.	Yes	11.3	239/256	2	1.26	19, 22
2EC	M/19	4.3/6.9	Neg.	Yes	17.9	263/292	9	2.80	19, 20, 22
3KS	F/17	4.6/6.4	Neg.	No	16.7	268/272	<2	6.93	17, 19
4RA	M/12	5.3/7.4	Pos.	Yes	19.2	275/290	1.4	7.65	13, 14, 15
5CDL	F/12	4.9/7.0	Neg.	Yes	12.4	135/166	3	7.53	12, 13, 15
6RC	F/12	?5/7.8	Neg.	Yes	+6.8	154/164	1.5	2.24	12, 13, 14
7GS	M/11	4.0/6.8	Neg.	Yes	11.0	233/490	4	4.20	11, 12, 14
8SB	F/10	4.1/9.7	Neg.	Yes	28.3	154/179	1.1	3.01	11, 12, 13
9LL	F/9/12	4.3/4.3	Neg.	No	—	—	—	7.57	9/12, 2, 3, 4, 5
10MB	F/6/12	6.8/6.8	—	No	—	—	—	—	10/12, 2, 3
11CTL	M/4/12	6.1/6.1	—	No	—	—	—	—	5/12, 1 1/2, 2 7/12
Normal values						60–175/ 250–400	5–24	9.8–21.6	

* The Pre-HTP Hgb is the mean of the observed values for 3 years prior to the HTP except for patients 9, 10, and 11, for whom it is the Hgb value prior to their initial transfusion (Start of HTP).

† After 1 to 2 years on HTP and prior to Vitamin E therapy.

173

TABLE 2. Chemical Analysis of Liver and Skin Biopsies [†]

Pt. No.	Age at Biopsy (yr)	Iron	Phosphorus	Copper	Zinc	Manganese	Magnesium
Liver							
Normal (mean) values (mg/100 g dry tissue)		131.0	660.0	2.8	28.0	0.61	74.0
2	19	4650.0	880.0	7.5	13.2	0.66	150.0
3	17	3450.0	1200.0	4.5	15.0	1.94	300.0
4	13	2496.0	820.0	6.9	16.0	0.48	32.0
5	12	2131.0	1110.0	11.3	33.0	0.47	88.0
6	12	2550.0	750.0	8.2	30.0	0.82	300.0
6 *	12	2635.0	675.0	8.5	33.0	0.93	246.0
7	11	3040.0	800.0	3.1	16.8	0.76	60.0
8	10	3894.0	940.0	2.9	13.2	0.66	132.0
8 *	10	3740.0	890.0	3.1	12.5	0.58	120.0
9	9/12	488.0	690.0	4.2	32.0	0.90	60.0
Skin							
Normal (mean) values (mg/100 g dry tissue)		3.8	80.0	0.24	2.0	0.04	17.4
1	19	42.0	385.0	1.54	5.6	0.21	28.0
2	19	32.0	640.0	1.20	4.8	0.40	48.0
2 *	19	34.2	590.0	1.70	5.1	0.09	12.0
3	17	40.5	400.0	1.50	5.0	0.01	30.0
4	13	40.4	360.0	0.90	3.5	0.06	13.8
5	12	24.0	165.0	0.07	3.3	0.06	18.9
6	12	9.0	490.0	0.45	1.9	0.05	18.6
7	11	18.0	150.0	0.27	1.2	0.01	15.0
8	10	29.0	350.0	0.53	3.6	0.20	20.4
8 *	10	43.0	365.0	0.50	4.2	0.20	20.0
9	9/12	11.8	110.0	0.10	2.4	0.03	5.9

* Additional sample from different area. † We are indebted for the chemical analyses to Dr. E. M. Butt and Mr. S. DiDio of the Department of Pathology, Los Angeles County General Hospital.

Light Microscopy

As is demonstrated in this section, hemosiderosis is regularly more severe peripherally in hepatic lobules, and fibrosis is also marked around the border of lobules. Since the grading vocabulary used in this study tends to give higher gradings of hemosiderosis than of fibrosis at the same age or in the same specimen, numerical gradings of degree of iron deposition or fibrosis in the various specimens, as given in the text and Tables 3 and 4, thus refer to the most severe degree of either process demonstrable in each specimen. Gradings of degree of hemosiderosis or fibrosis in the legends of illustrations, on the other hand, refer only to the degree illustrated by the figure.

IRON DEPOSITION. All liver biopsies contained increased amounts of iron, as diffuse cytoplasmic staining of hepatocytes, due to ferritin, and as hemosiderin granules of varying size. The sequential biopsies demonstrated the following pattern of iron deposition:

Stage 1. All patients less than 18 months of age showed fine granular iron deposition in parenchymal cells, more prominent toward the periphery of lobules, plus more diffusely aggregated hemosiderin granules in Kupffer cells and in portal areas.

Stage 2. In patients from 18 months of age to 24 through 36 months, there was more marked hemosiderin deposition in hepatocytes, as well as a further increase of iron in Kupffer cells and portal areas.

Stage 3. In patients from 24 to 36 months to 5 years, large hemosiderin "clumps," possibly in groups of macrophages located in the parenchyma between portal and central areas, were prominent (Fig. 1). Although such clumps persisted into terminal stages of disease, in stages 4 and 5 they were overshadowed by septal siderosis (Fig. 2).

Stage 4. All patients more than 5 years of age showed parallel increases of parenchymal cell and portal tract iron, as well as of iron within cells in developing fibrous bands. Parenchymal iron was greater in the periphery of lobules, or at the borders of cirrhotic nodules and micronodules (Fig. 3).

Stage 5. Patients aged 10 years or more showed end-stage disease, characterized by regenerative nodules and increased fibrosis. The iron-filled cells lacked recognizable cell borders. Some nodules bordered by fibrous bands had a low iron content and "fetal" two-cell-thick liver cords, typical of regenerative nodules (Fig. 4).

At all stages, no iron deposition was observed in the smooth muscle of vascular medias, whereas the endothelial cells of portal tract and other septal vessels were hemosiderotic in all specimens beyond stage 1. The amount of hemosiderin in the interlobular duct epithelium was minimal. More hemosiderin was present in Hering duct epithelium, but less than the amount seen in hepatocytes.

LIPOFUSCIN. No clear-cut relationship between the amount of lipofuscin and the degree of iron deposition in hepatocytes could be seen, although most biopsies showed more lipofuscin than normal. Lipofuscin was found in hepatocytes, in Kupffer cells, in the smooth muscle of large vessels, and in bile duct epithelium,

TABLE 3. Microscopic Findings in Liver Biopsies *

Pt. No.	Age at Biopsy (yr)	Iron Deposition	Fibrosis Degree and Pattern	Other Findings
1	19	3+, C+	3+, bridging	
	22	3+, C+	3+, bridging	EMH+
2	19	3+, C+	2+, septal	EMH+
	20	3+, C+	2+	EMH+
	22	3+, C+	1–2+	EMH+
3	17	2+, C+	+, bridging, interhepatocyte	
	19	2+, C+	2+, bridging	EMH+
4	13	3+, C+	3+, bridging	
	14	2–3+, C+	2–3+, bridging	EMH+
	16	3+, C+	3+, bridging	
5	12	3+, C+	2+, bridging	
	13	3+, C+	2+, bridging	
	15	3+, C+	3+, interhepatocyte	
	16	3+, C+	3+, portal	
6	12	3+, C+	3–4+, septal	
	13	3+, C+	3–4+, septal	
	15	3+, C+	4+	
7	11	2–3+, C+	+, portal	
	12	2–3+, C+	1–2+	
	14	2–3+, C+	1–2+	
	16	3+, C+	2–3+, portal interhepatocyte	
8	10	2–3+, C+	2–3+, portal	
	11	3+, C+	2–3+, bridging	EMH+
	13	3+, C+	2–3+	EMH+
	14	3+, C+	3–4+, bridging	
9	6/12	+	+, interhepatocyte	
	2	+	+, interhepatocyte	
	3	2+, C+	+, interhepatocyte, also septal	
	4	2+, C+	2+, septal	EMH 2+
	5	2+, C+	2+, septal, bridging	EMH 2+
10	1 1/12	—	±	
	2	2+	+, interhepatocyte	
	3	3+, C+	2+, portal	EMH 2+
11	5/12	+	+, portal, creeping	EMH+
	1 1/2	+	2+	
	2 5/12	3+, C+	2+, septal, interhepatocyte	EMH 3+

* C denotes intralobular aggregates of cells with unusually high iron content, presumably macrophages ("clumps") present (Figs. 1 and 2). Such aggregates were definitely present in 26 of 29 specimens obtained above the age of 3 years, and were probably present in all above the age of 2 5/12 years. Fibrosis is expressed as interhepatocyte, portal, creeping (extending from portal tracts into lobular parenchyma), or as bridging (from portal to central zones). Some variation in pattern from specimen to specimen may well reflect sampling error in needle biopsies, as well as progression of the fibrous process. Septal means that fibrous bands were present, but that the biopsy was not large enough to establish whether true bridging was present. When the pattern of fibrosis could not be established from the biopsy, only an estimate of severity (grade) is given.
EMH: extramedullary hemato(erythro)poiesis, graded 1–3+.

TABLE 4. Microscopic Findings in Liver Specimens (Autopsy)

Pt. No.	Age at Autopsy (yr)	Iron Deposition	Fibrosis Degree and Pattern	Other Findings
1	23	4+, C+	2+, bridging	EMH +, ferrocalcinosis, regenerative nodules
4	19	3–4+, C+	4+, bridging	"Alcoholic hyaline," regenerative nodules
6	14	2+, C+	3–4+, bridging	EMH +, regenerative nodules
8	16	4+, C+	4+, bridging	"Alcoholic hyaline," ferrocalcinosis, regenerative nodules
12	12	3+, C+	4+, bridging	EMH +, ferrocalcinosis, regenerative nodules
13	13	3+, C+	3+, bridging	EMH +, ferrocalcinosis, regenerative nodules
14	15	3+, C+	3+, bridging	Ferrocalcinosis (vascular), regenerative nodules
15	10	2–3+, C+	+, bridging	Regenerative nodules
16	9	2–3+, C±	2+, bridging	EMH 3+, ? regenerative nodules, congestive centrilobular necrosis
17	18	3+, C+	4+, bridging	Ferrocalcinosis, regenerative nodules
18	8 1/2	3+, C±	+, bridging ±	EMH +
19	4 1/2	2–3+	2+, bridging ±	EMH +, ferrocalcinosis (vascular)

as demonstrated by indirect aldehyde fuchsin stain or by autofluorescence under ultraviolet light.

FERROCALCINOSIS.   In stage 5 specimens, marked iron deposition in fibrous septa was associated with mineral deposition resembling that of Gandy-Gamna bodies. The ferrocalcinosis involved vessel walls as well as septal connective tissue (Figs. 3, 5, and 6).

FIBROSIS.

Stage 1.   Although the degree of fibrosis was slight in this age group, there was an increased amount of collagen around some hepatocytes. However, increased fibrosis of portal areas was present in only one of the three specimens from infants 18 months of age or younger. Electron microscopy (see next section) confirmed the presence of some degree of increased collagen deposition in the earliest biopsies studied (patients 9, 10, and 11 at 5, 9, and 10 months).

Stage 2.   Compared with stage 1, there was marked increase in fibrosis during this period, both around individual hepatocytes (Fig. 7) and by extension of fibrous connective tissue from portal areas into adjacent parenchyma (Fig. 8). Early stages of bridging of connective tissue from portal to central tracts were seen occasionally, with loss of the typical centrilobular position of some central veins.

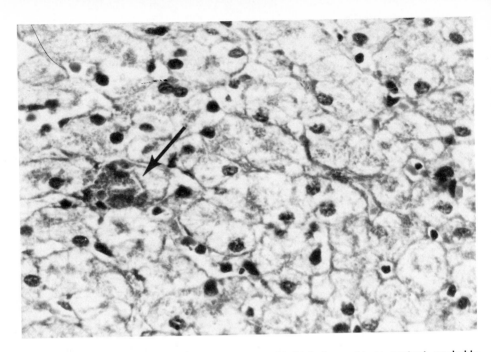

Fig. 1. Patient 9 at 4 years. Aggregate of cells with high hemosiderin content, probably macrophages (clump), within lobular parenchyma, with no associated fibrosis (arrow). Masson trichrome. × 600.

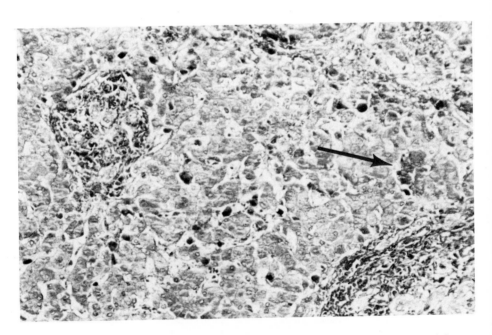

Fig. 2. Patient 14 at 15 years. Iron storage of stage 3 degree with fibrosis and hemosiderosis of portal tracts. Hemosiderin-laden Kupffer cells are numerous, and clumps suggesting aggregates of macrophages are seen within lobules (arrow). Masson trichrome. × 190.

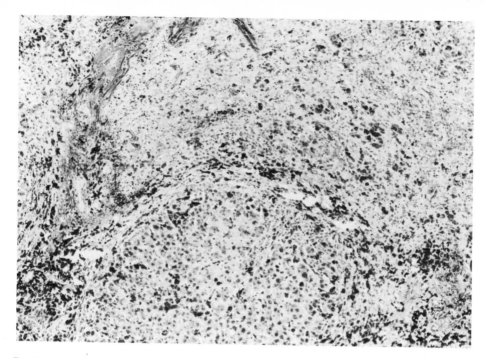

Fig. 3. Patient 8 at 15 years. Advanced stage 4 disease, with cirrhosis and marked hemosiderosis of septa and parenchyma, showing greater iron content of peripheral zones of parenchymal nodules. Ferrocalcinosis is visible in the connective tissue. H&E. × 75.

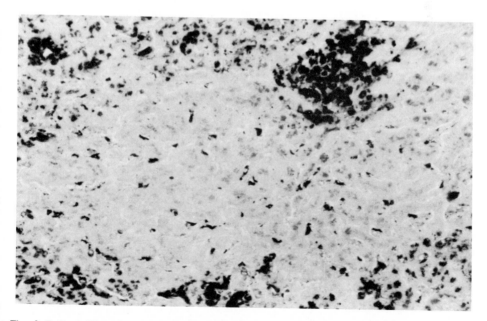

Fig. 4. Patient 15 at 10 years. Regenerative nodule in stage 5 disease, showing lower iron content of hepatocytes in the nodule compared to those in the adjacent parenchyma. Septal and Kupffer cell siderosis is severe. Note that the regenerative nodule grades into the adjacent liver parenchyma, without demarcation by fibrous tissue. Iron stain. × 150.

179

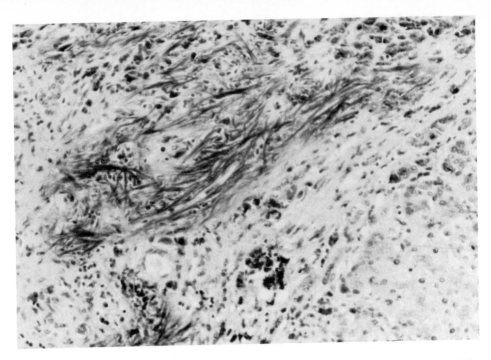

Fig. 5. Patient 8 at 15 years. Mineralization of septal connective tissue (ferrocalcinosis) in end-stage disease. The process tends to be central in fibrous septa; the mineral material stains for both iron and calcium. H&E. × 190.

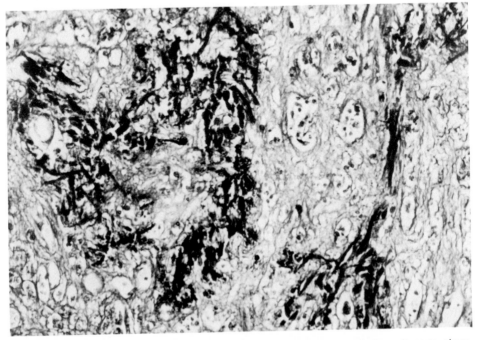

Fig. 6. Same specimen as in Figure 5. Ferrocalcinosis of septa in end-stage disease, showing positive silver stain. Reticulum stain. × 125.

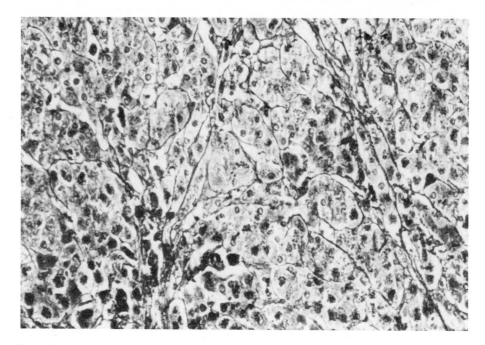

Fig. 7. Patient 9 at 4 years. Interhepatocyte collagen formation in stage 2 fibrosis. Iron granules are numerous in hepatocytes and Kupffer cells. Masson trichrome. × 125.

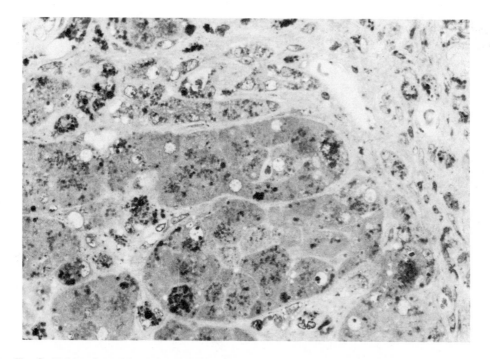

Fig. 8. Patient 8 at 15 years. Creeping of fibrous tissue from portal area into adjacent parenchyma, illustrating continued activity of this process in an advanced stage of disease. Epon embedding, Paragon (R) stain. × 450.

Stage 3.   Some differences in severity of the fibrotic process were noted between patients. In some, a lobular pattern was still preserved, but others showed impressive disruption of liver architecture and formation of micronodules (Fig. 9).

Stage 4.   The liver at autopsy or from late biopsies showed cirrhosis roughly correlated in severity with age and with iron content. Generally, central veins could no longer be identified at this stage, and whether their number was normal could not be determined.

Stage 5.   This differed from stage 4 by the greater amount and extent of fibrosis and the presence of apparent regenerative nodules. Marked bile duct proliferation was seen in most autopsy specimens.

Sections of liver from autopsies of five patients with chronic aplastic anemia treated by transfusions showed an overall iron content lower than that of patients with TM of the same age. More iron was located in the reticuloendothelial system (RES) than in parenchymal cells; and in none of the patients with aplastic anemia was fibrosis more advanced than stage 2.

Electron Microscopy

STAGE 1.   The following early changes occurred in patients 5 to 18 months of age. The three patients in this group were 5, 9, and 10 months old at the time their

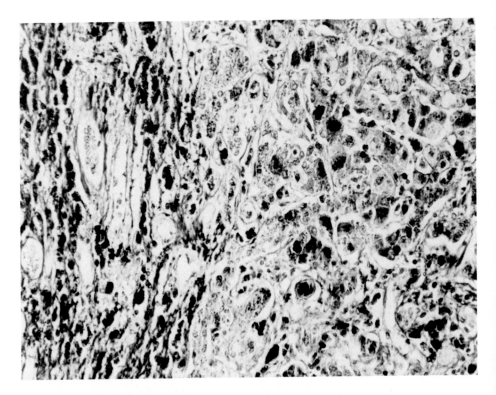

Fig. 9. Patient 4 at 16 years. Advanced stage 3 fibrosis, showing both interhepatocyte fibrosis and marked septal hemosiderosis and fibrosis. H&E. × 325.

first biopsies were taken. All three patients had normal general architecture and appearance of hepatic tissue at low magnifications, but higher magnifications disclosed both increased iron content of liver cells and excessive numbers of collagen fibers in two patients. Patient 10 had an increased amount of collagen, but iron was present only as rare ferritin molecules in the cell sap with minimal accumulation within secondary lysosomes.

Hepatocytes.

Cell Membrane.   The border facing the space of Disse showed a decrease or absence of microvilli over extended areas, associated with the increase in collagen fibers. In some areas where collagen filled the space of Disse, a thin layer of basement membrane-like material lay between the sinusoidal lining and the collagen fibers (Fig. 10). An increased amount of collagen was seen between individual hepatocytes, in areas adjacent to portal tracts, either as an exaggeration of the normal intercellular "pits" or as collagen bridging between two such pits (Fig. 11).

Cell Sap.   Ferritin was best identified when unstained sections were examined. Single molecules were randomly distributed throughout the cell sap, except for some increased concentration around secondary lysosomes. No abnormality

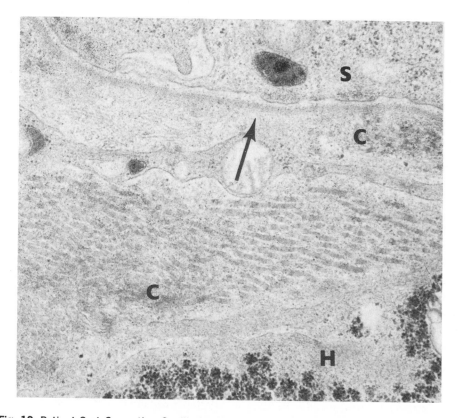

Fig. 10. Patient 9 at 6 months. Capillarization of sinusoids: Collagen (C) is present in the space of Disse. Between the hepatocyte (H) and a sinusoidal cell (S), a line of basement-membrane-like material can be seen (arrow). Uranyl acetate, lead citrate. × 30,000.

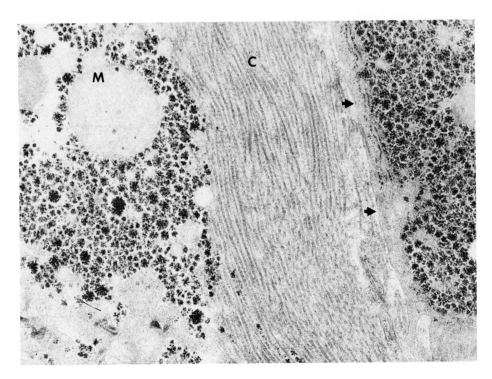

Fig. 11. Patient 11 at 5 months. The presence of interhepatocyte collagen (C) is accompanied by flattening or absence of microvilli (arrows). Uranyl acetate, lead citrate. × 18,000.

in glycogen, fat, or lipofuscin content was noted, and free (poly)ribosomes showed no visible changes of structure or amount.

Cytocavitary Network. Occasional hepatocytes showed a generalized dilatation of the smooth endoplasmic reticulum (SER), but in many cells the SER was normal, as was the rough endoplasmic reticulum (RER). No abnormalities of the Golgi apparatus were seen. Ferritin molecules were rarely identified in these structures.

Organelles. The mitochondria were normal and no ferritin molecules were seen within mitochondria. Microbodies were present in apparently increased numbers in a few cells. The most remarkable changes were seen in the lysosomes, with most hepatocytes showing an increased number of secondary lysosomes of variable appearance and size. The unstained and stained sections revealed these sections to contain iron in a variety of forms, as follows:

1. Ferritin arrays arranged in layers usually lay within round or oval structures, identified as secondary lysosomes. In stained sections, the ferritin molecules arranged in arrays could be seen in relation to a number of parallel single-layered membranes of medium electron density (Fig. 12), suggesting that the pattern of the arrangement of ferritin molecules is determined by these lamel-

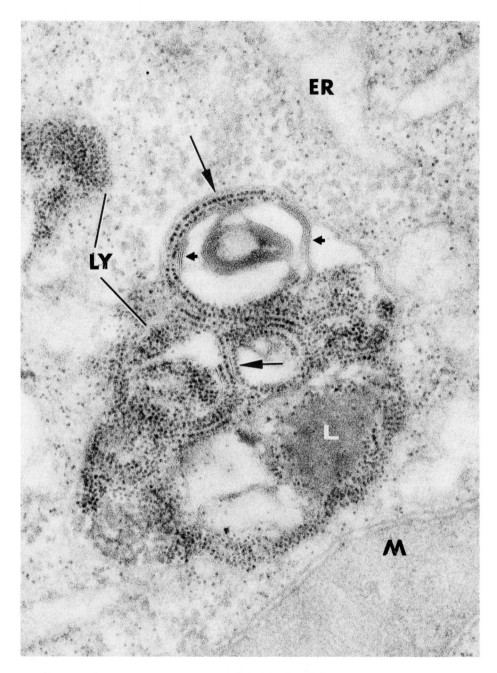

Fig. 12. Patient 9 at 4 years. Ferritin molecules within hepatocytes: Within lysosomes (LY) some of the ferritin molecules form arrays (large arrows) in relationship with parallel lamellae (small arrows). Lysosomes also contain lipid (L). Note the absence of ferritin from mitochondria (M) and endoplasmic reticulum (ER). Within the cell sap, ferritin molecules, in lesser concentration, are randomly distributed. M: normal mitochondrion. Uranyl acetate, lead citrate. $\times$ 120,000.

lar membranes. Ferritin arrays were seen in all biopsies at all stages of the disease, if iron overload was present. Lysosomes without ferritin molecules, but with the parallel lamellae, were seen in the 10-month-old patient in whom no iron overload was detected by either light or electron microscopic techniques.

2. Ferritin molecules without organized relation were seen in most lysosomes, either together with amorphous content in the centers of array-containing structures, or scattered within the lysosomes.

3. Paracrystalline arrangements. In occasional lysosomes, ferritin molecules were seen in a paracrystalline arrangement with a hexagonal pattern.

4. Hemosiderin. Whenever single ferritin molecules could no longer be clearly resolved as such, they were assumed to form what is generally termed hemosiderin. This aggregation of iron molecules presented as membrane-bound areas of varying electron-density, in some of which, several ferritin molecules could still be recognized, whereas others formed hemosiderin clumps of extreme electron density (Fig. 13).

Sinusoidal Cells.   In unstained sections, features differentiating the cells of this area could not be recognized. The majority of sinusoidal cells, probably Kupffer cells, showed marked increase in concentration of ferritin molecules, randomly dis-

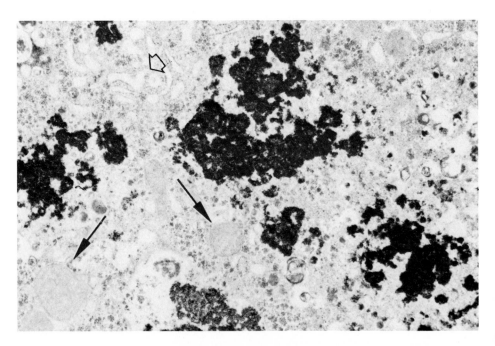

Fig. 13. Patient 5 at 16 years. Hemosiderin-laden lysosomes displace or replace much of the cytoplasmic contents of the hepatocyte. This cell shows signs of degeneration and no iron in mitochondria (large arrows), or in the dilated ER (small empty arrow), at this advanced stage of iron overload. Uranyl acetate, lead citrate. $\times$ 12,000.

tributed within the cell sap. A large amount of iron was seen in many siderosomes bounded by a triple-layered membrane. Within these membrane-bound structures (lysosomes-siderosomes), the ferritin molecules had a variety of forms, from individual molecules to hemosiderin aggregates. Array formation was not as conspicuous as in hepatocytes, but occasionally was seen. The absence of ferritin molecules from the mitochondria, SER, RER, and Golgi apparatus was very striking, because of the contrast to the large number in the cell sap and siderosomes.

Other Cells. Bile ducts and blood vessels of the portal area showed no abnormality except for some increase in iron-laden lysosomes in a few sections in which endothelial cells were seen.

STAGES 2 TO 5: LATE LESIONS. In general, as patients grew older their iron overload increased, as did the concentration of iron-laden lysosomes and the amount of collagen. This progression was impressive in patient 10 who had a nearly normal biopsy at 10 months but showed marked iron overload and increased number of collagen fibers at age 3 years. Although the number and electron density of lysosomes were increased in the later biopsies, the amount of ferritin in the cell sap seemed to be stable, as soon as the state of iron overload was reached. Thus no progressive increase in the concentration of ferritin molecules in the cell sap was noted, despite the increase in lysosomal iron in advanced stages of disease. Because of the presence of large amounts of hemosiderin in many hepatocytes, the normal hepatocyte ultrastructure was no longer recognizable. In the vicinity of hemosiderin-containing lysosomes, ferritin arrays were identical to those seen in earlier biopsies; the number of arrays was not greater than in cases with less advanced iron overload. In other cells, dilatation of RER, proliferation of SER, and increased autophagocytosis were seen.

Differences between patients in the pattern of collagen deposition were observed. All patients beyond infancy showed collagen fibers extending from portal tracts, but this was not paralleled by similarly progressive perihepatocyte collagen deposition. In four patients, large areas of intercellular collagen, as well as perisinusoidal collagen, were seen. In the other patients, even in advanced stages of cirrhosis, sinusoidal collagen deposition and intercellular fibrosis were present only in areas adjacent to fibrous septa.

In these advanced stages of disease, additional iron content in Kupffer cells was not recognized, although some iron-containing structures, possibly membrane bound, were observed within sinusoids, and the iron content of bile duct and vascular endothelial cells was increased.

Discussion

Light and electron microscopy of liver biopsies, as well as examination of autopsy material, confirmed that progressive fibrosis parallels the increased iron content of the liver in TM. A variety of mechanisms have been proposed to explain this complication of TM. The electron microscopic examination of biopsies from young patients was considered especially important in the attempt to resolve these questions, since the morphologic abnormalities were not obscured by the multitude of secondary mechanisms operative in TM.

Relationship Between Intracellular Iron, Cell Damage, and Fibrogenesis

STAGE 1. EM examination of the livers of small infants with TM provides no evidence of parenchymal cell necrosis or of sublethal cell damage preceding the onset of abnormal collagen deposition. When periportal areas showed an increase in collagen fibers in the space of Disse and in intercellular spaces, the hepatocytes in these areas showed no ultrastructural evidence of damage, except for reduction of microvilli adjacent to the collagen. In these early stages, there was no evident relationship between the iron content of parenchymal cells and the location of collagen deposition, as shown by the fact that cells with the largest number of iron-laden lysosomes were not necessarily adjacent to collagen deposits.

Increased iron content of hepatocytes did not change many ultrastructural features in the early stages of iron storage. This may be due to the efficiency of the iron-segregating mechanism in these cells, with progressive accumulation of ferritin molecules in round or oval lysosomal structures.

STAGE 2. Beyond early infancy, progressive iron overload is accompanied by some increase in autophagocytosis, by occasional dilatation of the RER, and by proliferation of the SER. These features are not specific to iron overload, but have been seen in a variety of conditions in which liver cells have altered metabolic activity.[1, 2] The iron-segregating mechanism of the hepatocytes is clearly very efficient, since the ferritin molecule concentration in the cell sap remains constant while the number of iron-laden lysosomes increases with the age of the patient.

STAGES 3 AND 4. When cirrhosis is fully established, the EM findings confirm those of light microscopy, in that hepatocytes near fibrous septa contain more hemosiderin-laden lysosomes than those elsewhere. Ultrastructural features of hepatocytes are essentially the same as in previous stages, except for an increased displacement of organelles by the large number of lysosomes. The proliferation of microvilli reported in cirrhosis of other types [3] was not present. In this stage, unusually extensive pericellular and sinusoidal fibrosis was observed in four patients in areas where parenchymal cells contained no more iron than those in adjacent, less fibrous areas. Intracellular collagen fibers [4] were not observed. Because of the patchy distribution, and its presence in only some of the patients, collagen deposition within the space of Disse, with "capillarization of sinusoids," [5] does not appear to be a primary pathogenetic mechanism in this cirrhosis, but it may play a role in later stages of disease.

STAGE 5. In the most advanced stage, when hepatocytes were filled with iron, most of the normal cell components appeared quantitatively deficient and replaced by lysosomes, with the ultrastructural appearance of the hepatocytes so altered that normal function would appear impossible. In this stage, occasional disintegrating hepatocytes could be seen (Fig. 13).

Kupffer Cells

The major finding in these cells is the very large concentration of iron in the cell sap and lysosomes. As in hepatocytes, the concentration of randomly dispersed ferritin molecules in the cell sap is similar in all cells from specimens beyond stage

1. These findings suggest that there is a specific level of cytoplasmic iron above which additional iron is not accumulated in the cell sap, but must be transferred into lysosomes.[6, 7] Iron-containing lysosomes are more numerous in Kupffer cells than in hepatocytes, especially in stages 1 and 2 when parenchymal iron overload is relatively mild. The lysosomes, usually called siderosomes within Kupffer cells and hematopoietic cells, also differ from hepatocyte lysosomes in that they form single round bodies instead of polycyclic structures and are bound by triple-layered membranes. Most siderosomes in the Kupffer cells contained hemosiderin only, and few have membranous material, lipid droplets, or single ferritin molecules. Only occasional single-layered lamellae with ferritin arrays, similar to those seen in hepatocytes, were found. However, the same basic intracellular iron transport route seems to be operative in both hepatocytes and Kupffer cells. The relative absence of ferritin molecules from mitochondria, SER, RER, and Golgi complex suggests that these organelles and the cytocavitary network do not play an important role in the segregation of iron. The ultrastructural observations suggest that ferritin molecules synthesized by free polyribosomes [8] in the cell sap enter secondary lysosomes by transmembranous movement, and are eventually aggregated as hemosiderin by digestion of their apoferritin coat.[7] It is also possible that transmembranous movement into lysosomes of the nonprotein iron moiety of ferritin occurs, followed by subsequent resynthesis of (holo)ferritin within the secondary lysosomes. This proposition implies that apoferritin reaches secondary lysosomes separately by the usual pathway of secretory proteins.[9]

Relationship between Sinusoidal Cells and Fibrogenesis

There is little agreement on the nomenclature, types, or functions of these cells. It has been suggested [10] that a perisinusoidal cell, located within the space of Disse, differs from endothelial cells, fibroblasts, fat-storing cells, and Kupffer cells and has a special function in fibrogenesis. Our observations confirm the presence of cells, apparently producing large amounts of collagen within both Disse's spaces and sinusoids, but we were not able to conclude which cells were most involved in the fibrogenic process. The cells apparently producing collagen did not contain conspicuous amounts of iron, and no increase of fat-storing cells was seen. No direct relationship between iron-laden Kupffer cells and increased fibrogenesis was identified, in that such Kupffer cells were seen in areas both with and without collagen fibers.

From the EM examination of these biopsies, it appears that the excessive collagen deposition seen in young patients is not the consequence of ultrastructurally identifiable liver cell injury, but may be the result of metabolic alterations in which iron plays a role.

By light microscopy, the earliest demonstrable features of hepatic fibrosis in these patients were portal fibrosis in one (patient 11) and interhepatocyte collagen deposition in others (patients 9 and 10). In several patients, interhepatocyte collagen was more marked in periportal zones, suggesting that "creeping" fibrosis from the edges of portal tracts was the source of the intralobular fibrosis, but in others (patients 2, 7, 14, and 19) varying numbers of small patches of intralobular fibrosis, apparently not in contact with the edges of portal tracts, were present. Proliferation of fibrous tissue in association with intralobular macrophage aggregates (clumps) was noted in several patients (patients 2, 4, 5, 7, and 14). The degree of fibrosis of the liver in these patients progressed steadily with age, and cirrhosis was present by age 5 years in one patient (patient 9). The exact mechanism of conversion of fibrosis to cirrhosis, defined as the presence of bridging between portal and central tracts by fibrous strands, could not be established. Neither creeping fibrosis from portal tracts, typically stellate in pattern, fibrosis associated with macrophage aggregates, nor enlargement and fusion of isolated patches of intralobular fibrosis, can be confidently regarded as the basic mechanism of bridging fibrosis. It is tempting to propose that the location of bridging fibrosis is dependent on the basic hemodynamic and functional anatomy of the hepatic acinus, as defined by Rapaport,[11] but data are not yet adequate to assess this concept.

In discussing the pathogenetic mechanisms in the cirrhosis of thalassemia, a distinction is made between primary factors (Fig. 14) and secondary factors (Table 5) operative in the genesis of this condition. A number of factors in each category, the existence of which seems to be supported by other data, will be discussed briefly.

TABLE 5. Possible Secondary Mechanisms in Hepatic Cirrhosis of Thalassemia

Process	Cause	Effect
Congestive failure	Anemia, myocardial hemosiderosis	Passive congestion of liver, liver cell necrosis
Reduced arterial perfusion of liver	Cirrhosis	Ischemic liver cell damage
Portal venous obstruction, liver	Cirrhosis	Ischemic, nutritional liver cell damage
Regenerative nodules	Cirrhosis	Ischemic liver cell damage
Bile duct proliferation	?	Increased portal fibrosis
Pancreatic atrophy and fibrosis, gastric mucosal and Brunner's gland siderosis	Hemosiderosis	Malabsorption, nutritional deficiencies
Hepatitis B infection	Transfusions	Chronic persistent or aggressive hepatitis
Chronic edema of liver	Cardiac dysfunction, cirrhosis	Fibrosis ("serous inflammation")
Septal ferrocalcinosis	? Parathyroid, thyroid hemosiderosis	? Vascular occlusions
? Splenectomy	Hypersplenism	? Increased hepatic parenchymal siderosis ? Decreased lysosomal hydrolases in portal vein blood

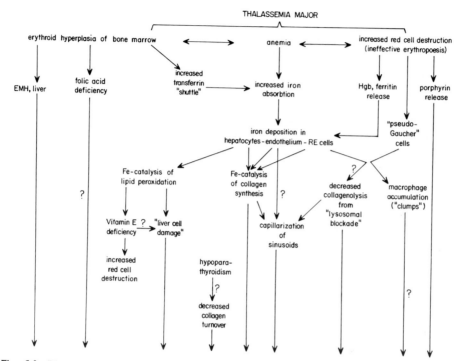

Fig. 14. Diagrammatic representation of primary factors presumed to be involved in the pathogenesis of cirrhosis in thalassemia major, and their interrelationships. EMH: extramedullary hematopoiesis; RE: reticuloendothelial; Hgb: hemoglobin; Fe: iron.

Primary Fibrogenic Mechanisms

Increased Iron Content of Liver

The early and progressive increase in iron stored in thalassemic livers has been repeatedly reported and is documented in our patients.

The description of mechanisms and routes by which iron reaches the various liver cells is beyond the scope of this chapter. However, it should be noted that thalassemic patients have a definitely increased iron absorption from the gut [12] in contrast to patients with other types of anemia (aplastic or hyporegenerative), which do not cause erythroid hyperplasia of the bone marrow and ineffective erythropoiesis. Since increased amounts of iron have been found in the livers of thalassemic patients who have received few or no blood transfusions, the secondary hemochromatosis can be due mainly to increased iron absorption, and not to the therapeutic transfusion regimen. This latter treatment has been shown to diminish iron absorption from the gut and to keep the total body iron burden [13] stable by reducing the excessive "transferrin shuttle" operative in ineffective erythropoiesis.

In addition to the transferrin-bound plasma iron that is delivered to hepatocytes or Kupffer cells, iron is thought to be available from increased breakdown of erythrocytes and immature red cells. Haptoglobin-bound hemoglobin, heme-hemopexin, and ferritin released during hemolysis of immature or mature red cells may be taken up predominantly by hepatocytes, increasing the parenchymal iron overload.[14] These mechanisms presumably contribute to the more severe hepatic damage of chronically anemic patients with erythropoietic hyperplasia, compared to those with hypoplastic bone marrow, as reported by others [15] and as confirmed in the material of this study. Splenectomy might reduce the importance of red cell destruction as a source of liver iron by reducing the flow of iron-containing substances in splenic vein blood.

Iron Overload—Iron Toxicity

Acute iron toxicity is a well-known entity. However, whether chronic iron overload can produce iron toxicity is controversial. It has been claimed that the liver can accommodate very large amounts of storage iron without alteration of its functions,[16] but other authors maintain that in the presence of iron the cell must adjust by attaining a new or altered steady state, similar, for example, to the sublethal injury of fat deposition.[17]

Iron is a weak fibrogenic factor, as is demonstrated by the difficulty of producing cirrhosis in animals by iron overload alone. Lisboa [18] reported the only successful such experiment, in which cirrhosis was found in dogs given large amounts of intravenous iron for long periods of time. However, cirrhosis can be produced with relative ease if the animals are also exposed to liver-damaging agents, such as ethionine [19] or carbon tetrachloride.[20] In humans, including thalassemics, the chronic iron toxicity is apparently enhanced by a variety of nutritional factors, some of which will be further discussed under "Secondary Mechanisms."

There is sufficient circumstantial evidence favoring an important role of iron in the pathogenesis of cirrhosis in hemochromatosis,[21, 22] but, as the evidence of cell toxicity of iron is inconsistent, emphasis is now being placed on the effect of iron at subcellular levels, leading to a concept of "organelle injury." [17] The influence of excessive iron on cell metabolism can be seen in several pathways.

IRON CATALYSIS OF COLLAGEN SYNTHESIS. The action of protocollagen proline hydroxylase, an enzyme necessary for the conversion of soluble precursor-collagen to mature and more insoluble collagen, is catalyzed by iron.[23] Excessive amounts of iron have been claimed to enhance this process. This pathogenetic step may be the single most important one in the cirrhosis of thalassemia, because the accumulation of both iron and collagen in the livers of these patients with this disease begins very early, before evidence of liver cell damage is demonstrable microscopically. Although fibrosis also occurs in some other hemosiderotic organs (eg, pancreas) in thalassemia, it is not prominent in others (eg, thyroid, parathyroid, pituitary). Therefore, attribution of hepatic cirrhosis to iron-catalyzed exaggeration of collagen synthesis would appear to require a proposition that different organs have a differing capacity to produce collagen following this stimulus.

IRON CATALYSIS OF LIPID PEROXIDATION.   It has been suggested that the effect of iron overload is caused by its ability to decrease the number of reducing equivalents within cells.[24] Also, hematin and other iron compounds appear to be the important catalysts of lipid peroxidation in vivo.[25, 26] Finally, it has been shown that iron overload induces relative deficiency of vitamin E,[27] which is recognized to function as a chain-breaking antioxidant. Increased lipid peroxidation may account for the increased lipofuscin seen in various cell types in patients with hemochromatosis and other iron-storage diseases.[25, 28, 29] Vitamin E deficiency of the patients in this study is documented by the low serum levels before supplementation (Table 1), by the transient response of the patients to supplemental vitamin E,[29] and by increased amounts of lipofuscin seen in hepatocytes, Kupffer cells, vascular smooth muscle, and other cell types. Increased lipid peroxidation, initiated by iron overload, with concomitant or secondary vitamin E deficiency, has been proposed to be a major mechanism of the liver cell damage considered by some workers to be necessary for explanation of the hepatic cirrhosis.[19, 30]

DECREASED COLLAGENOLYSIS FROM LYSOSOMAL BLOCKADE.   It has been proposed that pericellular collagen is normally turned over by the action of collagenases released by cells, and that a reduction in collagenase release would lead to fibrosis.[31, 32] It is possible that the massive accumulation of iron, and to a lesser degree of lipofuscin, in hepatocyte and macrophage lysosomes prevents the release of lysosomal collagenase. This mechanism is supported by the observation that liver fibrosis occurs in some other lysosomal storage diseases, such as Gaucher's, Niemann-Pick, and Hurler's diseases. The production of "pseudo-Gaucher cells" in TM, apparently as a result of overloading of the lysosomal pathway of globoside breakdown by the increased pace of destruction of erythroid cells, has been described.[33] Whether these macrophages also contribute to fibrous tissue production in TM is uncertain. The association of fibrosis with iron-laden macrophages in hemochromatosis, described by others, but without a specified mechanism for the relation,[34] is supported by the results of this study.

Thalassemia major differs from many other types of anemia, being a condition of early and severe hemolytic anemia with ineffective erythropoiesis. Some cirrhogenic factors may be related to these aspects of the disease.

Anemia

Table 1 shows that all patients in the study program had at some time very low hemoglobin levels. In addition to inducing increased iron absorption, such anemia might alter liver cell metabolism, and the proposition that hypoxia can be part of the pathogenic mechanism of cirrhosis has been made.[32, 35, 36] Doubts should be expressed as to the importance of this factor, since hepatic fibrosis of significant degree does not occur in patients with severe and long-standing tissue anoxia of other causes (eg, tetralogy of Fallot). In addition, protocollagen proline hydroxylase, considered to be important in collagen formation, is dependent on atmospheric oxygen for activity.[23] Therefore, tissue hypoxia theoretically might reduce collagen formation.

The hemolytic component of the anemia of TM may also be relevant to the hepatic fibrosis. An increased level of porphyrins in the red blood cells of patients with TM has been demonstrated by Sturgeon et al;[37] and toxic effects on the liver of porphyrins released from destroyed red cells may occur. The exact role of abnormal porphyrin metabolism, and its relationship to the increased iron stores found by Lundvall et al [38] and the micronodular cirrhosis found by Turnbull et al [39] in patients with porphyria cutanea tarda, is not known.

Another hemolysis-related factor may be uptake, by the RES through erythrophagocytosis, of large amounts of stromal residue, part of which may then serve as a substrate for collagen formation. Although it is generally considered that collagen is produced by fibroblasts, it is probable that other cells (macrophages, perisinusoidal cells, etc) take part in this process, and it has been proposed that the fibrogenic effect of iron is related to the presence of iron-laden macrophages that are attracted to and remain closely associated with the developing septa.[20] An anatomic relationship between such cells and collagen fibers has been shown,[40, 41] and it has been proposed that iron-laden macrophages act either as fibroblasts or as a mechanical scaffold for collagen deposition.[20] The possible role of lysosomal blockade in reducing collagen turnover by macrophages has already been discussed.

Of special interest is the folic acid deficiency found in these thalassemic patients before they entered the high transfusion program (Table 1). The low–folic acid levels are considered to be the result of relative deficiency due to hyperconsumption of folic acid, associated with the short life span of the erythrocytes and the hyperplastic bone marrow.[42] One of the study patients did not take the recommended folic acid supplement and developed a megaloblastic bone marrow (patient 4). The concept that folic acid deficiency may enhance fibrosis is supported by the observation that folic acid supplements impede the development of cirrhosis and the accumulation of iron deposits in the myocardium and pancreas of rats on a lipotropic-deficient, iron-rich diet.[43] Folic acid antagonist drugs have been proposed to cause cirrhosis in some children treated with these agents for acute leukemia.[44] Although low folic acid levels were found in our patients before therapy, it is difficult to evaluate the importance of this factor, since most of the patients entered the hypertransfusion program when their cirrhosis was already established.

Secondary Fibrogenic Mechanisms

In this group, we include pathogenetic processes secondary to the hepatic fibrosis or cirrhosis of TM, which enhance or exacerbate the pace or severity of the scarring processes. Although not primarily responsible for the cirrhosis described previously, these mechanisms may well contribute significantly to its severity, pattern, and course.

Circulatory Factors

These factors are thought to alter the normal pattern of hepatic blood flow, disturbing hepatocyte oxygenation and nutrition, and either enhancing fibrogenesis or inhibiting reparative processes.

CAPILLARIZATION OF SINUSOIDS. Formation of capillary-like sinusoid basement membranes has been reported by Schaffner and Popper [5] in hepatic cirrhosis. As is mentioned under the electron microscopic findings in our material, capillarization of sinusoids was not seen in all patients and was patchy in distribution when present. The importance of this factor is not clear at this moment.

PORTAL HYPERTENSION AND VENOUS OBSTRUCTION WITHIN THE LIVER. This may be the result of advanced hepatic fibrosis, and of compression of sinusoids by regenerative nodules, as well as of hepatic artery-portal vein shunts.[36]

REDUCED EFFECTIVE ARTERIAL INFLOW TO THE LIVER. This reduction can be due either to factors mentioned in the previous section, or to intrahepatic shunting of arterial blood to veins within the fibrous septa.[32]

PASSIVE CONGESTION OF THE LIVER. Heart failure due to myocardial hemosiderosis, with or without severe anemia, is a constant finding in patients with advanced TM.[45] Varying degrees of cardiac fibrosis were found in the autopsied patients, but frank liver cell necrosis due to passive congestion was recognized in only one patient (patient 16). This process should be considered a valid, but infrequent, contributor to hepatic fibrosis in patients of this type.

Nutritional Factors

Malabsorption and possibly more selective nutritional deficiency secondary to pancreatic atrophy and fibrosis, and possibly also secondary to gastric mucosal and Brunner's gland siderosis, deserve serious consideration as regards the pathogenesis of late features of TM. Pancreatic atrophy and fibrosis, of varying but typically of severe degree, was observed in all autopsied patients in this study. Pancreatic a(hypo)-chylia has been proposed to cause increased absorption of iron,[46] and pancreatic enzymes have been given orally to thalassemic patients in recent years, with the hope of reducing iron uptake. Deficiency of vitamin E and folic acid in the patients of this study has already been mentioned, but this is considered due, at least in part, to increased requirements for these vitamins and not to malabsorption. Clinical deficiency of the fat-soluble vitamins A, D, and K has not been demonstrated in the patients of this study, nor have low vitamin B_{12} levels been present, but much more detailed studies of absorption and balance of these vitamins, of essential fatty acids, of lipotropic factors, and of trace minerals are needed for evaluation of the effects of pancreatic atrophy and fibrosis of this type. The pancreatic atrophy may be partially responsible for clinical diabetes mellitus found in thalassemia,[47] and idiopathic hemochromatosis as well,[48] although iron-deposition in islet beta cells is probably more responsible for the diabetes. The effects of the severe hemosiderosis of gastric and Brunner's gland epithelium on absorption of iron or any of the other mentioned nutrients are not known.

Other Factors

FIBROSIS SECONDARY TO CHRONIC EDEMA. That chronic edema of hepatic connective tissue causes or exaggerates fibrosis is a long-standing concept, discussed extensively by Rössle in the past.[49] The extent to which it operates in cirrhosis, and whether it applies more to some types of portal hypertension—presinusoidal, sinusoidal, postsinusoidal, parasinusoidal—than others, is uncertain.

STROMAL PROLIFERATION IN RESPONSE TO BILE DUCT PROLIFERATION AND/OR TUBULOFORM DEGENERATION.   Connective tissue proliferation associated with and presumably secondary to bile ductule proliferation is well known in biliary cirrhosis. It has also been noted to occur in infantile polycystic disease, although primary abnormality of the connective tissue with secondary induction of bile duct growth has also been proposed to explain the latter disease.[50] Apparent ductule proliferation in the later stages of thalassemic cirrhosis has been described previously, and there seems no reason to doubt that some degree of stromal proliferation is associated with these ductular changes. It has been proposed that, in some form^c of cirrhosis, ductular proliferation is really pseudoductular proliferation of liver cell cords [51] and also that it is not a proliferative but a degenerative change (tubuloform degeneration).[52] To the extent that these two latter concepts are valid, one might expect stromal proliferation to be more associated with the former than with the latter. However, any contribution of this mechanism to the cirrhosis of TM would appear to occur only very late in the disease.

EFFECTS OF SPLENECTOMY.   Splenectomy has been proposed to affect the distribution of storage iron in TM, and splenectomized patients have been found to have more parenchymal iron than nonsplenectomized patients.[53] Other authors, however, have concluded that, although parenchymal siderosis was indeed heavier in splenectomized patients, this did not apparently affect the severity of fibrosis.[13] The present study does not add information regarding the claimed fibrogenic effect of splenectomy, since most of our patients were studied after splenectomy. In the few patients who had liver biopsies both before and after splenectomy, no clear-cut effect of the splenectomy was noted. The possible effect of splenectomy in reducing the flow of iron-containing red cell products from spleen to liver is discussed in a previous section in this chapter.

CHRONIC HEPATITIS AND/OR POSTHEPATITIC CIRRHOSIS DUE TO HEPATITIS B VIRUS INFECTION.   The occasional operation of this mechanism in patients of the type under discussion, who receive large numbers of blood transfusions over the course of years, is not surprising. Only one of the patients in this study (patient 4) was seropositive for hepatitis B virus, and histochemical study for the hepatitis B carrier state, using the sulfuric acid-permanganate aldehyde fuchsin stain,[54] gave negative results on all other patients. This low frequency of hepatitis B infection does not seem to be related to an inherent resistance of thalassemics to this hepatitis virus, since others have reported a high percentage of seropositive patients.[55]

SEPTAL FERROCALCINOSIS.   Possibly secondary to parathyroid and/or thyroid hemosiderosis, this has been seen in a number of patients in this study (Table 4 and Figs. 3, 5, and 6). The pathogenesis of the lesion is not known, but it has features of similarity to the condition called chondrocalcinosis or pseudogout,[22, 56] described in hemochromatosis, and may well have the same basis. A tentative proposal that the septal ferrocalcinosis is secondary to hypoparathyroidism appears warranted, but physiologic studies of the matter are needed, as is study of the effect of the regularly severe thyroid hemosiderosis on thyrocalcitonin production by the thyroid C cells. Whether the septal ferrocalcinosis can produce obstructive lesions of larger vessels—in effect, hepatic veno-occlusive disease—is not known. Comparable ferrocalcinosis has been observed in some of our patients also in kidney, heart, and lymph nodes.

Summary and Conclusions

The development of hemosiderosis and cirrhosis of the liver in children with thalassemia major was studied histologically and electron microscopically, in an effort to define the pathologic sequences and pathogenetic mechanisms responsible. Material from liver biopsies of patients obtained before or during treatment with a high-transfusion regimen showed that increased hepatic iron content and fibrosis are both present by age five months. No evidences that liver cell necrosis or regeneration precede the early stages of hepatic fibrosis in thalassemia were found. Pathogenetic mechanisms related to erythroid hyperplasia of bone marrow, extramedullary hematopoiesis, and increased red cell destruction (ineffective erythropoiesis) are analyzed, and the possible roles of vitamin E deficiency, iron-catalyzed collagen synthesis, macrophage proliferation, folic acid deficiency, and lysosomal blockade as contributors to the fibroplastic process in the liver in thalassemia are discussed.

The material offers new insights into the mechanisms of accumulation of ferritin into lysosomes and into routes of iron transport within cells. The ferritin level of liver cell sap appears to plateau, with subsequent iron accumulation causing progressively more lysosomal hemosiderin accumulation. Although no simple or precise mechanism for the severe cirrhosis present in all patients with thalassemia major above the age of five years has been identified, the conclusion that the process is primarily dependent on the hepatic hemosiderosis appears inescapable. Fibrosis affects some hemosiderotic organs in thalassemia (liver, pancreas), but not others equally iron-laden (thyroid). The evidence thus suggests that certain epithelial cells exercise a hitherto underemphasized form of control over collagen synthesis or turnover in their vicinity. Apparently, increased intracellular iron levels in some way derange this control mechanism; this derangement occurs before the plateau in cytoplasmic ferritin level seen with progressive iron overload is reached.

Acknowledgments

This work was supported in part by: General Clinical Research Center Grant No. MO1-RR-00086, General Research Support Grant No. 5-S01-RR-05469, Michael J. Connell Foundation of Los Angeles, and Southern California Chapter of the Cooley's Anemia and Blood Research Foundation for Children, Inc.

References

1. Schaffner F: Some unresolved ultrastructural problems encountered in the study of the liver and its diseases. In Schaffner F, Sherlock S, Leevy CM (eds): The Liver and Its Diseases. New York, Intercontinental Medical Book Corporation, 1974, pp 7–18

2. Trump BF, Dees JH, Shelburn JD: The ultrastructure of human liver cells and its common patterns of reaction to injury. In Gall EA, Mostofi FK (eds): The Liver. Baltimore, Williams & Wilkins, 1973, pp 80–120

3. Steiner JW, Jezequel AM, Phillips MJ, Miyai K, Arakawa K: Some aspects of the ultrastructural pathology of the liver. In Popper H, Schaffner F (eds): Progress in Liver Diseases. New York, Grune & Stratton, vol 2, 1965, pp 303–72

4. Gmelin K, Rossner JA, Feist D: Untersuchungen an Leberbiopsien bei Thalassemia Major. Verh Dtsch Ges Pathol 57:251, 1973

5. Schaffner F, Popper H: Capillarization of hepatic sinusoids in man. Gastroenterology 44:239, 1963

6. Sturgeon P, Shoden A: Hemosiderin and ferritin. In Wolman M (ed): Pigments in Pathology. New York, Academic Press, 1969, pp 93–113

7. Iancu TC, Neustein HB, Landing BH: The liver in thalassaemia major: Ultrastructural observations. In Ciba Found Symp on Iron Metabolism, Elsevier–Excerpta Medica, North Holland, Amsterdam, 1977 (in press)

8. Hicks SJ, Drysdale JW, Munro HN: Preferential synthesis of ferritin and albumin by different populations of liver polysomes. Science 164:584, 1969

9. Arborgh BAM, Glaumann H, Ericsson JLL: Studies on iron loading of rat liver lysosomes: Effect on the liver and distribution and fate of iron. Lab Invest 30:664, 1974

10. McGee JOD, Patrick RS: The role of perisinusoidal cells in hepatic fibrogenesis. Lab Invest 26:429, 1972

11. Rapaport AM: Anatomic considerations. In Schiff L (ed): Diseases of the Liver. Philadelphia, Lippincott, 1969, pp 1–49

12. Heinrich HC, Gabbe EE, Optiz KH, et al: Absorption of inorganic and food iron in children with heterozygous and homozygous B-thalassemia. Z Kinderheilkd, 115:1, 1973

13. Risdon AR, Barry M, Flynn DM: Transfusional iron overload: The relationship between tissue iron concentration and hepatic fibrosis in thalassemia. J Pathol 116:83, 1975

14. Cook JD, Barry WE, Hershko C, Fillet G, Finch CA: Iron kinetics with emphasis on iron overload. Am J Pathol 72:337, 1973

15. Bothwell TH, Finch CA: Iron Metabolism. Boston, Little, Brown, 1962, pp 364–434

16. MacDonald RA: Hemochromatosis: A perlustration. Am J Clin Nutr 23:592, 1970

17. Trump BF, Arstila AU: Cell injury and cell death. In Lavia MF, Hill RB (eds): Principles of Pathobiology. New York, Oxford, 1971, pp 9–95

18. Lisboa PE: Experimental hepatic cirrhosis in dogs caused by chronic massive iron overload. Gut 12:363, 1971

19. Golberg L, Smith JP: Iron overloading and hepatic vulnerability. Am J Pathol 36:125, 1960

20. Kent G, Volini FI, Minick OT, Orfei E, De La Huerga J: Effect of iron loading upon the formation of collagen in the hepatic injury induced by carbon tetrachloride. Am J Pathol 45:129, 1964

21. Grace ND, Powell LW: Iron storage disorders of the liver. Gastroenterology 64:1257, 1974

22. Powell LW: Hemochromatosis. In Becker FF (ed): The Liver: Normal and Abnormal Functions, Part A. New York, Marcel Dekker, 1974, pp 129–61

23. Prockop DJ: Role of iron in the synthesis of collagen in connective tissue. Fed Proc 30:984, 1971

24. Witzleben CL, Buck BE: Iron overload hepatotoxicity: A postulated pathogenesis. Clin Toxicol 4:579, 1971

25. Tappel AL: Vitamin E and free radical peroxidation of lipids. Ann NY Acad Sci 203:12, 1972

26. Wills ED: Mechanisms of lipid peroxide formation in tissues. Role of metals and hematin proteins in the catalysis of the oxidation of unsaturated fatty acids. Biochim Biophys Acta 98:238, 1965

27. Golberg L, Smith JP: Changes associated with the accumulation of excessive amounts of iron in certain organs of the rat. Br J Exp Pathol 39:59, 1958

28. MacDonald RA, Mallory GK: Hemochromatosis and hemosiderosis. Arch Int Med 105:686, 1960

29. Hyman CB, Landing BH, Alfin-Slater R, et al: dl-α-Tocopherol, iron, and lipofuscin in thalassemia. Ann NY Acad Sci 232:211, 1974

30. Trump BH, Valigorsky JM, Arstila AU, Mergner WJ, Kinney TD: The relationship of intracellular pathways of iron metabolism to cellular overload and the iron storage diseases. Am J Pathol 72:295, 1973

31. Hirayama C: Hepatic fibrosis: Biochemical considerations. In Schaffner F, Sherlock S, Leevy CM (eds): The Liver and Its Diseases. New York, Intercontinental Medical Book Corporation, 1974, pp 273–82

32. Popper H, Hutterer F: Hepatic fibrogenesis and disturbance of hepatic circulation. Ann NY Acad Sci 170:88, 1970

33. Zaino EC, Rossi MB, Pham TD, Azar HA: Gaucher's cells in thalassemia. Blood 38:457, 1971

34. Schaffner F, Popper H: Electron microscopy of liver. In Schiff L (ed): Diseases of the Liver. Philadelphia, Lippincott, 1969, pp 50–83

35. Popper H, Kent G: Fibrosis in chronic liver disease. Clin Gastroenterol 4:315, 1975

36. Leevy CM, Kiernan T: The hepatic circulation of portal hypertension. Clin Gastroenterol 4:381, 1975

37. Sturgeon P, Chen LPL, Bergren WR: Free erythrocyte porphyrins in thalassemia: Preliminary observations. Proceedings of the VIth International Congress of Hematology of the International Society of Hematology. New York, Grune & Stratton, 1958, pp 730–31

38. Lunvall O, Weinfeld A, Lundin P: Iron storage in porphyria cutanea tarda. Acta Med Scand 188:37, 1970

39. Turnbull A, Baker H, Vernon-Roberts B, Magnus IA: Iron metabolism in porphyria cutanea tarda and in erythropoietic protoporphyria. Q J Med 42:341, 1973

40. Oliver RAM: Siderosis following transfusion of blood. J Pathol Bact 77:171, 1959

41. Popper H, Hutterer F, Kent G, et al: Hepatic fibrosis. J Mount Sinai Hosp NY 25:378, 1958

42. Robinson MG, Watson JR: Megaloblastic anemia complicating Thalassemia Major. Am J Dis Child 105:275, 1963

43. MacDonald RA, Jones RS, Pechet GS: Folic acid deficiency and hemochromatosis. Arch Pathol 80:153, 1965

44. Hutter RVP, Shipkey FH, Tan CTC, Murphy ML, Chowdhury M: Hepatic fibrosis in children with acute leukemia. Cancer 13:288, 1960

45. Witzleben CL, Wyatt JP: The effect of long survival on the pathology of thalassemia major. J Pathol Bact 82:1, 1961

46. Murray JM, Stein N; Does the pancreas influence iron absorption? Gastroenterology 51:694, 1966

47. Lassman MN, O'Brien RT, Pearson HA, et al: Endocrine evaluation in thalassemia major. Ann NY Acad Sci 232:226, 1974

48. Dymock IW, Cassar J, Pyke DA, Oakley WG, Williams R: Observations on the pathogenesis, complications and treatment of diabetes in 115 cases of haemochromatosis. Am J Med 52:203, 1972

49. Rössle R: Entzündungen der Leber. In Henke F, Lubarsch O (eds): Handbuch der Speziellen Pathologischen Anatomie und Histologie. Berlin, Springer, vol. 5, 1930, pp 243–505

50. Nathan M, Batsakis JC: Congenital hepatic fibrosis. Surg Gynecol Obstet 178: 1033, 1969

51. Baggenstoss AH: Morphological features: Their usefulness in the diagnosis, prognosis, and management of cirrhosis. Clin Gastroenterol 4:227, 1975

52. Klein KM, Becker FF: Hepatitis. In Becker FF (ed): The Liver: Normal and Abnormal Functions, Part B. New York, Marcel Dekker, 1975, pp 627–45

53. Berry CL, Marshall WC: Iron distribution in the liver of patients with thalassemia major. Lancet 1:1031, 1967

54. Gerber MA, Hadziyannis S, Vernace S, Vissoulis C: Incidents and nature of cytoplasmic hepatitis B antigen in hepatocytes. Lab Invest 32:251, 1975

55. Stamatoyannopoulos G: Discussion. In Zaino EC (ed): Third Conference on Cooley's Anemia. Ann NY Acad Sci 23:361, 1974

56. Dymock IW, Hamilton EBD, Laws JW, Williams R: Arthropathy of hemochromatosis. Ann Rheum Dis 29:469, 1970

CYSTADENOFIBROMA, ADENOFIBROMA, AND MALIGNANT ADENOFIBROMA OF THE OVARY

BERNARD CZERNOBILSKY

The ovarian neoplasms that are being classified as cystadenofibroma, adenofibroma, and malignant adenofibroma originate from the germinal epithelium of the ovary,[1] and thus belong to the group of tumors of surface-epithelial and ovarian-stromal origin also known as tumors of müllerian derivation.[2] Wolfe and Seckinger[3] distinguished five subgroups of these neoplasms, namely: surface, intraovarian, conjoined surface-intraovarian, coincidental serous cystoma-ovarian fibroma, and fibroadenocarcinoma or fibrocystadenocarcinoma. Each of these subgroups was further qualified as cystic, solid, or semisolid.

While the evidence supporting the histogenesis of the numerous ovarian neoplasms from the germinal epithelium and underlying stroma varies from merely circumstantial to fairly conclusive, the origin of the adenofibromatous tumors from ovarian elements can be traced most easily.[1] Nevertheless, in spite of the obvious histogenesis of these neoplasms, they occupy an equivocal position among ovarian tumors. While some consider them as mere variants of serous cystadenomas and of other common epithelial tumors of the ovary,[4, 5] I believe that their characteristic macro- and microscopic pathologic, as well as clinical, features justify a separate listing of these neoplasms.

Cystadenofibroma

Since one frequently observes papillary projections arising from the surface in the normal ovary (Fig. 1), it is advisable not to make a diagnosis of cystadenofibroma if the lesion measures less than 1 cm in diameter. This criterion is, however, not uniformly accepted. Thus, while in Scott's[1] and Czernobilsky et al's series[2] these tumors varied in size from 1 to 20 cm with a mean of 9 cm in diameter, Malloy et al[6] do include the tiny cortical projections with the cystadenofibromas. Consequently the reported incidence of these tumors varies considerably. In Czernobilsky et al's series, they constituted 46.5 percent of all benign serous tumors.[2] Bilaterality ranges from 5.8 percent to 15 percent.[7]

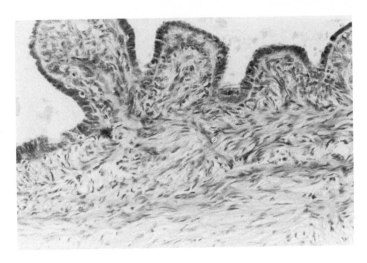

Fig. 1. Surface of normal ovary showing small papillary projections lined by germinal epithelium with underlying stroma. H&E. × 250.

These are cystic, occasionally multiloculated tumors containing serous, clear fluid. The cyst wall may present solid nodular thickenings. On gross examination, these tumors are characterized by firm, short, and rounded papillary projections often arranged in tight clusters, arising from the inner lining of the cyst (Figs. 2 and 3). This is in contrast to the papillary projections of serous cystadenomas which are softer, more elongated, and occupy larger areas of the cyst lining.

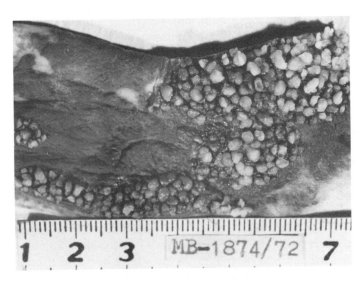

Fig. 2. Gross appearance of inner surface of cystadenofibroma showing tight clusters of firm, short, rounded papillary structures. (From Czernobilsky et al: Cancer 34:1971, 1974. Courtesy of J.B. Lippincott Co.)

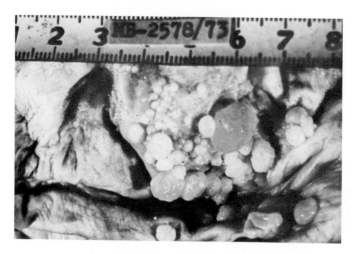

Fig. 3. Close-up of papillae of cystadenofibroma demonstrating some of the commonly observed swollen, edematous formations.

On microscopic examination, the stroma of the papillary projections of the cystadenofibromas is made up of fibrous tissue of varying cellularity ranging from highly cellular to hyalinized areas. Severe stromal edema is a frequent finding (Figs. 4 and 5). A striking feature is a narrow, acellular zone of connective tissue, corresponding to the tunica albuginea ovarii, situated between the epithelial lining cells and the main stroma of the papillae (Fig. 6). This was present in almost one-third of Czernobilsky et al's cases.[2] Since this zone is a normal feature of the ovarian cortex (Fig. 7), its presence in the cystadenofibroma provides additional

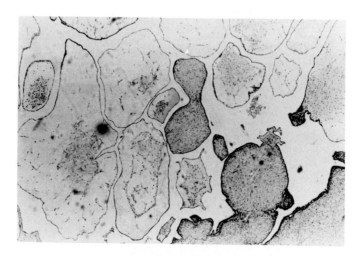

Fig. 4. Microscopic appearance of papillary structures of cystadenofibroma showing both fibrous and markedly edematous components. H&E. $\times$ 40.

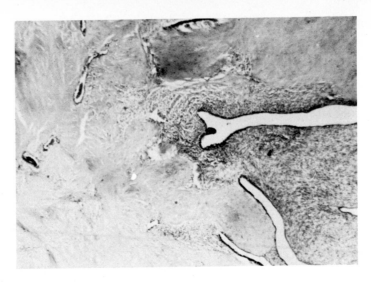

Fig. 5. Detail of stroma in papillae from cystadenofibroma showing hyalinized area. H&E. × 100. (From Czernobilsky et al: Cancer 34:1971, 1974. Courtesy of J.B. Lippincott Co.)

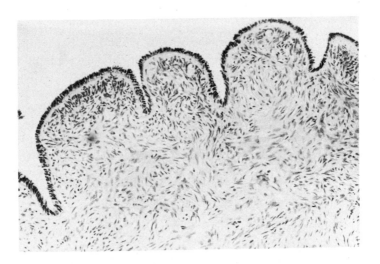

Fig. 6. Papillae of cystadenofibroma showing acellular zone underneath surface epithelial lining. H&E. × 200.

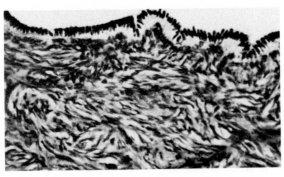

Fig. 7. Normal ovary with acellular tunica albuginea underneath surface epithelium. H&E. × 100. (From Czernobilsky et al: Cancer 34:1971, 1974. Courtesy of J.B. Lippincott Co.)

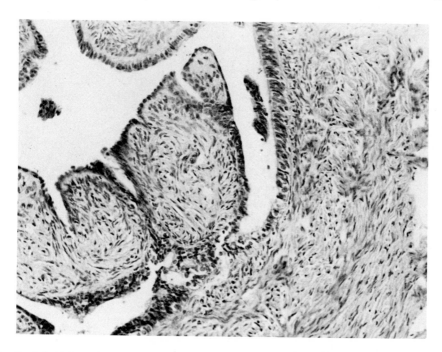

Fig. 8. Cuboidal and columnar epithelial cells lining papillae of cystadenofibroma. H&E. × 200.

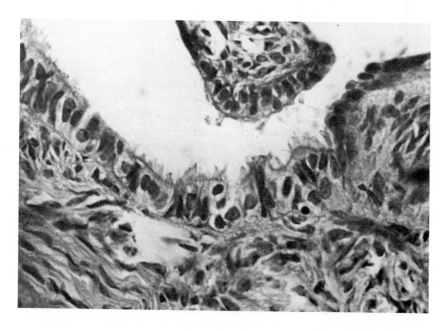

Fig. 9. Ciliated cells with interspersed clear cells similar to oviduct epithelium lining cystadenofibroma. H&E. × 400. (From Czernobilsky et al: Cancer 34:1971, 1974. Courtesy of J.B. Lippincott Co.)

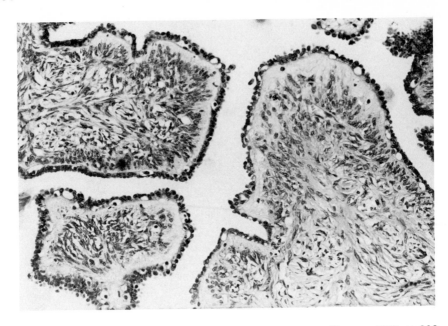

Fig. 10. Hobnail-type cells among epithelial lining of cystadenofibroma. H&E. $\times$ 200.

evidence linking this neoplasm to the normal ovarian cortex. As in other papillary tumors, psammoma bodies are occasionally observed.[2]

The predominant epithelial cells lining the cyst and its papillae in cystadenofibromas are cuboidal and columnar cells (Fig. 8). Cilia, droplet secretion, and scattered clear cells can also be present, often giving the lining of these cysts an appearance strikingly similar to that of the fallopian tube (Fig. 9). Hobnail-type cells can also be present (Fig. 10). Since such admixtures of epithelial cells are common in ovarian tumors of müllerian derivation, and since the predominant cells in cystadenofibromas are usually the serous cuboidal and columnar ones, I see no need to subdivide these neoplasms into serous, mucinous, endometrial, and clear cell groups as it was done in the International Histological Classification of Ovarian Tumors by the World Health Organization.[8] This would only be justified if in some of these tumors the nonserous epithelial elements constitute the only, or at least the predominant, feature, something which I have not yet encountered. The luminal border of the epithelial cells stains positively with alcian blue and PAS before and after diastase digestion, which are reactions similar to those observed in other ovarian neoplasms of surface epithelial origin.[5] In contrast to papillary serous cystadenomas, multilayering, tufting, atypism, or mitotic activity of the epithelial lining indicative of borderline malignancy have not been observed in cystadenofibromas (Table 1).

Ultrastructural studies of the epithelial lining cells of cystadenofibromas revealed mature, frequently ciliated cells with numerous supranuclear mitochondria and cross-striated ciliary rootlets. The picture is similar to that of oviduct mucosa (Fig. 11).[9]

According to Scott,[1] over 90 percent of patients with cystadenofibromas are

**TABLE 1. Microscopic Features of 34 Cystadenofibromas
and 39 Cystadenomas** *

Features	Cystadenofibroma (Number of cases)	Cystadenoma (Number of cases)
Papillary projections	34	14
Epithelial lining		
Cuboidal	34	39
Columnar	22	20
Cilia	11	10
Hobnail	7	8
Clear	4	1
Pseudostratification	6	8
Psammoma bodies	10	5
Tufting	—	6
Atypism	—	5
Mitoses	—	5
Borderline malignancy	—	3
Stroma		
Spindle cells	34	32
Collagen	27	28
Hyaline	15	3
Edema	18	10
Subepithelial acellular layer	11	1

* Each tumor presents more than one cell type.
From Czernobilsky et al: Cancer 34:1971, 1974. Courtesy of J.B. Lippincott Co.

40 years or older. This was not borne out by Czernobilsky et al's series,[2] where the patients' ages ranged from 15 to 65, with a mean of 30.7 years. The most common presenting symptom is that of abdominal pain, although abnormal vaginal bleeding also seems to occur frequently.[1, 2, 6, 10-15] The most likely explanation of the latter is estrogen production by functional steroidogenic cells present in the stroma of the neoplasm.[10, 12, 15, 16] This may have been the cause in a number of cases of abnormal endometrial proliferation,[10, 15] although Scott[1] doubts such endocrine activity. Pleural effusion has also been reported in some cases.[14]

Since cystadenofibromas are benign tumors, surgical removal of the involved ovary with conservation of the uterus and the opposite ovary constitutes adequate therapy. The gross appearance of the neoplasm with its characteristic clusters of small, round, firm papillary projections should enable the pathologist in most instances to reach the correct macroscopic diagnosis when called upon to perform a frozen section. The latter will confirm the diagnosis. This is of primary importance, since in contrast to papillary serous cystadenomas which frequently are of the borderline variety justifying a more radical therapeutic approach, a correct diagnosis of cystadenofibroma in the operating room might save the patient unnecessary extensive surgery.

Adenofibroma

This is the solid counterpart of the cystadenofibroma in which the stromal elements predominate. In the past, it has been described together with the cyst-

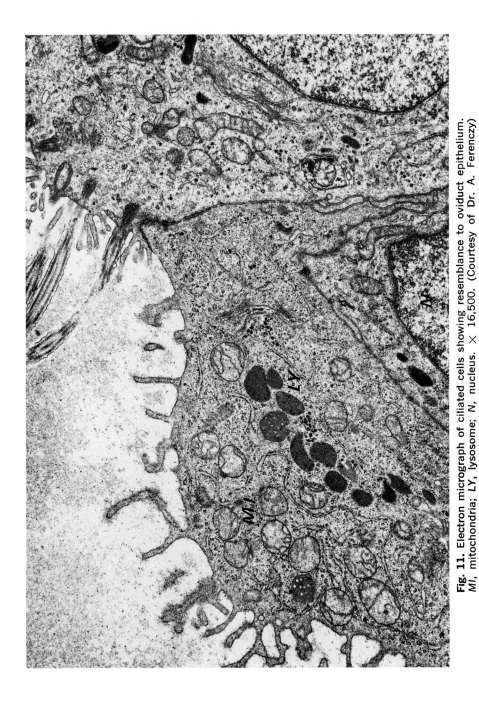

Fig. 11. Electron micrograph of ciliated cells showing resemblance to oviduct epithelium. MI, mitochondria; LY, lysosome; N, nucleus. × 16,500. (Courtesy of Dr. A. Ferenczy)

adenofibroma,[7, 17] as well as treated as a separate entity.[10, 14, 18] Although the adenofibroma appears to have the same origin as the cystadenofibroma, it should be separately discussed by virtue of its macro- and microscopic characteristics, as well as its malignant potential.

Here, as in the cystadenofibroma, lesions of less than 1 cm in diameter should not be considered as neoplastic, but may represent normal nodularity of the ovarian surface. The size of this tumor varies from 1 to 15 cm in diameter, with about 20 percent of bilaterality.[10]

Grossly, these smooth and encapsulated neoplasms resemble other benign solid ovarian tumors such as thecomas, fibromas, or Brenner tumors. On cut section, they are solid or predominantly solid with small cysts scattered throughout the stroma (Fig. 12).

On microscopic examination, the fibrous stroma varies from highly cellular to almost acellular, hyalinized areas. The glandular components may be lined by the same epithelia present in cystadenofibromas, namely cuboidal, columnar, ciliated, as well as scattered clear and hobnail cells with the first two types predominating (Figs. 13 to 15). As it becomes obvious from these illustrations, this tumor can occasionally simulate the parvilocular cystoma variant of clear cell carcinoma [19] as well as cystic types of Brenner tumors. However, as higher magnifications reveal in the clear cell carcinoma, most of the epithelial cells are of the clear or hobnail type with atypical features (Fig. 16), while Brenner tumors with cystic structures usually demonstrate the typical solid epithelial Brenner nests in at least some areas.

In some instances, the glandular components of the adenofibroma may demonstrate crowding and bizarre shapes which are most probably the result of proliferative activity (Fig. 17). These may perhaps represent borderline lesions, but our present state of knowledge does not enable us to establish any such clinicopathologic correlations at this time. The term "proliferating adenofibroma" may suit this type of neoplasm for the time being at least.

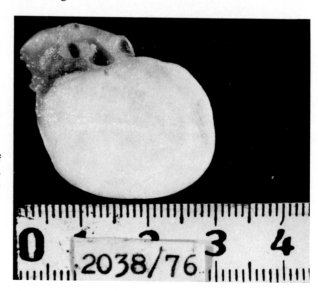

Fig. 12. Gross photograph of adenofibroma showing solid, whitish, cut surface of tumor.

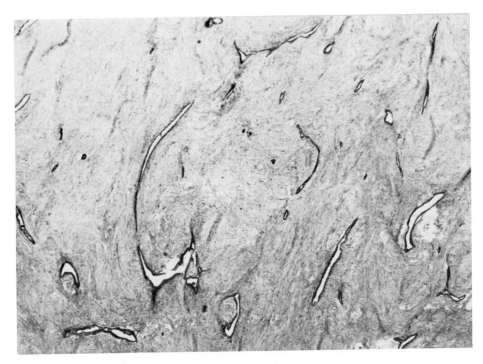

Fig. 13. Compressed slit-like glandular spaces in adenofibroma with poorly cellular stroma. H&E. × 29. (From Czernobilsky: In Blaustein (ed): Obstetrics and Gynecologic Pathology, 1977. Courtesy of Springer Verlag)

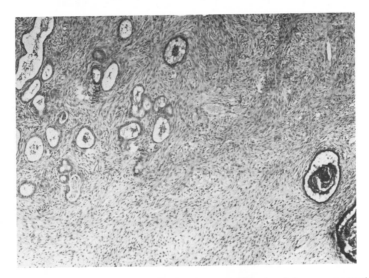

Fig. 14. Adenofibroma showing fairly cellular stroma with glandular components lined by cuboidal epithelium. H&E. × 100. (From Czernobilsky: In Blaustein (ed): Obstetric and Gynecologic Pathology, 1977. Courtesy of Springer Verlag)

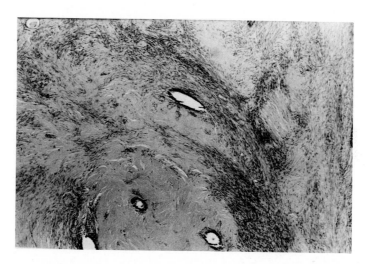

Fig. 15. Adenofibroma with predominantly hyalinized stroma. H&E. $\times$ 100.

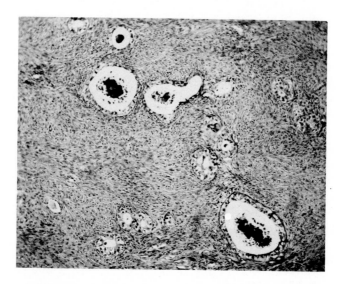

Fig. 16. Parvilocular cystoma variant of ovarian clear cell carcinoma showing resemblance to adenofibroma. Closer scrutiny reveals a predominantly atypical clear cell and hobnail-type epithelial lining. H&E. $\times$ 70. (Courtesy of Dr. H. J. Norris)

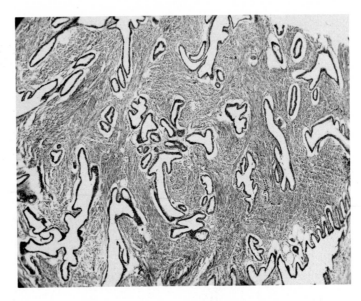

Fig. 17. Adenofibroma showing irregularly budding glandular spaces within fibrous stroma, possibly justifying the term "proliferating adenofibroma." H&E. × 100. (Courtesy of Dr. H. J. Norris)

Because of the lack of uniform criteria of adenofibromas and the fact that in some publications these lesions are discussed together with cystadenofibromas,[7, 17] their incidence is difficult to ascertain, but adenofibromas are most definitely much less frequent than the cystadenofibromas. In Timonen and Purola's series,[10] adenofibromas constituted 0.68 percent of all benign ovarian tumors. Among the 34 cystadenofibromas in our series, we found only 2 instances with solid nodular thickening within the cyst wall, but not a single predominantly solid tumor warranting a diagnosis of adenofibroma.[2]

Adenofibroma is a neoplasm characteristically in older individuals, with 50 percent of the neoplasms occurring in patients over the age of 50.[10] The clinical picture is similar to that of other benign solid ovarian tumors and depends mostly on the size of the lesion. In addition to the presence of an abdominal mass and pain, vaginal bleeding possibly related to estrogenic activity of stromal cells has been described.[10, 11, 14] The lesion is perfectly benign and thus necessitates only a conservative surgical approach.

Malignant Adenofibroma

Since by the generally accepted definition, the malignant adenofibroma contains malignant epithelial and not malignant stromal elements, it would have been more correct to designate this tumor as an adenocarcinofibroma. It certainly seems to be one of the rarest neoplasms of the female genital tract, with only about 30 tumors reported in the literature.[10, 11, 14, 20]

Grossly, these neoplasms are usually similar to the benign adenofibromas, but

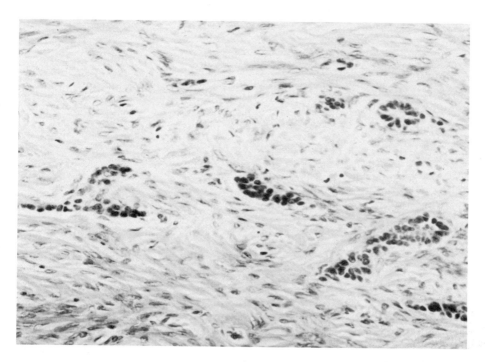

Fig. 18. Malignant adenofibroma showing benign fibrous stroma infiltrated by malignant epithelial components. H&E. × 110. (From Czernobilsky: In Blaustein (ed): Obstetric and Gynecologic Pathology, 1977. Courtesy of Springer Verlag)

occasionally are of softer consistency than the latter. They are primarily solid tumors in which frequently small cystic spaces can be identified. Six of the reported cases have been bilateral, and in some instances the contralateral ovary contained a benign adenofibroma.[10, 11]

As in the benign adenofibromas and cystadenofibromas, the epithelial cells lining the cystic spaces of the malignant adenofibroma vary and may include serous, mucinous, ciliated, vacuolated, and hobnail-type cells. Naturally, in the malignant tumors, these cells may show multilayering, atypism, mitotic activity, but particularly invasion of the stroma (Fig. 18). However, it is a difficult task to reach the diagnosis of malignant adenofibroma in the absence of histologic elements of a benign adenofibroma within the same tumor. As in the benign adenofibroma, the differential diagnosis between malignant adenofibroma and the parvilocular cystoma variant of the clear cell carcinoma may be particularly problematic. Malignant Brenner tumors can also simulate malignant adenofibromas, and so can endometrioid carcinomas with a dense fibrous stroma. However, close examination of these neoplasms will usually reveal their characteristic histologic features which differ from those of the malignant adenofibroma. In addition, a careful study of numerous sections of malignant adenofibromas will often demonstrate areas of typical benign adenofibroma, obviously facilitating the correct diagnosis of the former.

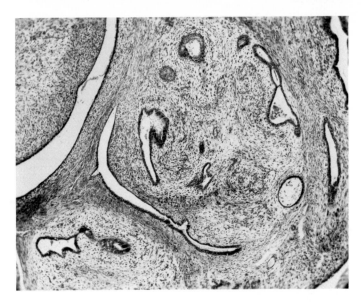

Fig. 19. Ovarian tumor showing benign glandular structures surrounded by sarcomatous stroma, similar to the müllerian adenosarcoma of the uterus. H&E. × 42. (Courtesy of Dr. H. J. Norris)

Norris [21] has observed some adenofibromas with obvious malignant change of the stromal elements (Fig. 19). These lesions are similar to the müllerian adeno-sarcomas of the uterus described by Clement and Scully.[22] It follows that the rare ovarian carcinosarcomas and mixed mesodermal tumors in which both glandular and stromal elements are malignant,[23] may actually be derived from adenofibromas, constituting the ultimate type of malignancy that this lesion can achieve.

The treatment of choice of malignant adenofibromas is total hysterectomy with bilateral salpingo-oophorectomy. Postoperative radiation and chemotherapy have been added in some cases.[10, 11] This appears to be a very malignant neoplasm, with 5 patients dying within one year following surgical removal of the tumor.[10, 14]

Conclusion

The characteristic macro- and microscopic features of the cystadenofibroma make it the prototype of ovarian tumors of surface epithelium and stromal origin. Although frequently presenting a variety of epithelial lining cells which is a feature of all of the ovarian epithelial neoplasms, the predominant cell is cuboidal. It thus is similar to the so-called serous epithelial tumors of the ovary. Nevertheless, the cystadenofibroma should be separately listed because of its special features and its unequivocal benign nature. This is in contrast to the nonfibromatous papillary serous cystadenomas that frequently are of borderline malignancy.

The adenofibroma is the solid counterpart of the cystic tumor. It too is com-posed of epithelial-lined structures and fibrous stromas, but it lacks a predominant cystic cavity and the typical papillary projections of the cystadenofibroma. The differential diagnosis between this neoplasm and certain types of Brenner tumors or the parvilocular cystoma variant of the clear cell carcinoma may occasionally prove to be problematic.

The rare malignant adenofibroma is a neoplasm in which the epithelial elements only are malignant. Hence, this tumor too must be differentiated from other malignant epithelial neoplasms with fibrous stroma, such as the malignant Brenner tumor, certain types of endometrioid carcinoma, and above all, the parvilocular cystoma. The presence of areas of benign adenofibroma in the vicinity of the malignant lesion will obviously facilitate reading the correct diagnosis.

Recently, some malignant adenofibromas in which the stromal rather than the epithelial components are malignant have been observed. In these rare cases, the tumor is similar to the müllerian adenosarcoma described in the uterus. Cases in which both epithelial and stromal components are malignant are known as ovarian carcinosarcomas and mixed mesodermal tumors.

Finally, it should be pointed out that cystadenofibromas and adenofibromas are by no means exclusively found in the ovary. They have also been described in other genital organs of müllerian derivation, such as the uterine cervix, endometrium, and fallopian tubes.[24-27]

References

1. Scott RB: Serous adenofibromas and cystadenofibromas of the ovary. Am J Obstet Gynecol 43:773, 1942
2. Czernobilsky B, Borenstein R, Lancet M: Cystadenofibroma of the ovary. A clinicopathologic study of 34 cases and comparison with serous cystadenoma. Cancer 34:1971, 1974
3. Wolfe SA, Seckinger DL: Varied anatomical types of ovarian adenofibroma. A proposed classification. Am J Obstet Gynecol 99:121, 1967
4. Kraus FT: Gynecologic Pathology. St. Louis, Mosby, 1967, p 333
5. Scully RE: Recent progress in ovarian cancer. Hum Pathol 1:73, 1970
6. Malloy JJ, Dockerty MB, Welch JS, Hunt AB: Papillary ovarian tumors. I. Benign tumors and serous and mucinous cystadenocarcinomas. Am J Obstet Gynecol 93:867, 1965
7. Hertig AT, Gore H: Atlas of Tumor Pathology. Section IX. Fascicle 33, Tumors of the Female Sex Organs. Part 3. Tumors of the Ovary and Fallopian Tube. Washington, DC, Armed Forces Institute of Pathology, 1961, p 118
8. Serov SF, Scully RE, Sobin LH (eds): International Histological Classification of Tumours, No. 9. Histological Typing of Ovarian Tumours. Geneva, World Health Organization, 1973, p 17–18
9. Ferenczy A, Richart RM: The Female Reproductive System. Dynamics of Scan and Transmission Electron Microscopy. New York, Wiley, 1974, p 287
10. Timonen S, Purola E: Adenofibroma and cystadenofibroma of the ovary. Ann Chir Gynaecol Fenn 56, Suppl 154:5, 1967
11. Compton HL, Fink FM: Serous adenofibroma and cystadenofibroma of the ovary. Obstet Gynecol 36:636, 1970
12. Daley D, Harrison CV, Millar WG: A case of cystadenofibroma of the ovary. J Obstet Gynaecol Brit Commonwealth 57:408, 1950
13. McNulty RY: The ovarian serous cystadenofibroma. A report of 25 cases. Am J Obstet Gynecol 77:1338, 1959
14. Rothman D, Blumenthal HT: Serous adenofibroma of the ovary. Report of five cases with malignant change in one. Obstet Gynecol 14:389, 1959

15. Herman G: Cystadenofibroma of the ovary. Comments on hormonal aspects. Am J Obstet Gynecol 99:117, 1967

16. Papadaki L, Beilby JOW: Ovarian cystadenofibroma: A consideration of the role of estrogen in its pathogenesis. Am J Obstet Gynecol 121:501, 1975

17. Novak ER, Woodruff JD: Novak's Gynecologic and Obstetric Pathology with Clinical and Endocrine Relations, 7th ed. Philadelphia, Saunders, 1974, pp 373–374

18. Morris JM, Scully RE: Endocrine Pathology of the Ovary. St. Louis, Mosby, 1958, p 131

19. Czernobilsky B, Silverman BB, Enterline HT: Clear cell carcinoma of the ovary. A clinicopathologic analysis of pure and mixed forms and comparison with endometrioid carcinoma. Cancer 25:762, 1970

20. Minkowitz S, Cohen HM: Adenocarcinoma within serous cystadenofibroma of the ovary. NY State J Med 66:527, 1966

21. Norris HJ: Personal communication, 1976

22. Clement PB, Scully RE: Müllerian adenosarcoma of the uterus. A clinico-pathologic analysis of ten cases of a distinctive type of müllerian mixed tumor. Cancer 34:1138, 1974

23. Czernobilsky B, LaBarre CG: Carcinosarcoma and mixed mesodermal tumor of the ovary. A clinicopathologic analysis of 9 cases. Obstet Gynecol 31:21, 1968

24. Abell MR: Papillary adenofibroma of the uterine cervix. Am J Obstet Gynecol 110:990, 1971

25. Vellios F, Ng ABP, Reagan JW: Papillary adenofibroma of the uterus: A benign mesodermal mixed tumor of müllerian origin. Am J Clin Pathol 60:543, 1973

26. Kanbour AI, Burgess F, Salazar H: Intramural adenofibroma of the fallopian tube. Light and electron microscopy. Cancer 31:1433, 1973

27. Grimalt M, Arguelles M, Ferenczy A: Papillary cystadenofibroma of endometrium: A histochemical and ultra structural study. Cancer 36:137, 1975

THE SMALL CELL LESION OF MAMMARY DUCTS AND LOBULES

CYRIL TOKER AND JUDITH D. GOLDBERG

In his text on *Neoplastic Diseases* (1919), Ewing illustrated a distinctive lesion of the mammary lobules, which he considered to be precancerous.[1] Two decades later, Foote and Stewart [2] designated this lesion "lobular carcinoma in situ," in the belief that it represented a preinvasive carcinoma rather than a precancerous condition. More than half a century has elapsed since Ewing's original illustration, but agreement does not yet exist with regard to the prognostic significance and therapeutic implications of this entity. Neither is it to be anticipated that such agreement is imminent.

It is the purpose of this chapter to review the authors' experience with this lesion—an experience that now spans a period of 30 years—and to survey the pertinent literature on the subject.

Normal Mucosal Structure and the Differentiation of Dysplastic from Nondysplastic Proliferations

The normal mammary tubule, whether acinus or duct, is lined by a double-layered epithelium (Fig. 1).[3, 4] The superficial layer is composed of columnar or cuboidal eosinophilic cells. The basal layer contains crescentic cells with clear cytoplasm. The eosinophilia, uniformity, and compactness of the superficial layer contrast with the loose texture, variability, and light staining of the basal zone. The polarity of the cells forming these layers is, furthermore, dissimilar. Thus, the long axes of the superficial cells are perpendicular to the basement membrane, while those of the basal clear cells are, generally, parallel to that structure. Disturbance of normal mucosal stratification and polarity is characteristic of dysplastic epithelial proliferations, which impose a certain homogeneity upon the tubular lining.

The ultrastructural features of normal mammary epithelium have been described elsewhere.[4] Suffice it to observe here that the superficial eosinophilic cells exhibit marked electron density, while the basal clear cells present an electron-

217

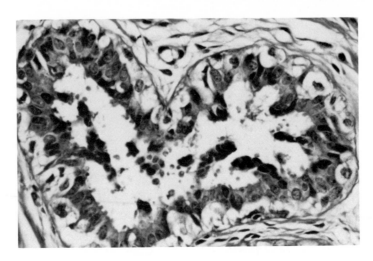

Fig. 1. Normal mammary acinus, showing double-layered mucosa. H&E. × 320.

lucent cytoplasm containing many fine fibers (Fig. 2). The basal clear cells differ from typical myoepithelial cells, and the relationship between these two cell types is uncertain.

Proliferations of the mammary epithelium may be divided into dysplastic and nondysplastic categories. The term "dysplastic" is employed to denote the possession of a malignant (invasive) potential. As will be discussed later, however, recognition of the precise morphologic stage at which this potential has been transformed into an actual capability is uncertain. Nondysplastic proliferations lack a malignant (invasive) potential, although they may evolve into benign neoplasms. We believe that these two pathways (dysplastic and nondysplastic) are quite distinct from one another, even though, on occasion, dysplastic changes may supervene in a process that was originally nondysplastic.

The principles of structural organization which permit a distinction between dysplastic and nondysplastic proliferations apply without regard to size of the participating cells (ie, whether large or small). Such proliferations, whether dysplastic or nondysplastic, may assume one or more of three fundamental growth patterns—the solid (aglandular), the cribriform (glandular), and the papillary. These forms may be present in combination, particularly when the process is nondysplastic. In this chapter, we shall be concerned solely with solid (aglandular) proliferations composed of small cells.

The direction of the (solid) dysplastic proliferation is toward uniformity, toward homogeneity, of the cellular mass. The nondysplastic theme, by contrast, is one of irregularity and disarray. Thus, the dysplastic cells are seen to assume polygonal or spherical configurations (Figs. 3 and 4), losing the normally pronounced distinction between their long and short axes. As their number increases, apolar sheets are formed (Figs. 4 and 5). The resulting diffuse masses, whether within lobules or ducts, are devoid of organization. Nondysplastic aggregates of solid type do not exhibit loss of cellular polarity. Long and short axes remain

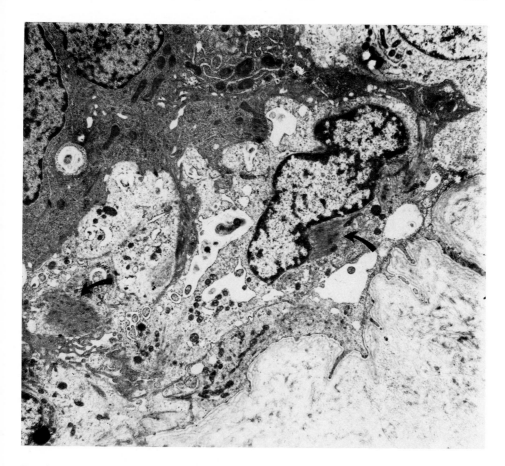

Fig. 2. Electron micrograph of normal mammary acinus showing basal clear cell and part of overlying eosinophilic cell. Fascicles of fine fibers (arrows) are seen within the cytoplasm of the basal clear cell. $\times$ 4600.

distinct. The cells are elongated and are arranged haphazardly (Fig. 6). This is the pattern commonly observed within lobules, where the volume of cells is small. As the cell population increases, the (solid) nondysplastic proliferation develops a trabecular construction. This is the pattern commonly observed within ducts (Fig. 7). The trabeculae, separated by narrow clefts, are disposed irregularly at various angles to one another. They are composed of columnar or cuboidal cells arranged in single- or double-layered rows. Stromal cores containing blood vessels may be observed within the lesion; they are usually effaced in the more advanced dysplastic multiplications.

It should be noted that the recognition of a trabecular composition may be difficult—particularly when the trabeculae are compressed and the intervening clefts are obscured. The problem may be resolved by the preparation of further sections, which, if obvious clefts are revealed, will often expose the trabecular character of the lesion.

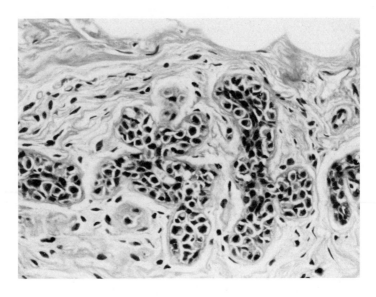

Fig. 3. Early dysplastic proliferation of solid type. Round, basally located, small cells of myoepithelial type occupy individual lacunae. H&E. × 200.

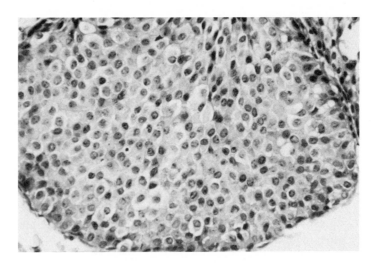

Fig. 4. Advanced dysplastic lesion of solid type. Polygonal small cells of myoepithelial type form an apolar sheet. H&E. × 200.

Distinction between dysplastic and nondysplastic proliferations is qualitative, not quantitative, and the stigmata of each category are imprinted upon it from the earliest morphologic stages. As the cellular multiplication proceeds, a progressive quantitative augmentation occurs, but the essential structural traits that were evident at the inception of the process are retained.

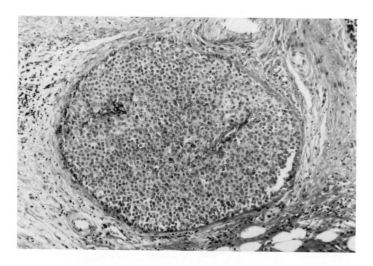

Fig. 5. Low-power micrograph of dysplastic (solid) proliferation in duct. The cells are round and form a diffuse, apolar sheet. H&E. × 80.

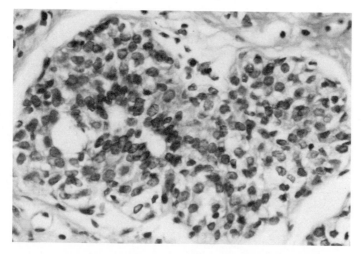

Fig. 6. Nondysplastic (solid) proliferation in acinus. The cells are elongated. H&E. × 320.

The Small Cell

It is appropriate, at this juncture, to define "small cell." Nuclei generally range from a diameter approximately equal to that of the erythrocyte—some 8 μm —to approximately double that size (Figs. 8 to 10). Smaller nuclei tend to pyknosis, larger nuclei exhibit a more lightly staining vesicular appearance. With regard to cytoplasmic structure, two distinct varieties of small cell may be encoun-

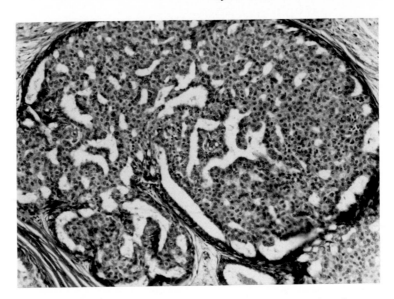

Fig. 7. Nondysplastic lesion of solid type in duct. The cells form trabeculae separated by serpiginous clefts. H&E. × 80.

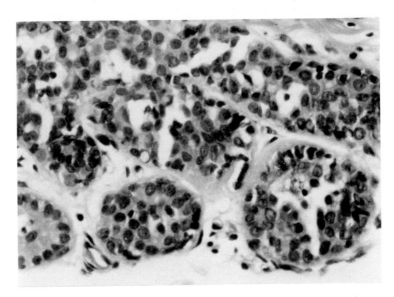

Fig. 8. Small cells of syncytial type. Cytoplasm is scanty, and cell membranes are indistinct. Nuclei are pyknotic. H&E. × 320.

tered. The first variety (Figs. 8 and 9), which we have designated the syncytial form, presents central nuclei surrounded by scanty cytoplasm. Cell membranes are indistinct, the cells merging in a syncytial fashion. The second variety (Fig. 10), which we have termed the myoepithelial form, exhibits eccentric nuclei and a relatively large amount of eosinophilic cytoplasm. Cell boundaries are usually

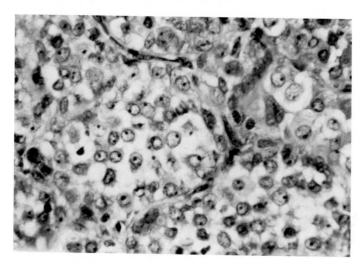

Fig. 9. Small cells of syncytial type. Nuclei are larger than in Figure 8, and vesicular. Cytoplasm is scanty. H&E. × 320.

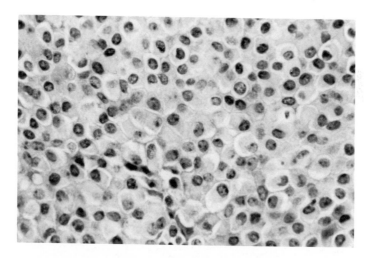

Fig. 10. Small cells of myoepithelial type. Nuclei are eccentric, and there is abundant eosinophilic cytoplasm. Cell membranes are distinct. H&E. × 320.

discernible, and these cells are often located in isolated lacunae, separate from their neighbors (Fig. 3). Their appearance is distinctly myoid. Admixtures of these cell types may occur.

Mitotic activity is slight and usually encountered only when nuclei are in the larger size range. Small cell populations may contain cells of different sizes, but their configuration (spherical or polygonal) is similar, with the result that a characteristic sense of uniformity is conveyed. Large cell lesions, by contrast, display huge nuclei, abundant cytoplasm, mitotic activity, and profound variations in cell size and shape (Fig. 11).

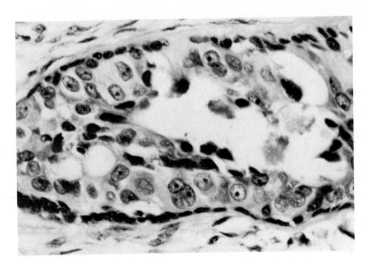

Fig. 11. Intraductal large cell tumor. Cells are large. Nuclei are large and pleomorphic. H&E. × 320.

Both large and small cell proliferations may occur concurrently in different areas of the same breast. It would appear, furthermore, that small cells may enlarge beyond the range recorded. Figure 12 illustrates cells larger than those previously depicted, which do, nevertheless, exhibit the characteristic uniformity of a small cell population. There is, in addition, evidence to suggest that small cells may undergo transformation to a large cell form. Thus, Figure 13 illustrates large cells within the substance of a small cell lesion. No independent large cell tumor was

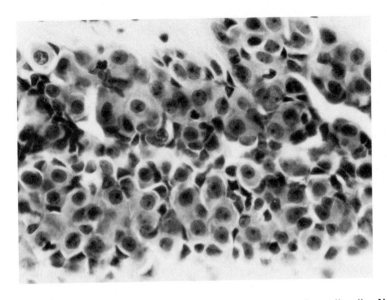

Fig. 12. Relatively large cells that still belong to the category of small cells. Note uniformity of shape and size. H&E. × 320.

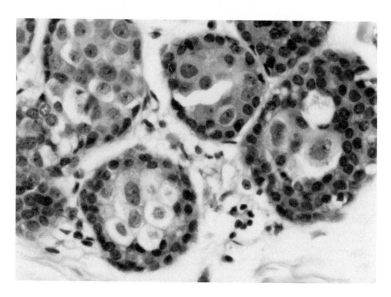

Fig. 13. Large cells seen within the center of small cell aggregates. These large cells are believed to have resulted from enlargement of the surrounding small cells. H&E. × 320.

present, and the integration of the large and small cells certainly suggests that the former were derived from the latter. It is our belief that some large cell tumors are derived from preexisting small cell lesions. Small cells that have invaded the connective tissues present morphologic features identical to those that may be observed in the intralobular or intraductal populations (Fig. 14).

The histogenesis of the small cell remains uncertain. As will be described in the next section, they appear to arise within the basal layer. Ultrastructural

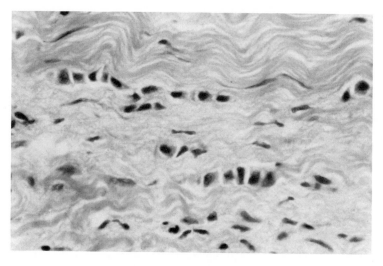

Fig. 14. Infiltrating small cell carcinoma. Characteristic trabeculae are seen. H&E. × 320.

study of small cell tumors has yielded equivocal results.[5] The cells have been found to contain cytoplasmic fibers, but they were not considered to be of myo-epithelial origin. It is these authors' belief that the small cells, either wholly or in part, are derived from the basal clear cells illustrated in Figures 1 and 2, but this opinion awaits confirmation. Finally, it should be observed that small cells may undergo mucinous transformation, resulting in a signet-ring type of cell.

"Lobular Carcinoma in Situ"

Recognition of the "lobular carcinoma in situ" as a cancerous proliferation was tardy. The reason for this delay is to be found in the absence from this tumor of the two morphologic features that have, for decades, provided the basis for a malignant diagnosis in in situ lesions of the breast, ie, bizarre cytology and a cribriform growth pattern. There has been little difficulty in the recognition of in situ carcinomas that present the classic cytologic stigmata of malignancy—nuclear abnormalities, pleomorphism, and mitotic activity. Where the in situ growth comprised small cells of innocuous appearance, the familiar cribriform (honeycomb) pattern of the carcinoma has long provided the criterion for a diagnosis of malignancy. The "lobular" tumor, however, possesses neither of these features. It is composed of cells that lack the usual cytologic features of carcinoma, and the growth pattern is solid, devoid of the characteristic circular fenestrae seen in the cribriform type. Once the small cells have invaded the connective tissues, their cancerous nature is, of course, revealed, the innocuous aspect notwithstanding.

Recognition of the lobular component of this solid small cell tumor,[2] for it is the lobular component that is the more conspicuous, has been followed by a division of in situ breast carcinomas into two categories according to location. The "lobular" tumor was differentiated from the "ductal" tumor, and involvement of the mammary tree at sites other than those conforming to this system of classification was considered to be secondary extension. Thus, involvement of the ducts by "lobular" tumor was regarded as a manifestation of spread from a lobular site. Invasion of the connective tissues by small cells was designated as "invasive lobular carcinoma." On the other hand, involvement of lobules by "intraductal" tumors (large cell) was again regarded as a function of spread within the mammary channels, and invasive large cell tumors are referred to as invasive "duct" carcinomas.

There is little basis for such a regional concept, which evolved from the original recognition of the small cell lesion in a lobular location. It is our belief that the primary distinction between these forms of in situ breast cancer must be made on the basis of cell type and not on the basis of geography. Thus, we have observed many examples of in situ small cell tumors in which the ductal involvement was equal to, or exceeded, the lobular component. We have observed examples of in situ small cell tumors in which no lobular component was detected at all, the lesion being entirely ductal (Fig. 15). We see no justification for the assumption that a solely lobular origin existed under these various circumstances; and no basis for the designation of invasive small cell carcinomas, in which the in situ changes involve ducts to a degree equal to or greater than lobules, as "invasive lobular carcinoma." Neither do we believe that the lobular involvement seen in large cell

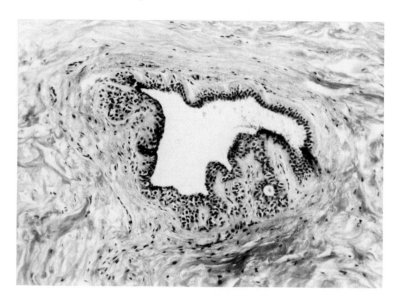

Fig. 15. Early, ductal, small cell lesion. The proliferation is basal and inconspicuous. H&E. × 80.

"intraductal" tumors must invariably be a function of secondary extension from the ducts.

We prefer, therefore, to designate the "lobular carcinoma in situ"—"small cell in situ carcinoma of solid type" (or for brevity, "in situ small cell carcinoma") and "invasive lobular carcinoma"—"invasive small cell carcinoma." "Intraductal" tumors are, similarly, designated "large cell tumors" irrespective of their location in ducts or lobules.

Finally, it should be observed that the identification of a particular channel as a duct, ductule, or acinus may be tenuous, if not impossible, after the accumulating tumor cells have produced an appreciable degree of distention. Only in the less advanced stages of the process can a particular lesion be classified as ductal or lobular with reasonable certainty. Even within the lobule itself, the problem remains as to whether the involvement is of the acinar elements or of the secretory (terminal) ductule. These difficulties provide additional justification for the designation of in situ tumors according to cell size.

Evolution of the Small Cell Lesion

The dysplastic changes with which we are concerned represent a continuous and insensible gradation that extends from the earliest basal alteration to gross distension of the affected channel. The extent of the cellular accumulation may, however, vary appreciably in different areas of the same biopsy or mastectomy specimen.

The dysplastic proliferation appears to commence in the basal layer (Figs. 3, 15 to 17). At low magnification, the affected channel displays abnormal cellularity,

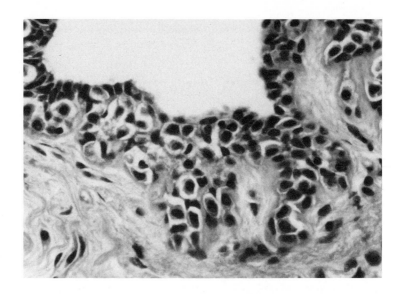

Fig. 16. High-power micrograph of Figure 15. The small cells are of myoepithelial type. The proliferation is basal, and many cells occupy individual lacunae. H&E. × 320.

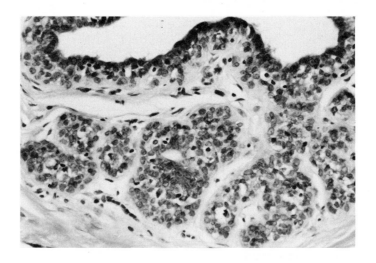

Fig. 17. Early small cell lesion. Cells are syncytial. The basally located small cells are beginning to form sheets. Acini remain elongated and angular. H&E. × 200.

usually distinctly basal in location (Fig. 15). It should be emphasized that detection of the dysplastic lesion is most readily accomplished under the very low power objective (× 2.5), at which magnification the crowded tubule contrasts noticeably with the surrounding ducts and lobules. The dysplastic cells become rounded, and, in the case of the myoepithelial form, frequently occupy individual lacunae in the basal layer (Figs. 3 and 16). Cells of syncytial type, even at this early stage, may fuse to form sheets (Fig. 17). The condition of the superficial layer of the normal mucosa varies. This layer may persist, undergoing progressive attenuation, atop the proliferating basal cells (Fig. 16) until it is ultimately effaced. In the case of a syncytial cell population, however, the superficial layer often disappears at an early phase, the characteristic normal stratification into two dissimilar strata being lost; a single or double row of syncytial cells is seen lining the acinus or duct (Figs. 18 and 19). A characteristic homogeneity of the lining is produced. The configura-

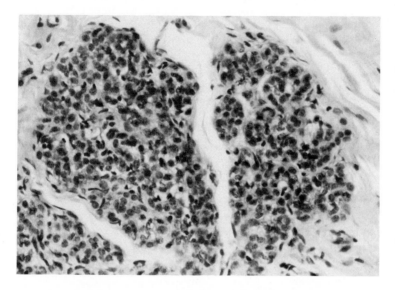

Fig. 18. Early small cell lesion. Normal mucosal architecture has been effaced. The acini are lined by rows of small cells. H&E. × 200.

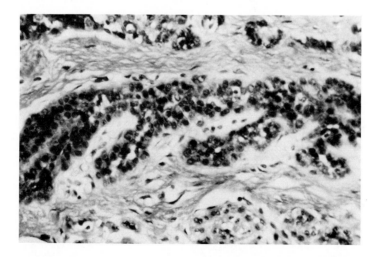

Fig. 19. Early small cell lesion in duct. The normal mucosa has been replaced by rows of small cells. H&E. × 200.

tion of the affected channel has not yet been significantly altered. The narrow, elongated, angular outline of the normal tubule is retained. (This angulation, this tortuosity, is progressively dissipated in more advanced proliferations as cellular accumulation distends the channel.) The lumen has not yet been encroached upon. This early stage of the process is most apt to be overlooked. The lesions are focal, may be few in number, and are extremely inconspicuous (Figs. 3, 15 to 17).

Continued accumulation of small cells leads to increasing distension of the affected tubule. At low magnification, the crowded duct or lobule stands out darkly (Fig. 20). Some angularity or tortuosity of the tubules may persist, but they are

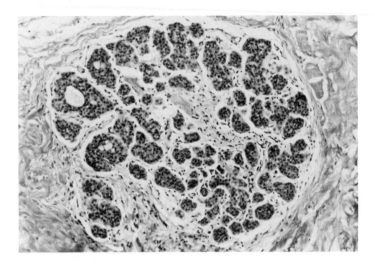

Fig. 20. Low-power micrograph of more advanced small cell lesion. The acini are crowded, and distension has begun. H&E. × 80.

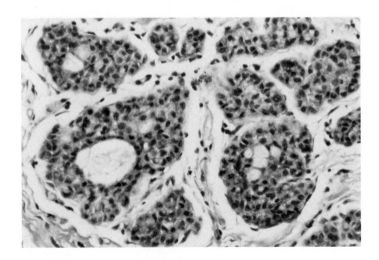

Fig. 21. High-power micrograph of Figure 20. The acini are distended by sheets of cells. H&E. × 200.

beginning to assume a globular shape (Figs. 20 and 21). The polygonal or spherical cells are disposed in sheets (Fig. 21). Within these sheets, the nuclei may occasionally be aligned in circular rows, forming small rosettes; these structures may represent an attempt to form rudimentary lumina. The lumen of the channel may be occluded, but may still be discernible (Fig. 21).

The ultimate expression of the dysplastic multiplication is illustrated in Figures 22 through 24. Tubules, distended by apolar sheets of cells, present globular outlines. Lumina have usually disappeared, and no more than an occasional vestige of

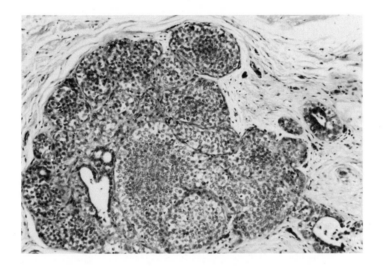

Fig. 22. Advanced small cell lesion. The acini are globular, distention is extreme, and septa separating acini are being obliterated. H&E. × 80.

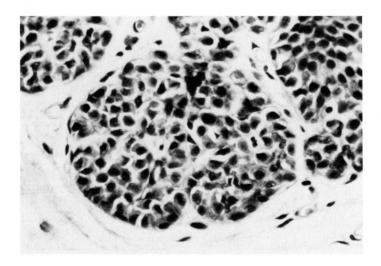

Fig. 23. High-power micrograph of advanced small cell lesion. The acinus is globular, and the basement membrane is indistinct. H&E. × 320.

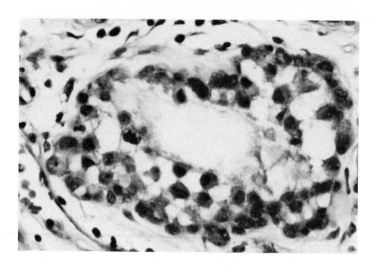

Fig. 24. Advanced small cell lesion showing dissociation of cells. H&E. × 320.

the preexisting normal mucosal lining is visible. Dissociation of the neoplastic cells may be evident, the spherical or polygonal cells floating widely separate from one another in loosely textured sheets (Fig. 24). Basement membranes intervening between individual acini may be obliterated, and they may fuse with one another, the entire lobule being converted into a conglomerate mass. Ultimately, the enveloping basement membranes disintegrate and infiltration supervenes. A cellular fibroblastic reaction surrounding the duct or lobule is a disturbing feature, for it may portend imminent infiltration. When, however, a small cell lesion develops in an area of sclerosing adenosis, cellular fibrosis surrounding the affected channels may be related to the preexisting sclerotic process.

Occurrence of Small Cell Lesions

Sections from breast tissue removed for reasons other than invasive carcinoma during the period from 1946 to 1975, inclusive, at the Mount Sinai Hospital, New York, have been reviewed by the author. These specimens were excised primarily for fibrocystic disease; but breast tissue removed together with fibroadenomas and tissues excised during mammoplasty have been included. All specimens found to contain invasive carcinomas, or predominantly large cell in situ carcinomas, have been excluded. Fibroadenomas submitted without surrounding breast tissue are not included.

During this 30-year period, specimens from 4400 patients were received and have been examined. Review of these sections revealed 211 patients with dysplastic small cell proliferations of all grades of severity (4.8 percent). Bilateral lesions were encountered in 8 patients, but systematic biopsy of both breasts has not been performed in this institution. For the period from 1946 to 1967, when it was customary to prepare no more than 1 or 2 blocks per specimen, the occurrence rate of small cell lesions was 2.7 percent of biopsies performed. From 1968 onward, the number of blocks embedded has been progressively increased. A minimum of 5 blocks is now taken per specimen (unless the totally embedded tissue is insufficient for this number); and, if there is reason to suspect the presence of a dysplastic lesion (contralateral carcinoma, suspicious but indefinite structural changes in the initial sections), 10 or 20 blocks may be processed. As may be observed from Table 1, the average occurrence rate during the years 1968 to 1975 was found to be 7.8 percent, with a maximum yield during 1974 of 14.3 percent. We ascribe the higher occurrence rate during these years to improved detection, resulting from more adequate sampling of the tissues, and from increased familiarity with the morphology of the early lesions. Even these occurrence rates probably reflect underestimates, for it is likely that some lesions were overlooked. The focal, and highly limited, nature of the involvement in many instances must be emphasized. We have encountered examples in which lesions have been detected in as few as 1 or 2 of as many as 10 or 20 blocks. The involvement, furthermore, may be highly restricted even in the section in which it is found, affecting no more than a single duct or lobule, or part thereof. Thorough sampling and careful attention to the early basal alterations are mandatory if the lesions are to be identified. The florid examples are conspicuous and will not escape detection, but the initial basal changes are unobtrusive and are not, we believe, being accorded the recognition that they deserve. Thus, occurrence rates of 2.5 percent or lower have been recorded in the literature.[6-8] We suspect that the disparity between these figures and our own reflects a disparity in detection rather than a disparity in occurrence.

Systematic biopsy of the contralateral breast was not performed in these patients. However, McDivitt et al [9] concluded from their studies that positive biopsies of the contralateral breast were to be expected in excess of 30 percent of patients.

TABLE 1. Occurrence of Small Cell Lesions at The Mount Sinai Hospital, 1946–75

Year of Biopsy	No. of Pts. Biopsied *	No. of Pts. with Small Cell Lesions	% of Pts. with Small Cell Lesions
1946–67	2594	71	2.7
1968–75	1806	140	7.8
1968	219	11	5.0
1969	152	11	7.2
1970	174	12	6.9
1971	193	10	5.2
1972	203	13	6.4
1973	219	19	8.7
1974	272	39	14.3
1975	374	25	6.7
Total	4400	211	4.8

* Eight patients had bilateral biopsies at Mount Sinai. Each biopsy is counted in the year in which it occurred.

Location of the Lesions Within the Breast

We have not recorded the particular quadrant(s) of the breast in which the lesions were situated. From the investigation of 9 resected breasts, Lambird and Shelley [7] claimed that the lesions are located mainly in the upper quadrants, beneath the periphery of the areola. Although their examination was detailed, it is doubtful whether any conclusion can be derived from so small a number of specimens. McDivitt et al [9] refer to the affection of multiple quadrants in their fascicle on breast tumors.

Concomitant Changes in the Breast

Small cell lesions may occur in breasts within which no other appreciable abnormality is seen, or in breasts that exhibit varying degrees of nondysplastic epithelial proliferation (eg, papillomatosis, sclerosing adenosis). The small cell changes may be found in areas unaffected by such proliferations, or may be present within them. In view of the indefinable nature of these nondysplastic proliferations, it is virtually impossible to arrive at any conclusion with regard to the relationship between these processes. Epithelial proliferation is so common within the breast that a decision as to what is, or is not, abnormal may be highly arbitrary. Consequently, any attempt to compare the occurrence of small cell lesions in normal breasts as opposed to those with abnormal epithelial multiplications becomes exceedingly difficult, if not impossible. Suffice it to observe that only 13.0 percent of patients surveyed exhibited significant degrees of (nondysplastic) epithelial proliferation in addition to their small cell lesions.

Calcification is not a frequent finding in the actual small cell lesion, having been detected in only 17 percent of patients. The actual occurrence may be somewhat greater than this, for it is not improbable that some fine calcifications were overlooked. Even, however, if this possibility is taken into consideration, it is doubtful whether the occurrence of radiologically detectable calcifications in these lesions exceeds 50 percent. Dependence, therefore, upon mammography for the detection of small cell lesions in either the patient or the specimen will result in a substantial deficit. Thus, Hutter [10] recorded positive mammograms in only 37 out of 87 patients with positive histologic findings. Although specimen radiography may be employed to confirm the presence in the excised tissue of calcifications seen in the clinical mammogram, it cannot replace adequate random sampling in the selection of material for histology.

Calcifications in small cell lesions were unrelated to the dimension of the lesion. Some calcifications, furthermore, may well have anteceded the dysplastic proliferation, for they are commonly observed in nondysplastic processes, and may, on occasion, merely have been included in the dysplastic mass as it effaced the preexisting lining.

Involvement of fibroadenomas has been observed but rarely, occurring in only 6 cases. However, it should be noted that fibroadenomas have not been systematically surveyed in this study. They have only been included when an appreciable quantity of breast tissue was submitted together with the fibroadenoma. The breast tissue, and not the fibroadenoma, has been the primary object of our investigation.

Prognosis of Patients with Small Cell Lesions on Biopsy

Description of Cases Followed for Prognosis

A series of 209 patients with small cell lesions identified at one or more biopsies during the period from 1946 to 1975 at the Mount Sinai Hospital, New York, were followed for the development of invasive breast cancer in the ipsilateral or contralateral breast. Of these patients, 11 had bilateral biopsies performed either at Mount Sinai (8 patients) or at Mount Sinai and other institutions (3 patients). In addition, 20 of these women had a contralateral mastectomy for invasive cancer prior to the biopsy that identified the small cell lesion. In fact, 70 percent of these contralateral mastectomies occurred 5 years or less prior to the biopsy, with an average of 5.4 years (standard deviation, 5.3 years).

Age Distribution at Biopsy

The age distributions for patients found to have small cell lesions at biopsy are given in Table 2 for those patients with and without prior contralateral mastectomy. Haagensen [11] reported a similar age distribution for patients with (presumably) all forms of breast cancer treated at Columbia-Presbyterian Medical Center, New York, although he observed a lower proportion (27 percent) of women in the age group 40 to 49 than we find (42 percent).

Our 178 patients without prior contralateral mastectomy were on the average 48.7 years of age at the time of biopsy and were found to be significantly younger than those 20 women with prior contralateral mastectomy (average age, 54.9 years, student's $t_{196} = 2.6$, $p < 0.01$).

It is well known that women who have had breast cancer may have an in-

TABLE 2. Age Distribution at Biopsy for Patients with Small Cell Lesions *

Age at Biopsy (yr)	Pts. with No Prior Contralateral Mastectomy		Pts. with Prior Contralateral Mastectomy		All Pts.	
	NO.	%	NO.	%	NO.	%
20–29	3	1.7	—	—	3	1.5
30–39	23	12.9	—	—	23	11.6
40–49	76	42.7	8	40.0	84	42.4
50–59	55	30.9	2	10.0	57	28.8
60–69	13	7.3	8	40.0	21	10.6
70–79	5	2.8	2	10.0	7	3.5
80–89	3	1.7	—	—	3	1.5
Total	178	100.0	20	100.0	198	100.0
Average	48.7		54.9		49.5	
Standard error of mean	0.7		2.8		0.7	

* Patients with bilateral biopsies not included.

creased risk of developing breast cancer in the remaining breast. Lewison and Neto [12] reported that 7 to 10 percent of women with breast cancer eventually develop a contralateral lesion.

Since those women who have undergone prior contralateral mastectomy are also older than those without prior contralateral mastectomy, we will consider the two groups separately in further analysis. Patients with bilateral biopsy are also considered separately, since these patients also represent a subgroup with possibly different risk (average age at first biopsy was 49.2 years, standard error of mean, 4.6 years; 73 percent under age 50).

Classification of Small Cell Lesions in Relation to Prognosis

Before we proceed to examine the incidence of invasive breast cancer in patients with small cell lesions, it is appropriate to consider the question of classification as it relates to prognosis. Small cell lesions vary quantitatively and, to a lesser extent, qualitatively from one another. We may, therefore, seek parameters within the group that might be associated with subsequent events. Alternatively, no such attempt may be made. The latter approach has been adopted by those who employ a single designation—either, for example, lobular carcinoma in situ, or lobular neoplasia—in all instances, irrespective of dimension; thereby assuming from the outset prognostic homogeneity for the entire group.

The relationship of lesion size to prognosis does, however, still remain an important, if unresolved, aspect of the problem. Conventional thought holds that the neoplastic transformation of epithelium at any site commences with an initial phase of dysplasia (implying an invasive potential, but not an invasive capability). The process may be arrested at the dysplastic stage, or may progress to the stage of in situ carcinoma (implying an invasive capability). The in situ carcinoma may regress, remain dormant, or, at any time, rupture the basement membrane and invade the connective tissues. Distinction between dysplasia and in situ carcinoma is dependent upon morphologic parameters relating to the number and cytology of the proliferating tumor cells.

Examination of breasts resected for invasive tumors occasions some doubt as to the invariability of the dysplasia–in situ carcinoma sequence presented here. Invasive tumors are often encountered in which the in situ changes are inconspicuous (no more than dysplasia), raising the possibility that invasion may supervene at any stage in the evolution of the in situ lesion, whether it be morphologically dysplasia or in situ carcinoma. Progression to a morphologic in situ carcinoma may not be a prerequisite for infiltration, even though it may be correct that the in situ carcinoma may be more likely to invade than the morphologically less advanced dysplasia. It is even conceivable that the florid dimensions of the in situ carcinoma may, on occasion, have resulted from an ability of the host to contain the lesion within the basement membrane. If this were true, some in situ carcinomas might actually be less dangerous to the patient than the morphologically less impressive dysplasia.

If this thesis is to be tested in the area of mammary small cell lesions, quantity rather than quality of the participating cells would have to form the basis for appraisal. Whereas a limited degree of cytologic variation does occur, the profound cytologic aberrations encountered within in situ changes in other epithelia (eg, squamous epithelium) are not seen. We are thus concerned here essentially with a question of cell numbers. Evaluation of the total cell population present—as indicated by the total extent of ductal and lobular involvement—has not been attempted. Comparative evaluation has been restricted to the dimension attained by the lesion at the site of maximum cellular accumulation. Initial attempts [13] relied upon visual estimates expressed in a simple grading system. This method was, however, seriously deficient in reproducibility.

We have, therefore, more recently essayed, by means of a micrometer placed in the microscope ocular, to measure the square area at the site of greatest cellular accumulation—an indication of cell numbers at that site. The largest, completely involved, spherical, discrete duct or acinus encountered in all sections was measured in two diameters at right angles to one another. The product of these two measurements, expressed in thousands of square micrometers ($10^3 \mu m^2$), was taken as an index of square area, and indirectly of cell numbers, at that location. Where no suitable cross section was observed, a longitudinally sectioned channel was selected —the square of the transverse diameter being utilized. Although far from precise, it is felt that this method is superior to visual estimation of maximum lesion size, and furthermore, that it does provide a more reliable basis for communication with other observers. The system of grading, or the designations dysplasia and in situ carcinoma are no longer employed. All instances are classified as small cell lesions and assigned a numerical value according to the criteria outlined earlier in this section.

The distribution of small cell lesions according to maximum lesion size (MLS) is shown in Table 3 for all patients without bilateral biopsy and for all patients without bilateral biopsy or prior contralateral mastectomy. The median MLS in both groups was $5.6 \times 10^3 \mu m^2$; however, the variability in MLS at biopsy was large, ranging from 0.6 to $412.5 \times 10^3 \mu m^2$.

The 20 cases with prior contralateral mastectomy have an average MLS of $6.6 \times 10^3 \mu m^2$, which is smaller than the average MLS of 13.1 for the 178 cases with no prior contralateral mastectomy ($t_{196} = .76$, $0.2 \leq p \leq 0.3$). While this difference is not statistically significant at the 0.05 level, this observed difference does serve to suggest again that those patients with prior contralateral mastectomy should be considered as a separate subgroup. In addition, these patients may be more likely to undergo biopsy at an earlier stage than noncancer patients, because they are already under continuing medical care.

No associations between age and MLS at biopsy were found in these various subgroups of patients when the data were analyzed using a variety of methods. For example, for the 198 patients without bilateral biopsies, the correlation coefficient between age and MLS was -0.06. Table 4 shows this lack of association for the group without bilateral biopsies or prior contralateral mastectomies. Note, however, that those 20 cases with a prior contralateral mastectomy were older at biopsy and had smaller MLS than the remaining group.

Cumulative Probabilities of Developing Invasive Breast Cancer

The probabilities of developing invasive breast cancer simultaneously with or subsequent to a breast biopsy and diagnosis of small cell lesions were evaluated using life-table methods,[14] which take into account the length of follow-up for each patient. All patients in this series were followed for periods up to 20 years subsequent to biopsy. The average length of follow-up to first diagnosis of invasive breast cancer in either breast (excluding those patients with prior contralateral mastectomy or bilateral biopsy) was 6.05 years (95 percent confidence limits

TABLE 3. Size of Small Cell Lesion at Biopsy *

Maximum Lesion Size ($\times 10^3 \ \mu m^2$)	Pts. with No Prior Contralateral Mastectomy		Pts. with Prior Contralateral Mastectomy		All Pts.	
	NO.	%	NO.	%	NO.	%
Under 1	5	2.8	—	—	5	2.5
1– 1.9	16	9.0	3	15.0	19	9.6
2– 2.9	20	11.2	5	25.0	25	12.6
3– 3.9	30	16.9	1	5.0	31	15.7
4– 4.9	12	6.7	1	5.0	13	6.6
5– 5.9	19	10.7	3	15.0	22	11.1
6– 6.9	12	6.7	—	—	12	6.1
7– 7.9	12	6.7	1	5.0	13	6.6
8– 8.9	5	2.8	—	—	5	2.5
9– 9.9	5	2.8	1	5.0	6	3.0
10–14.9	14	7.9	3	15.0	17	8.6
15–19.9	5	2.8	1	5.0	6	3.0
20–39.9	16	9.0	1	5.0	17	8.6
40 or larger	7	3.9	—	—	7	3.5
Total	178	100.0	20	100.0	198	100.0
Average	13.1		6.6		12.4	
Standard error of mean	2.6		2.8		2.0	

* Patients with bilateral biopsies not included.

TABLE 4. Age by Size of Lesion at Biopsy *

Age (yr)	Size of Lesion ($\times 10^3 \ \mu m^2$)			TOTAL
	UNDER 5.0	5.0–9.9	10.0 OR LARGER	
Under 50	43	31	28	102
50 or older	39	22	15	76
Total	82	53	43	178

$$\chi\frac{2}{2} = 1.90 \quad 0.5 \geq p \geq 0.25$$

* Bilateral biopsies and prior contralateral mastectomies not included.

[C.L.], 5.08 to 7.02 years) with 50 percent of the cases followed for longer than 3.9 years.

Cumulative probabilities of surviving free of invasive breast cancer in both breasts, in the ipsilateral, and in the contralateral breast for periods of up to 20 years were computed for the 178 patients without bilateral biopsy or prior contralateral mastectomy, for the 11 patients with bilateral biopsy, as well as for those 20 patients with prior contralateral mastectomy. In addition, these probabilities were derived for the 165 patients without a contralateral mastectomy at the time of biopsy.

The data were also stratified by age at biopsy and lesion size in order to examine the effects of these factors on prognosis.

All instances of noninvasive breast cancer, deaths or losses to follow-up, and live withdrawals due to the cutoff date for analysis (Jan. 1, 1976) are included as withdrawals in the survival analysis.* One year intervals are used to develop the cumulative probabilities of developing invasive breast cancer.

Results

The 20-year cumulative risk of developing a first invasive breast cancer in either breast among 178 women with small cell lesions without prior contralateral mastectomy or bilateral biopsy is .28 or 28 percent with 95 percent C.L. from 17 to 39 percent. Table 5 and Figure 25 show the cumulative probabilities of invasive

* Eleven patients were lost to follow-up and 12 died prior to any diagnosis of invasive breast cancer.

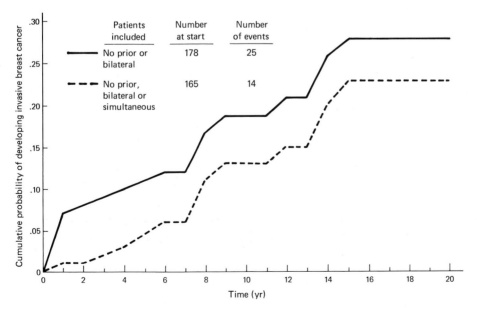

Fig. 25. Cumulative probabilities of developing a first invasive breast cancer in women with small cell lesions.

TABLE 5. Probability of Developing Invasive Breast Cancer in at Least One Breast Following Biopsy for Small Cell Lesion *

Period After Biopsy (yr)	No. of Cases at Start	No. with Breast Cancers in Interval	Withdrawn in Interval	Proportion with Breast Cancer in Interval	Cumulative Proportion Free of Breast Cancer ($\hat{P}$)	Cumulative Probability of Breast Cancer ($1 - \hat{P}$)	Standard Error of P
0– 1	178	12	29	0.07	0.93	0.07	0.0204
1– 2	137	1	20	0.01	0.92	0.08	0.0215
2– 3	116	1	20	0.01	0.91	0.09	0.0230
3– 4	95	1	6	0.01	0.90	0.10	0.0248
4– 5	88	1	9	0.01	0.89	0.11	0.0267
5– 6	78	1	10	0.01	0.88	0.12	0.0290
6– 7	67	0	7	0.0	0.88	0.12	0.0290
7– 8	60	3	10	0.05	0.83	0.17	0.0384
8– 9	47	1	4	0.02	0.81	0.19	0.0417
9–10	42	0	1	0.0	0.81	0.19	0.0417
10–11	41	0	1	0.0	0.81	0.19	0.0417
11–12	40	1	2	0.03	0.79	0.21	0.0456
12–13	37	0	2	0.0	0.79	0.21	0.0456
13–14	35	2	1	0.06	0.74	0.24	0.0532
14–15	32	1	3	0.03	0.72	0.28	0.0568
15–16	28	0	4	0.0	0.72	0.28	0.0568
16–17	26	0	4	0.0	0.72	0.28	0.0568
17–18	22	0	1	0.0	0.72	0.28	0.0568
18–19	21	0	2	0.0	0.72	0.28	0.0568
19–20	19	0	3	0.0	0.72	0.28	0.0568
20 and longer	16	—	16	—	—	—	—

* Excluding prior contralateral mastectomy and bilateral biopsy.

breast cancer for this group. Eleven of the invasive tumors were contralateral growths that were resected simultaneously with the biopsy that detected the small cell lesion in the ipsilateral breast. Note that the remaining cases of invasive breast cancer occurred throughout the first 15 years of the observation period (column 3, Table 5). For those 165 patients who were free of any simultaneous contralateral tumor, either invasive or noninvasive, at the time of biopsy, the 20-year cumulative risk of developing a first invasive breast cancer in either breast is 23 percent with 95 percent C.L. 11 to 35 percent. The incidence curve is also given in Figure 25 for this group.

Table 6 gives the cumulative risk of invasive cancer in the ipsilateral breast for the 178 women without prior contralateral mastectomy or bilateral biopsy. The 20-year cumulative incidence for the ipsilateral breast is 19 percent, 95 percent C.L., 8 to 30 percent. Comparable rates are given in Table 7 for the contralateral breast. The cumulative incidence of invasive breast cancer for the contralateral breast is 14 percent, 95 percent C.L., 6 to 22 percent. There is no difference between 20-year risks to the ipsilateral and contralateral breasts (normal deviate $z = 0.74$, $p = 0.46$). Figure 26 compares the cumulative incidences of invasive breast cancer for the ipsilateral and contralateral breasts.

Prognosis for patients without prior contralateral mastectomy or bilateral biopsy by age is given in Table 8, since the risk of developing breast cancer increases with age,[15] and the women under age 50 at biopsy were followed for slightly longer periods of time in this study. While the numbers of events are small in each subgroup, and the rates therefore unstable, the 15-year cumulative risk of develop-

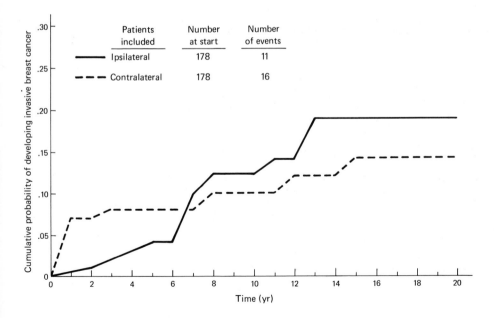

Fig. 26. Cumulative probabilities of developing ipsilateral or contralateral invasive breast cancer in women with small cell lesions.

TABLE 6. Probability of Developing Ipsilateral Invasive Breast Cancer Following Biopsy for Small Cell Lesion *

Period After Biopsy (yr)	No. of Cases at Start	No. with Breast Cancers in Interval	Withdrawn in Interval	Proportion with Breast Cancer in Interval	Cumulative Proportion Free of Breast Cancer ($\hat{P}$)	Cumulative Probability of Breast Cancer ($1 - \hat{P}$)	Standard Error of $\hat{P}$
0– 1	178	0	31	0.0	1.00	0.0	—
1– 2	147	0	24	0.0	1.00	0.0	—
2– 3	123	1	23	0.01	0.99	0.01	0.0089
3– 4	99	1	9	0.01	0.98	0.02	0.0137
4– 5	89	1	9	0.01	0.97	0.03	0.0178
5– 6	79	1	10	0.01	0.96	0.04	0.0218
6– 7	68	0	7	0.0	0.96	0.04	0.0218
7– 8	61	3	11	0.05	0.90	0.10	0.0356
8– 9	47	1	4	0.02	0.88	0.12	0.0401
9–10	42	0	1	0.0	0.88	0.12	0.0401
10–11	41	0	1	0.0	0.88	0.12	0.0401
11–12	40	1	2	0.03	0.86	0.14	0.0450
12–13	37	0	2	0.0	0.86	0.14	0.0450
13–14	35	2	1	0.06	0.81	0.19	0.0545
14–15	32	0	3	0.0	0.81	0.19	0.0545
15–16	29	0	2	0.0	0.81	0.19	0.0545
16–17	27	0	4	0.0	0.81	0.19	0.0545
17–18	23	0	1	0.0	0.81	0.19	0.0545
18–19	22	0	2	0.0	0.81	0.19	0.0545
19–20	20	0	4	0.0	0.81	0.19	0.0545
20 and longer	16	—	16	—	—	—	—

* Excluding prior contralateral mastectomy and bilateral biopsy.

TABLE 7. Probability of Developing Contralateral Invasive Breast Cancer Following Biopsy for Small Cell Lesion *

Period After Biopsy (yr)	No. of Cases at Start	No. with Breast Cancers in Interval	Withdrawn in Interval	Proportion with Breast Cancer in Interval	Cumulative Proportion Free of Breast Cancer ($\hat{P}$)	Cumulative Probability of Developing Breast Cancer ($1 - \hat{P}$)	Standard Error of $\hat{P}$
0– 1	178	11	24	0.07	0.93	0.07	0.0193
1– 2	143	1	22	0.01	0.93	0.07	0.0204
2– 3	120	1	22	0.01	0.92	0.08	0.0219
3– 4	97	0	6	0.0	0.92	0.08	0.0219
4– 5	91	0	10	0.0	0.92	0.08	0.0219
5– 6	81	0	10	0.0	0.92	0.08	0.0219
6– 7	71	0	8	0.0	0.92	0.08	0.0267
7– 8	63	1	10	0.02	0.90	0.10	0.0267
8– 9	52	0	4	0.0	0.90	0.10	0.0267
9–10	48	0	1	0.0	0.90	0.10	0.0267
10–11	47	0	3	0.0	0.90	0.10	0.0267
11–12	44	1	2	0.02	0.88	0.12	0.0333
12–13	41	0	2	0.0	0.88	0.12	0.0333
13–14	39	0	1	0.0	0.88	0.12	0.0333
14–15	38	1	4	0.03	0.86	0.14	0.0404
15–16	33	0	2	0.0	0.86	0.14	0.0404
16–17	31	0	5	0.0	0.86	0.14	0.0404
17–18	26	0	2	0.0	0.86	0.14	0.0404
18–19	24	0	2	0.0	0.86	0.14	0.0404
19–20	22	0	18	0.0	0.86	0.14	0.0404
20 and longer	18		20	—	—	—	—

* Excluding prior contralateral mastectomy and bilateral biopsy.

ing a first invasive breast cancer $(1 - P_{15})$ for the 102 women under age 50 is 23 percent (95 percent C.L., 9 to 37 percent). Seven of the 10 events in this subgroup occurred after the first year of follow-up. The corresponding incidence for women 50 to 64 at biopsy is somewhat greater, 33 percent with 95 percent C.L., 13 to 53 percent. Six of the 11 events in this age group occurred after year 1. This risk of developing invasive cancer is not significantly greater among the 50 to 64 year olds than among the younger women $(Z = 0.81, p = 0.42)$.

The risk of developing invasive cancer in the ipsilateral and contralateral

TABLE 8. Cumulative Probabilities of Developing Invasive Breast Cancer Within *t* Years After Diagnosis of Invasive Breast Cancer $(1 - \hat{P}_t)$ by Age at Biopsy and by Maximum Lesion Size *

Age at Biopsy		FIRST INVASIVE CANCER	IPSILATERAL INVASIVE CANCER	CONTRALATERAL INVASIVE CANCER
Under 50:	Number in group	102	102	102
	Number of events	10	7	5
	$1 - \hat{P}_5$ (s.e.)	0.05(0.026)	0.02(0.019)	0.03(0.018)
	$1 - \hat{P}_{10}$ (s.e.)	0.13(0.048)	0.10(0.046)	0.06(0.031)
	$1 - \hat{P}_{15}$ (s.e.)	0.23(0.069)	0.20(0.070)	0.09(0.044)
50–64:	Number in group	64	64	64
	Number of events	11	4	7
	$1 - \hat{P}_5$ (s.e.)	0.16(0.036)	0.06(0.040)	0.11(0.042)
	$1 - \hat{P}_{10}$ (s.e.)	0.25(0.079)	0.16(0.079)	0.11(0.042)
	$1 - \hat{P}_{15}$ (s.e.)	0.33(0.103)	0.16(0.079)	0.18(0.141)
65 and over:	Number in group	12	12	12
	Number of events	4	0	4
	$1 - \hat{P}_1$ (s.e.)	0.35(0.141)	—	0.35(0.141)
Maximum Lesion Size $(\times 10^3 \; \mu m^2)$				
<5.0:	Number in group	82	82	82
	Number of events	9	4	6
	$1 - \hat{P}_5$ (s.e.)	0.10(0.041)	0.05(0.035)	0.05(0.026)
	$1 - \hat{P}_{10}$ (s.e.)	0.19(0.068)	0.14(0.068)	0.09(0.045)
	$1 - \hat{P}_{15}$ (s.e.)	0.25(0.080)	0.14(0.068)	0.15(0.068)
5.0–9.9:	Number in group	53	53	53
	Number of events	7	3	5
	$1 - \hat{P}_5$ (s.e.)	0.08(0.039)	0	0.08(0.039)
	$1 - \hat{P}_{10}$ (s.e.)	0.17(0.071)	0.10(0.066)	0.08(0.039)
	$1 - \hat{P}_{15}$ (s.e.)	0.24(0.093)	0.17(0.094)	0.16(0.082)
≥10.0:	Number in group	43	43	43
	Number of events	9	4	5
	$1 - \hat{P}_5$ (s.e.)	0.16(0.062)	0.04(0.036)	0.13(0.055)
	$1 - \hat{P}_{10}$ (s.e.)	0.22(0.079)	0.10(0.070)	0.13(0.055)
	$1 - \hat{P}_{15}$ (s.e.)	0.38(0.117)	0.28(0.127)	0.13(0.055)

Event spans the FIRST INVASIVE CANCER, IPSILATERAL INVASIVE CANCER, and CONTRALATERAL INVASIVE CANCER columns.

* Patients with prior contralateral mastectomy or bilateral biopsy excluded.
s.e., standard error.

breasts by age at biopsy is also shown in Table 8 for the group of 178 patients. Women under 50 have a slightly lower 15-year cumulative risk of invasive breast cancer for the contralateral breast—9 percent with 95 percent C.L., 0 to 18 percent —than for the ipsilateral breast—20 percent with 95 percent C.L., 6 to 34 percent. The women aged 50 to 64 have equivalent ipsilateral and contralateral risks at this latter level (Table 8).

Prognosis is also examined in relation to maximum lesion size at biopsy (small, under $5.0 \times 10^3 \mu m^2$; moderate, 5.0 to $9.9 \times 10^3 \mu m^2$; large, greater than or equal to $10.0 \times 10^3 \mu m^2$). Results are shown in Table 8 for the group of 178 women. The 15-year cumulative risk of developing a first invasive cancer in either breast for women with small lesions is 25 percent (95 percent C.L., 8 to 42 percent), equivalent to the risk for the 53 women with moderate-size lesions. The elevated risk for the 43 women with large lesions, 38 percent with 95 percent C.L., 15 to 41 percent, is not significantly different from the risk for women with small lesions ($Z = 0.83$, $p = 0.41$). The cumulative risks are also given by lesion size for the ipsilateral and contralateral breasts separately.

Examination of these 15-year cumulative probabilities suggests that the lesion size is not related to the risk of subsequent invasive cancer, although the risks may be slightly greater in the ipsilateral breast in women with large lesions (greater than or equal to $10.0 \times 10^3 \mu m^2$).

Prognosis of Patients with Prior Contralateral Mastectomy or Bilateral Biopsy

In the group of 20 cases with prior contralateral mastectomy, 2 subsequent ipsilateral invasive breast cancers were identified at 6 and 15 years after biopsy. The median follow-up period for this subgroup was 2 years with an average of 3.4 years of observation. Of those 11 cases with bilateral biopsies, 3 had simultaneous bilateral mastectomies for noninvasive cancer, and 3 subsequent invasive mastectomies were performed in this group with a 12-year cumulative rate of developing invasive breast cancer in 1 breast of 36 percent.

Discussion

McDivitt et al [9] reported a 20-year cumulative risk of invasive breast cancer in the ipsilateral breast of 35 percent in a series of 40 patients, most of whom were followed for longer than 10 years. Hutter et al [15] reported that 15 of 46 patients with lobular carcinoma in situ subsequently developed 20 cancers within 4 to 27 years (14/40 [35 percent] ipsilateral, 6/46 [13 percent] contralateral). Actuarial estimates of cumulative risk are not reported, however. On the other hand, Wheeler et al [16] reported a 20-year cumulative ipsilateral rate of 4.4 percent (95 percent C.L., 0 to 13 percent) based on 1 event in 25 women and a 20-year cumulative contralateral rate of 11.7 percent (95 percent C.L., 0 to 26 percent) based on 3 events in 32 women.

This considerably larger series of 178 patients (exclusive of those with bilateral biopsy or prior contralateral mastectomy) followed at Mount Sinai Hospital for periods up to 20 years have a 20-year risk of developing invasive breast cancer in one or both breasts of 28 percent (95 percent C.L., 17 to 39 percent). There is no difference between the rate of 19 percent (95 percent C.L., 8 to 30 percent) in the contralateral breast and 14 percent (95 percent C.L., 6 to 22 percent) in the ipsilateral breast. While no statistically significant differences (at the 0.05 level) were found in prognosis with respect to age or size of lesion at time of biopsy, there may be an elevated risk of a first invasive breast cancer in either breast of women over 50 and in women with large lesions.

Further data may indicate that younger women (under 50 at diagnosis) have a poorer prognosis for the ipsilateral breast and that women with large lesion size (greater than or equal to $10 \times 10^3 \mu m^2$) may also have a poorer prognosis for the ipsilateral breast.

The average follow-up in this series was 6 years, with half the population followed for 3.9 years or less. The invasive carcinomas observed in this series were detected throughout the period of follow-up. As additional patients accrue and as follow-up periods on our current patients lengthen, the interpretation of these results may then become clear because the estimates of risk will become more precise.

It should be noted that the cases described here represent a selected group on whom biopsies were performed for some medical reason and in whom small cell lesions were therefore diagnosed. As such, this group may represent a subgroup of patients at greater risk of invasive cancer than those patients in whom the fortuitous diagnosis of small cell lesion was never made because no biopsy was ever performed. For example, the relative risk of developing breast cancer in 5 years is 2.1 times greater for women reporting a history of breast lump at an initial screening examination than for women not reporting this symptom (adjusted for age at screening and parity.[17]) It is also possible, however, that the observed prognosis in this series may represent the true course of this disease.

In addition, no information was available for these patients with respect to other potential risk factors for the development of breast cancer, such as age at first pregnancy, parity, and administration of hormones.

The 25 cases of first invasive breast cancer observed in this series of 178 patients represent an incidence of invasive breast cancer 15.4 times greater than the expected incidence of 1.6 cases computed from the Connecticut Cancer Registry data [18] for a population with the same age composition and years of exposure to risk. Note, however, that women harboring small cell lesions are not necessarily comparable to the general population of women at risk of developing breast cancer, on which the Connecticut data are based.

Histology of Invasive Tumors in Patients with Small Cell Lesions

As may be noted from Table 9, less than 50 percent of all invasive tumors were composed solely of small cells. These purely small cell cancers were usually trabecular (Fig. 14). In some instances, glandular differentiation was present. A majority, however, of the invasive tumors encountered in these patients exhibited large cell elements, with or without associated small cell populations. The large cell category thus comprises tumors composed solely of large cells, and composite tumors containing both small and large cells. Some of the large cells, as mentioned

**TABLE 9. Invasive Carcinomas in Patients with Small Cell Lesions
Classified by Cell Size**

Location and Timing	Small	Large	Unknown	Total
Subsequent ipsilateral	7 (43.8)	8 (50.0)	1 (6.3)	16
Prior contralateral	7 (35.0)	10 (50.0)	3 (15.0)	20
Simultaneous contralateral	6 (54.6)	5 (45.4)	—	11
Subsequent contralateral	—	5 (100.0)	—	5
Total	20 (38.5)	28 (53.9)	4 (7.7)	52

Percentages given in parentheses.

previously, may have resulted from the enlargement of preexisting small cells; others may have had independent origins. These large cell tumors exhibited, again, trabecular formations with, in some instances, glandular differentiation. It is noteworthy that even in the ipsilateral breast, large cell tumors were encountered in numbers at least equal to small cell tumors. The presence, therefore, of a small cell lesion does not necessarily signify that a subsequently developing invasive tumor will be of small cell type. The small cell lesion may evolve directly into a subsequently appearing small or large cell invasive tumor, or may, on other occasions, be no more than a harbinger denoting the action of a carcinogen that may ultimately evoke an invasive cancer derived from a different source.

Conclusion

The uncertain behavior of the in situ lesion, wherever it be located, must impose considerable restraints upon the therapist. Insofar as the breast is concerned, the risk of subsequent invasive carcinoma would appear to be of the order of 19 percent in the ipsilateral breast, with an almost equivalent risk to the contralateral side. Although the risk would appear to be somewhat greater than that to which the general population is exposed, there must be serious question as to whether ablative surgery can be justified on the basis of present evidence; more particularly since it is impossible to predict which breast will be affected by the subsequent invasion. Although available data are not yet sufficient for a definitive statement on the relationship, if any, between lesion size and prognosis, there is at present no firm evidence to support the belief that the quantitatively greater lesion is more dangerous than the lesser. There can, therefore, be no present basis for the division of the lesions into the categories of dysplasia and in situ carcinoma, with the implied differences in prognosis inherent in these terms. Therefore, until definite evidence to the contrary is obtained, it is appropriate that a single designation should be applied to the entire group, irrespective of dimension. Terminology is a matter of individual choice. We prefer the designation "in situ small cell lesion" or "in situ small cell tumor" to that of "in situ small cell carcinoma" because the term is less forceful, and less likely to produce an overreaction on the part of either clinician or patient.

The development of invasive carcinoma is an event that may occur over a period of many years. It is evident that prolonged periods of time may be involved.

These time factors call, again, for a conservative approach in the elderly and for those patients with concomitant disease. They call, too, for prolonged observation. This consideration may be overlooked by the clinician, who may monitor the patient intensively in the initial months or years after detection of the lesion, only to diminish his vigilance as time passes without further developments. Furthermore, prolonged observation is mandatory, if valid information is to be accumulated in relation to the incidence of subsequent invasive cancer in these patients.

Many decades have passed since Ewing illustrated the distinctive lobular change that he considered to be precancerous, and since Foote and Stewart set forth the concept of "lobular carcinoma in situ." Yet many problems pertaining to the pathogenesis and prognosis of this enigmatic lesion remain unresolved. The paucity of cases in any one facility remains a limiting factor in statistical evaluation. It is doubtful whether further advances in our understanding will be achieved by the endeavors of single observers in single institutions. The accumulation of data adequate for satisfactory statistical analysis will, we believe, require a collaborative effort of national dimension.

References

1. Ewing J: Neoplastic Diseases, 1st ed. Philadelphia, Saunders, 1919
2. Foote FW, Stewart FW: Lobular carcinoma in situ: A rare form of mammary cancer. Am J Pathol 17:491, 1941
3. Toker C: Some observations on Paget's disease of the nipple. Cancer 14:653, 1961
4. Toker C: Observations on the ultrastructure of a mammary ductule. J Ultrastruct Res 21:9, 1967
5. Tobon H, Price HM: Lobular carcinoma in situ: Some ultrastructural observations. Cancer 30:1082, 1972.
6. Giordano JM, Klopp CT: Lobular carcinoma in situ: Incidence and treatment. Cancer 31:105, 1973
7. Lambird PA, Shelley WM: The spatial distribution of lobular in situ mammary carcinoma: Implications for size and site of breast biopsy. JAMA 210:689, 1969
8. Andersen JA: Lobular carcinoma in situ: A long-term follow-up in 51 cases. Acta Pathol Microbiol Scand [A] 82:519, 1974
9. McDivitt RW, Stewart FW, Berg JW: Atlas of Tumor Pathology, Second Series. Fascicle 2, Tumors of the Breast. Washington, DC, Armed Forces Institute of Pathology, 1968
10. Hutter RVP, Snyder RE, Lucas JC, Foote FW, Farrow JH: Clinical and pathologic correlation with mammographic findings in lobular carcinoma in situ. Cancer 23:826, 1969
11. Haagensen CD: Diseases of the Breast, 2nd ed. Philadelphia, Saunders, 1971
12. Lewison EF, Neto AS: Bilateral breast cancer at The Johns Hopkins Hospital. Cancer 28:1297, 1971
13. Toker C: Small cell dysplasia and in situ carcinoma of the mammary ducts and lobules. Mt Sinai J Med NY 40:780, 1973
14. Chiang CL: Introduction to Stochastic Processes in Biostatistics. New York, J Wiley, 1968
15. Hutter RVP, Foote FW, Jr: Lobular carcinoma in situ: Long-term follow-up. Cancer 24:1081, 1969.
16. Wheeler JE, Enterline HT, Roseman JM, et al: Lobular carcinoma in situ of the breast: Long-term follow-up. Cancer 34:554, 1974

17. Shapiro S, Goldberg J, Venet L, Strax P: Risk factors in breast cancer—a prospective study. IARC Scientific Publications No. 7, Host Environment Interactions in the Etiology of Cancer in Man. International Agency for Research on Cancer, Lyons, France, 1973, pp 169–82
18. Doll R, Payne P, Waterhouse J (eds): UICC. Cancer Incidence in Five Continents. New York, Springer-Verlag, 1966

APPLICATIONS OF PLASMA—THROMBIN CELL BLOCK IN DIAGNOSTIC CYTOLOGY

Part I: Female Genital and Urinary Tracts

ETTORE DE GIROLAMI

During the past 25 years, the ever increasing use of diagnostic cytology as a screening method has demonstrated the possibility of uncovering occult neoplasia in tissues that appear entirely normal on clinical examination. The discovery of malignant cells in such cases has necessitated a change in the histologic methods required to prove the malignant nature of the disease and to determine whether the lesion was infiltrating or preinvasive. For instance, the "ring" or "cone" biopsy with serial sections has been developed, and experienced cytologists can usually predict with a high degree of accuracy that cancer will be found by the pathologist if enough sections are cut. Through the application of cellular diagnosis, a new phase of cancer study was brought into the realm of diagnosis and research.

It is through the method of cytologic smears that early detection of malignancy is performed today throughout the world. However, the spontaneous detachment of cells from tissues does not necessarily occur as single cells, but more often as clusters of cells. Therefore, when smears are prepared, cells are artificially separated. This altered relationship among cells is more readily observed in fresh material obtained from the endometrium, sputum, bronchial washings, gastric washings, voided urine, bladder washings, effusions, and breast needle aspirations. Our first observation of this problem dates back to 1964 [1] when we were studying endometrial material obtained from over 500 women treated with norethynodrel plus mestranol. We then noticed that it was difficult and often impossible to phase the endometrium correctly since only cell characteristics were available for study. Furthermore, diagnoses like cystic, adenomatous, or atypical hyperplasia were impossible to make on the basis of the examination of single cells. We then thought that instead of separating the cells by preparing smears, it would be justifiable to apply the principle of blood clotting to the material obtained. In such a way, the intercellular relationships and morphologic features of tissues in human organs could be maintained. Thus, we decided to cover the material obtained from the endometrium with several drops of plasma, and to that, we added a few drops of thrombin in order to entrap cells within the artificial blood clot. The clot was then fixed in 15 percent formalin, processed in paraffin, and stained like a tissue specimen.

Since 1964, we have been applying this procedure of plasma–thrombin cell block not only to endometrial specimens but also to urine, gastric washings, effusions, sputum, and bronchial washings, varying slightly the original method when necessary. The object of this chapter is to present our findings after more than 10 years of experience and to emphasize the advantages of studying clusters of cells rather than isolated cells in the diagnosis of neoplastic or other pathologic processes.

Materials and Basic Methods

Plasma

The plasma can be obtained from the blood bank or from the coagulation division of a laboratory. Preferably, it should be refrigerated at 4 C. Pooled plasma can be used.

Thrombin

The thrombin solution may be made from powdered thrombin, commercially available in vials of 1000 or 5000 NIH U.* In preparing solutions of thrombin, saline or distilled water should be used. The amount of diluent depends upon the degree of thrombin activity desired. For the cell block technique, we have found it satisfactory to use a solution that was prepared by adding 1 ml of saline or distilled water to each 1000 units. The thrombin solution, if stored near the freezer unit of the refrigerator, retains its clotting properties for at least 1 month. Since its activity decreases with time, it is advisable to test it periodically by combining two drops of plasma with two drops of thrombin in a watchglass and checking the clot formation time, which should occur within approximately 30 seconds.

If the thrombin activity decreases, larger amounts of solution will then be needed to form a clot with plasma. The sample for study can be fluid or more formed specimens, such as endometrium or mucoid material from sputum.

All fluids (urine, voided or catheterized; washings of bronchi, bladder, stomach, endometrium; effusions and breast needle aspirations) are treated in similar fashion. The sample is centrifuged for about 10 minutes at 1500 to 2000 rpm. After the supernatant fluid is decanted (for bronchial and gastric washings, see specific method), the centrifuged sediment is drained by gently inverting the glass tube on a filter paper so that the last drop of supernatant is absorbed, leaving a dry sediment. To the sediment within the test tube, three or four drops of plasma are added. The specimen is gently detached from the bottom of the tube with a

* Bovine thrombin, topical from Parke, Davis and Co., Detroit, Michigan, or the Upjohn Co., Kalamazoo, Michigan.

wooden applicator stick so as to obtain proper permeation of the plasma. Three or four drops of thrombin are then added, using the applicator stick in the same manner. The plasma–thrombin mixture is allowed to clot; this usually takes 1 or 2 minutes; otherwise let the tube stand for about 10 minutes (Fig. 1C). Occasionally, it is necessary to add more plasma or thrombin. When a small amount of fluid is sent to the laboratory, such as washings or catheterized urine from renal pelvis or needle aspirations from breast cysts, it is helpful to use a blood bank serofuge tube so that the tiny amount of sediment can be concentrated in the bottom of a

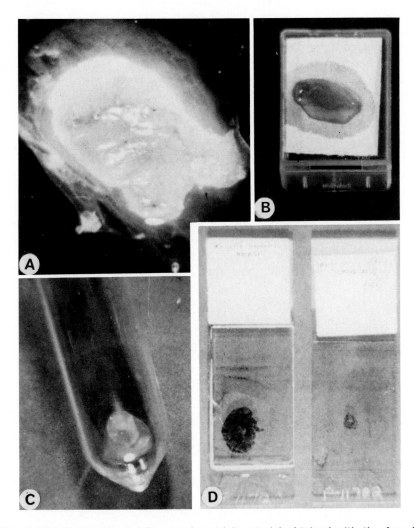

Fig. 1A. Artificial clot prepared from endometrial material obtained with the Ayre brush using the plasma–thrombin cell block (PTCB). **B.** Clot prepared from a urine sediment in receptacle lined with filter paper. **C.** Typical PTCB in conical centrifuge tube prepared from urine sediment. **D.** Two sections of PTCB. The left slide is the first of 200 sections from a bladder-washing sediment, and the right one is the last section.

small tube. If the sediment is minimal, add only one drop of plasma and one drop of thrombin. Ideally, the size of the clot should be proportional to the quantity of the sediment available; otherwise, the sediments become excessively diluted, risking difficulty in locating the specimen in the paraffin block.

The clot containing the entrapped sediment is now carefully transferred to a paraffin receptacle, the bottom of which is lined with a piece of filter paper (Fig. 1B). The use of filter paper seems to be essential, because the protein within the clot will become firmly attached to the paper during fixation, thus protecting the specimen from getting lost during processing. The clot is then stained with a drop of eosin to allow easier identification at the time of paraffin embedding and cutting. The receptacle is closed and then placed into a beaker containing 15 percent formalin along with the other tissue specimens to be processed. At least 30 minutes should be allowed for clot fixation (Fig. 2).

The method of preparing cell blocks of more formed specimens such as endometrium or sputum will be described later in this chapter.

For the embedding of cell blocks, the following precautions should be taken:

1. Remove cell block receptacle from the melted paraffin beaker.
2. On opening the receptacle, the cell block clot will be found attached to the filter paper liner.
3. By folding the filter paper convexly, the clot should be easily raised, removed, and transferred to the embedding surface.
4. Continue routine embedding procedures as used for histologic preparations. Tissue sections of cell blocks are cut 4 μm thick and stained with the Papanicolaou technique; two slides are usually prepared routinely. Recently, we have found it useful for diagnosis to stain an extra slide with hematoxylin and eosin, and if special stains are needed, the paraffin block is available (Fig. 1D).

The cell block slides should be screened as smears using 10× objective. Although the material is all concentrated in a small area, low-power examination with a 4× objective is not advisable. In fact, the preparation is really a combination of a smear and a tissue section with isolated cells and fragments of tissue. Consequently, the proper approach to reading the slide is by systematic screening.

In our experience, we have noticed that in the beginning technicians may be reluctant to look at cell block slides. Cytotechnicians are accustomed to read smears and are not familiar with tissue sections. At first, we have found it convenient to prepare routine smears and cell blocks simultaneously and to look at both preparations side by side.

When cytologists and cytotechnicians gain some familiarity in reading cell blocks, they will find themselves greatly rewarded and more secure in the diagnosis. This is because they will find that the preservation of cells or clusters is vastly superior to that seen with smear preparations, especially when there is blood, inflammation, or necrosis.

In order to minimize difficulties in microscopic reading, we would advise that, after deparaffinization, cell blocks be stained with the Papanicolaou technique,

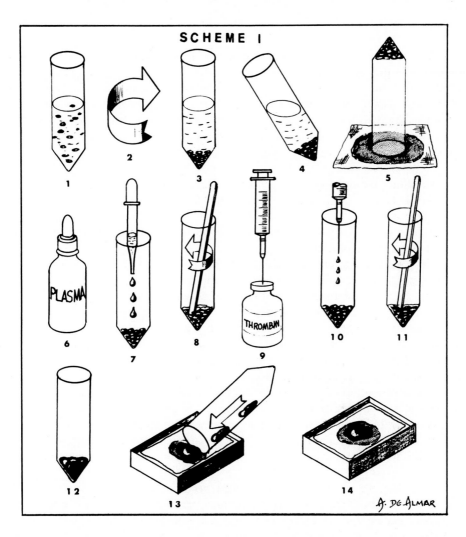

SCHEME I

Fig. 2. Technique for preparing plasma–thrombin cell blocks. 1. Fluid sample. 2. Centrifuge. 3. Sediment forms. 4. Decant supernatant. 5. Dry excess supernatant over filter paper. 6. Plasma. 7. Add 3 drops of plasma to sediment. 8. Gently stir with wooden applicator stick to permit the plasma to permeate the sediment. 9. Thrombin with syringe. 10. Add 3 drops of thrombin. 11. Gently stir the sediment with wooden applicator stick to allow thrombin to form clot. 12. Clot forms. 13. Transfer clot to receptacle. 14. Clot ready to be processed.

and that the slides be included in the same staining rack with routine smears. With experience, different staining techniques could be applied. The use of hematoxylin and eosin in staining cell blocks seems potentially useful in laboratories lacking cytotechnicians and where the pathologist may be required to screen all cytologic material.

General Information

The application of cell block techniques to cytologic material derived from body fluids and other sources has been under study since the beginning of the century. Various modifications have been proposed, all aiming toward better tissue sections.[2-9] Since 1964, this laboratory has been preparing the majority of the material submitted for cancer detection using the plasma–thrombin method.

The advantages in using the plasma–thrombin cell block procedure over the conventional cytologic method include the following:

1. The entire sediment is entrapped and available for study.
2. The sediment is concentrated in a small area, thus permitting faster microscopic study.
3. As a result of formalin fixation, the nuclear and cytoplasmic details are similar to those of tissue sections.
4. Since sections are cut uniformly at 4 μm, there is no cellular overlapping and the specimen is evenly distributed throughout the sections.
5. The presence of blood and other debris, which makes reading of cytologic slides difficult, is not a problem.
6. In cases of low-grade malignancy, because cellular cohesion is greatest, more clusters of cells are seen, whereas in conventional cytologic specimens, contacts between cells are destroyed artificially, thereby increasing the complexity of diagnosis (eg, benign papillomas and papillary carcinoma of the bladder).
7. The preservation of isolated normal and malignant cells is excellent.
8. Because a paraffin block is available, we can perform serial sections, special stains, and keep material at hand if further studies are necessary.
9. The cell block preparation is particularly useful in those centers where cytotechnicians are not available and the pathologist must read his own slides.

Two features of this technique which need to be emphasized are that cell block preparation takes as long as routine paraffin sections (12 hours), and secondly, that the final cell block slide may at times show clusters of cells that look more like a histologic section than a smear.

Specific Organ Systems

Endometrium

The ordinary vaginal smear is clearly not adequate for detecting endometrial carcinoma. Ayre,[10] in an effort to improve the accuracy of the cytodiagnosis of endometrium, designed an endometrial brush to be used routinely as a simple office technique. Boutselis and Ullery [11] described a cannula for obtaining endometrial material for cytologic studies. Gravlee [12] has been using a negative pressure irrigation technique for detecting endometrial lesions, and Jensen,[13] an endometrial aspiration cannula. Similar procedures with a satisfactory diagnostic accuracy have been described by different authors, some using the Gravlee Jet Washer,[14-18] others the Vabra Aspirator described by Jensen,[19-26] and others with different methods.[27-30] We have been using these approaches of direct endometrial study since 1964, first with the Ayre brush,[10] * then the Jet Washer,[12] and later the Vabra Aspirator of Jensen.[13] Applying the plasma–thrombin technique, we have modified the original way of preparing the samples. Our main purpose was to see if we could study clusters rather than separate cells, so as to try to detect precancerous conditions of the endometrium (eg, adenomatous hyperplasia and atypical hyperplasia). In using the Ayre endometrial brush, we [1] use the following technique: After removing the brush from the uterus, the endometrial tissue is expressed from the bristles with a glass slide onto a second glass slide (Figs. 3A, B, and 4), two or three drops of plasma are placed on the surface of the tissue, and then two or three drops of thrombin are added; these two solutions permeate the tissue and form a clot in less than a minute (Fig. 1A). This clot is then transferred to a paraffin receptacle, the bottom of which is lined with filter paper. The clot is stained with a drop of eosin, and then the receptacle is closed and placed into a beaker containing 15 percent formalin. Our first results with the Ayre brush were published 10 years ago,[1] and we continued to use this procedure for several years until the brush ceased to become commercially available. After 1971, we started to receive material obtained with the jet irrigation method described by Gravlee.[12] † A variety of techniques have been used for preparing material obtained with jet irrigations.[14-18] It is possible to use the plasma–thrombin method on centrifuged specimens obtained from a Gravlee washing of the uterine cavity (Fig. 3C and Fig. 4). We have been satisfied with the results obtained using this procedure. Due to the size and poor flexibility of the cannula, however, it may be difficult to insert it into the endocervical canal, particularly in postmenopausal women.

Recently, we have been receiving endometrial samples that were obtained with the Vabra Aspirator described by Jensen.[13] This unit has the advantage that the cannula is thin and easily inserted through a stenotic endocervical canal. The patient may experience only a transient cramping discomfort, and abundant endometrial tissue can be obtained for processing. The disadvantage of this method may be in the cost of the disposable unit, but its accuracy according to our experience is comparable to a conventional curettage. Several articles have appeared in the literature using the Vabra Aspirator ‡ techniques.[19-26]

To perform our own modification of the procedure described in previous publications (Fig. 4), we need the entire instrument including the plastic container and the aspiration metallic cannula, after which the following technique is used:

1. Fill a large conical centrifuge tube with 40 ml of saline.
2. Cover tightly the two pressure-equalizing holes with a tape.
3. Remove the plastic cap, and to the site connected with the vacuum source, attach a 2-inch-long rubber tube that is attached to a 12 ml syringe.

---

* Clay Adams Inc., New York, N.Y.
† Available from Upjohn Co., Kalamazoo, Mich.
‡ Available from Cooper Laboratories, Inc., Parsippany, N.J.

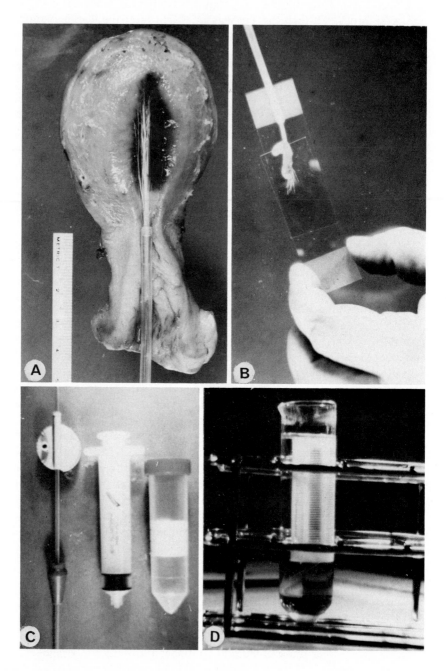

Fig. 3A. Endometrial brush with bristle exposed in uterine cavity. **B.** Expression of endometrial tissue from bristle of brush onto glass slide. **C.** Gravlee Jet Washer set. **D.** Plastic filter of Vabra Aspirator in conical centrifuge tube containing saline, after centrifugation.

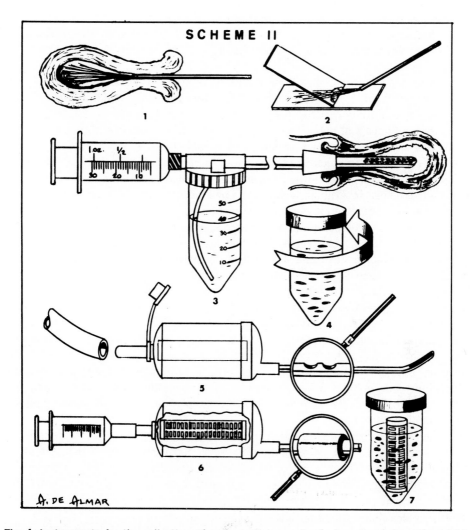

Fig. 4. Instruments for the collection of endometrial sample. 1. Ayre brush in endometrial cavity. 2. Expression of endometrial tissue from bristle. 3. Gravlee Jet Washer in endometrial cavity. 4. Washed fluid is centrifuged and processed with plasma-thrombin. 5. Vabra Aspirator showing left to right spout to be attached to suction pump, tubular chamber with filter inside, cannula with magnification of suction release holes. 6. Cross section of Vabra Aspirator showing left to right syringe with rubber tube attached to spout, filter in tubular chamber, with magnification of taped suction release holes to allow aspiration of saline. 7. Conical centrifuge tube containing saline, filter, and tissue fragments.

4. Place the cannula in a centrifuge tube, and suction saline into container. Lift out, shake well, and expel. Repeat the procedure until all fragments are removed.
5. Transfer the cylindrical plastic filter into a centrifuge tube, since it usually catches fragments of tissue.
6. Centrifuge the material up to 2000 rpm for 10 minutes.
7. Decant the supernatant, and add plasma and thrombin to the sediment as previously indicated (Fig. 3D and Fig. 4).

The quality of cell block preparation obtained using the Ayre brush, the Gravlee Jet Washer, and the Vabra Aspirator are comparable. However, with the Vabra, a more consistent quantity of material is available for study. Material prepared with the cell block technique is similar to a routine histologic section of endometrium and sometimes results in a combination of small clusters of cells and larger tissue fragments. Using the plasma–thrombin technique, we never noticed any difficulty due to the presence of red blood cell contamination, nor have we had difficulty in evaluating the specimen because of the intense background staining that is often seen in Nucleopore membrane filter preparations.

According to Bibbo et al,[15] using the Gravlee Jet Washer, the best specimens were obtained with the regular cell smear, the Millipore preparation ranked second, and Nucleopore third. The histologic material had a higher percentage of inadequate specimens than the cytologic material. Their results differed from those of So-Bosita et al,[18] who reported the highest incidence of accurate diagnosis using cell block preparations. Harris et al,[17] after comparing their results with the cell block preparations performed with plasma–thrombin and with those with the 3 percent agar technique, came to the following conclusions: When adequate material was present in the endometrial Jet Wash sample both methods were equally satisfactory, but when only minute microscopic tissue fragments were present, the 3 percent agar method proved superior; and when the sample was scanty and visible tissue fragments were not present, the plasma–thrombin method proved superior.

Our own experience, based on applying the plasma–thrombin technique to material obtained from the endometrial brush, the Gravlee Jet Washer, and the Vabra Aspirator was that we obtained practically the same results whether we had small fragments, scanty material, or large amounts of material. When the sample was taken with the Ayre brush, the amount of material obtained from the bristles was usually minimal, and the plasma–thrombin cell block still provided excellent results for us, especially if compared to cytologic smears. When the plasma–thrombin technique was applied to satisfactory material obtained from the Jet Washer, it usually seemed sufficient for diagnosis. Certain difficulties in obtaining an adequate sample may arise when dealing with patients with atrophic endometrium or with a stenotic cervical os. In these cases only an endocervical sample was often obtained. Using the Vabra Aspirator, there was a higher incidence of good samples of endometrium, possibly because of the thinner metallic cannula.

The Ayre wooden spatula was devised for the purpose of scraping cells directly from the squamocolumnar junction of the cervix and offers the advantages of the direct approach to the developing lesion. After a number of years of experience, we feel confident of being able to detect early malignancy and in anticipating premalignant changes so as to follow the patient, if necessary, until surgery is needed. This can be done with conventional cytologic smears by identifying cells of severe inflammation, mild or severe dysplasia, and carcinoma.

Using a direct approach to endometrial lesions through endometrial devices, cytology alone is incapable of giving comparable results to those obtained with cervical smears because (a) the tissue is obviously different (one is squamous, the other is columnar with glands dispersed within a more or less loose stroma), and (b) the uterine cervix is visible and relatively easy to approach with direct scraping, while the endometrium is more remote. For these reasons, we have tended to disregard the usefulness of cytologic smears from endometrial samples, and we have attempted to search for a method to view these specimens in a way that would be as comparable as possible to a histologic section. We first achieved this aim in applying the principle of blood clotting (plasma–thrombin) to samples obtained with the Ayre brush and later with the Vabra Aspirator. The plasma–thrombin clot does in fact keep all the material together. In addition, when the specimen is placed in formalin, the fixation of the plasma proteins is especially helpful in maintaining the endometrial fragments together, so that the cell block sections are very similar to tissue sections. We would agree with So-Bosita et al [18] that the cell block method is more reliable than endometrial smears in reflecting the histologic status of the endometrium.

In our experience, the endometrial specimens were obtained mainly from patients in the childbearing age in order to detect ovulation (Fig. 5A) and from postmenopausal women to exclude premalignant or malignant lesions (Fig. 5B and C). In cases of adenocarcinoma of endometrium, the cell block section frequently shows tissue fragments (Fig. 5E) and sometimes only small clusters of malignant cells that are well preserved (Fig. 5D). Failure in obtaining acceptable preparations seems most often due to the method of collecting the specimens. We reached this conclusion because material obtained with Vabra Aspirator yields cell block sections that are quantitatively superior.

In conclusion, we underscore the importance of detecting precancerous lesions of the endometrium today, when the number of postmenopausal women treated with hormones has increased greatly, and this can best be done with histologic or histologiclike preparations. Regardless of the office method used in collecting endometrial specimens, the availability of histologiclike section is ideal. We have documented that the plasma–thrombin cell block technique serves this purpose.

Urinary System

Exfoliative cytology, as an effective method for the detection of urothelial tumors, has not received the same acceptance as in other organs because reliable slide preparations are difficult to obtain; urine hypertonicity frequently causes cell degeneration; and low-grade malignant cells may be indistinguishable from normal cells lining the bladder wall.

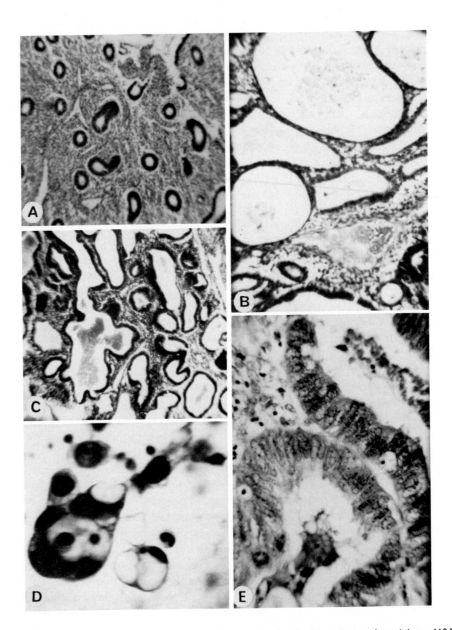

Fig. 5A. PTCB prepared from Gravlee Jet Washer sample. Proliferative endometrium. H&E. × 110. **B.** PTCB prepared from a sample obtained with Ayre endometrial brush. Cystic hyperplasia. H&E. × 102. **C.** PTCB prepared from Vabra Aspirator. Adenomatous hyperplasia. H&E. × 72. **D.** PTCB prepared from endometrial brush. Cell clusters of adenocarcinoma. Papanicolaou [Pap] stain. × 600. **E.** PTCB prepared from Vabra Aspirator. Adenocarcinoma of endometrium. Notice well-defined nuclear detail. Pap stain. × 290.

Most laboratories in this country and abroad that have reported the use of various cell preparations following Papanicolaou's technique have found the major problem to be the lack of adequate numbers of cells to examine following fixation and staining. In fact, there is a tendency for the cells to wash off the slide during the fixation and staining procedure because urine is lacking in mucus, which is necessary for cells to stick to the glass slide. In order to overcome this problem of cell adhesiveness, a variety of techniques have been proposed by different authors.[31-53]

In all the various methods, basic cytologic procedures, utilizing Papanicolaou's technique, were employed and isolated cells were the main object of study. More recently, Harris et al,[8] in reviewing the application of several techniques to urinary cytology, described a cell block preparation that makes use of 3 percent agar. Since 1965, our laboratory has been actively engaged in preparing a cell block technique for urine, bladder washings, and kidney irrigation through a method based on infiltrating the sediment with plasma–thrombin as described previously in this chapter.

The early morning sample of voided urine (200 to 300 ml) is considered satisfactory. In sediments containing heavy amounts of urates, the clotting seems to be more difficult. In catheterized specimens, if the sample is small (less than 3 ml), we advise the use of a blood bank serofuge tube for concentrating the sediment. Bladder washings are obtained by irrigation with 50 to 75 ml of sterile saline solution; thereafter, the bladder was emptied. Renal pelvis specimens are similarly collected using only 10 ml of sterile saline. If this fluid appears cloudy after collection, the sediment usually contains a good amount of cellular material. Occasionally, for therapeutic reasons, the bladder or renal pelvis is washed with thiotepa. Because the thiotepa solution seems to facilitate desquamation of malignant urothelial tissue, more material is present in this cell block preparation. However, the cells undergo morphologic changes caused by the chemical action of the drug. Renal pelvic washings with thiotepa are obtained in the following manner: 60 mg of thiotepa are dissolved in 30 ml of sterile distilled water. Next, 10 ml are instilled in the renal pelvis through the urethral catheter and held there for a period of 10 minutes. This solution of thiotepa is withdrawn from the renal pelvis by suction and replaced by another 10 ml, which is also allowed to remain in the renal pelvis for 10 minutes. The procedure is repeated a third time. All the specimens are centrifuged separately, and three different cell blocks are prepared. In this way, we have been following patients—one of them for a period of several years—treated medically for urothelial tumors of the bladder and of the renal pelvis.[54]

Much time and effort have been spent in trying to correlate the various clinical and pathologic classifications in use for malignant urothelial tumors. Though there is still obvious disagreement, one of the fundamental problems is to decide when certain histopathologic characteristics can predict malignant behavior. In low-grade epithelial tumors especially, morphology should run parallel to clinical findings. In our experience, continued follow-up of patients with cytologic study of the urine is of great value in predicting prognosis, particularly in low-grade malignancy. Even if urinary cytology is currently not accepted as a reliable screening method for early detection of urothelial tumor, cytodiagnosis still has an incomparable value in following these patients, since these tumors are characteristically recurrent and multicentric.

The traditional cytologic criteria for the diagnosis of inflammatory lesions and of low- and high-grade transitional tumors are summarized in Table 1. For the number of years that we have followed these criteria, we have found that, with the exception of those tumors classified as grades III and IV, the correct diagnosis was often impossible. The plasma–thrombin technique, which we originally had been using for endometrial specimens for some years, seemed ideally suited to improve our cytodiagnostic acumen in the study of urine sediment.[54, 55] The advantages of using the plasma–thrombin procedure in urine sediment are the same as previously described. Furthermore, in cases of low-grade malignancy (papilloma and papillary carcinoma), because cellular cohesion is greatest, more clusters of cells are seen, whereas in conventional cytologic specimens, contacts between cells are destroyed artificially, thereby increasing the complexity of diagnosis. The microscopic diagnosis of cell block sections not only requires cytopathologic knowledge but also a certain familiarity with the histopathology of the urinary tract. During the years that we have been studying samples obtained from the urinary tract, we have formulated and followed a convenient cytohistologic set of criteria for diagnosis which is summarized in Table 2.

TABLE 1. Cytologic Characteristics of Urothelial Lesions

	Inflammation		*Transitional Cell Carcinoma*	
	ACUTE	CHRONIC	GRADE I	GRADE II–IV
Grade of Exfoliation	+	++++	++	+++
Cytoplasmic characteristics				
Volume	+−	++++	++	+++
Polymorphism	+	+++	+	+++
Irregular border	+	++	+	+++
Degeneration	+++	+		+
Staining	Variable in accordance to cellular viability			
Vacuoles		+++		+
Basophilic inclusions	+	++		(+)
Nuclear characteristics				
Polynuclei		+++		+
Volume		+++	+	+++
Shape		+		+++
Chromatin clumping	Pyknosis	Regular and large granules	Coarse reticulum	Irregular and coarse reticulum
N/C * ratio		−	(+)	+++
Mitosis				++
Number of nucleoli		++	+	++
N/n † ratio				++

* Nuclear/cytoplasmic.
† Nuclear/nucleolar.

TABLE 2. Characteristics of Transitional Cell Carcinoma in Cell Block

	Grade I	*Grade II*	*Grade III*	*Grade IV*
Cellular exfoliation	+	++	+++	+++
Cellular polymorphism		+	++	+++
Nuclear volume and hyperchromatism		+	+++	+++
Small clusters	+	+	++	+
Large clusters with central vessel	+	++	+	
Free cells		+	+++	+++
Cellular cohesion	+++	++	+	+
Mitosis		+	++	++
Palisading	+++	+		
Scallops		++	+	
Cytoplasmic eosinophilia			+	+++
Pearl formation				(+)

A certain number of isolated urothelial cells, originating from the superficial layer of the transitional epithelium, are normally exfoliated daily. These so-called umbrella cells overlie four or five layers of pear-shaped cells, which may assume a cuboidal or flattened shape depending on the state of distention of the bladder. When specimens are obtained from bladder washings, especially in individuals harboring a certain degree of inflammation, the cell block sections may show fragments of normal transitional cell mucosa (Fig. 6A). The presence of neutrophils, blood, and increased exfoliation of superficial cells seems to be a very reliable index in diagnosing acute inflammation (Fig. 6B). Trichomonads can be seen in cell blocks of voided urine specimens (Fig. 6C).

We recently had occasion to examine the urine of an 8-year-old girl from Angola. Her main complaint was painless hematuria. The cell block of voided urine revealed the presence of several well-preserved *Schistosoma haematobium* (Fig. 7A, C through E). Surrounding the parasites, several giant cells and clusters of eosinophils were also noticed (Fig. 7B).

In cases of transitional cell tumors, the sections of the plasma–thrombin cell block usually show an abundant number of desquamated cells (Fig. 8). In cases of grade I transitional cell carcinoma (so-called benign papilloma), because of the degree of intercellular adhesiveness, the malignant cells have the tendency to desquamate in clusters. Frequently, the cells are aligned in a palisade (Fig. 9A), with a central capillary core surrounded by elongated cells with oval-shaped nuclei (Fig. 9B). In preparations of grade II transitional cell carcinoma (so-called papillary carcinoma), the cellular exfoliation is increased. The cells desquamate singly, in small or large clusters, with or without centrally placed blood vessels. If fragments of tissue with a papillary pattern are seen, they are characterized by a central vascular core surrounded by irregularly distributed cells (Fig. 9C). These features are usually diagnostic for a papillary bladder tumor. Clusters of cells with a papillary arrangement and a central vascular core are mainly seen only in grade I and grade II transitional cell tumors. At times, small compact clusters without central vascular core can be seen (Fig. 9D). These fragments show loss of cellular polarity, nuclear hyperchromasia, and occasional mitotic figures. A

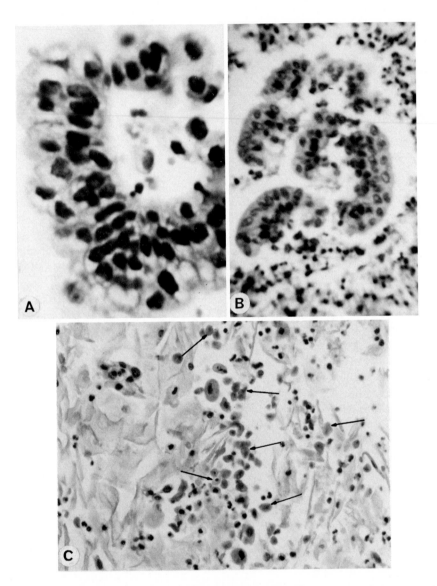

Fig. 6A. PTCB of voided urine. Fragment of normal urothelial mucosa showing umbrella cells at the periphery and pear-shaped cells in deeper layers. Pap stain. × 370. **B.** PTCB of voided urine. Clusters of urothelial cells surrounded by inflammatory cells. Pap stain. × 190. **C.** PTCB of voided urine. On the left are squamous epithelial cells and in the center are numerous *Trichomonas vaginalis* (arrows) with a few urothelial cells. H&E. × 180.

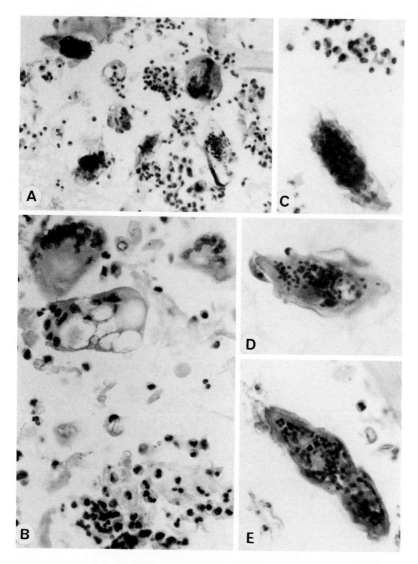

Fig. 7A. PTCB of voided urine. S. *haematobium* with giant cells and clusters of inflammatory cells. H&E. × 145. **B.** PTCB of voided urine, same as 7A. Notice three giant cells and marked eosinophilic reaction. H&E. × 325. **C–E.** Voided urine PTCB. S. *haematobium* three high-power views. Notice the good preservation of the parasite. H&E. × 315.

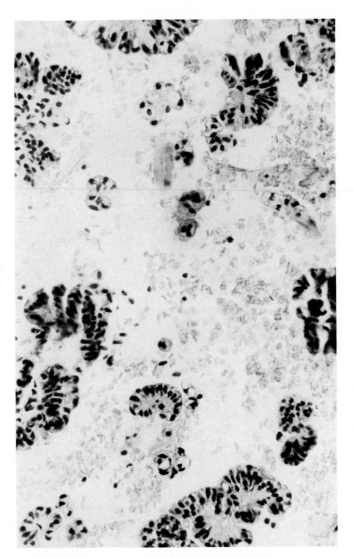

Fig. 8. PTCB of voided urine. Several papillary clusters without a central vascular core in a case of transitional cell carcinoma, grade II. Pap stain. × 162.5.

Fig. 9A. (See facing page) PTCB of voided urine. Clusters of urothelial cells aligned in a palisade as in grade I transitional cell carcinoma. Pap stain. × 130. B. PTCB of voided urine. Central vascular core surrounded by palisade alignment of urothelial cells with oval hyperchromatic nuclei as in papillary transitional cell carcinoma, grade I. Pap stain. × 465. C. PTCB of bladder washing. Large fragment with vascular central core surrounded by multiple layers of irregularly distributed urothelial cells with nuclear hyperchromasia as seen in papillary transitional cell carcinoma, grade II. Pap stain. × 127.5. D. PTCB of voided urine. Scattered small and large clusters without a central vascular core showing cells irregularly distributed as in grade II transitional cell carcinoma. Pap stain. × 185.

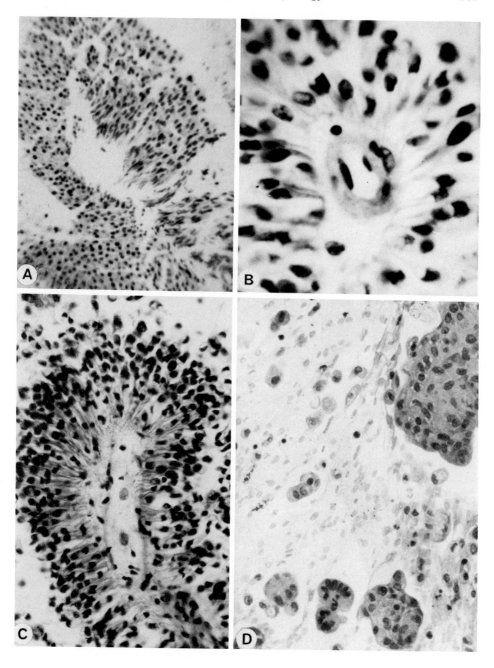

scalloped distribution of the outside layer with the irregular polarity of the remaining inner cells is characteristic (Fig. 10A and B).

In grade III transitional cell carcinoma, because the cellular cohesion is decreased, one of the striking features is the marked increase of isolated malignant cells similar to what is often observed in smear preparations (Fig. 10C). Sections of cell blocks may show marked cellular exfoliation, polymorphism, nuclear hyperchromatism, and mitotic figures (Fig. 10D). Occasionally, if the tumor is very friable, small and large clusters of cells are present. In transitional cell carcinoma grade IV (squamous cell carcinoma) as in grade III carcinoma, the cellular cohesion is minimal, resulting in abundant exfoliation of single cells, which differ from grade III carcinoma cells because their cytoplasm is eosinophilic and the nucleus shows severe hyperchromasia (Fig. 11A). In these cases, pearls, tadpoles, and spindle-shaped, highly eosinophilic cells may be present (Fig. 11B).

A total of 484 patients with a urinary disorder have had cytodiagnostic tests over the past 10 years as part of the routine work-up. Of these, 315 were male and 169 were female. All had at least one cytologic test. Those with positive biopsies have been followed with serial cytologic analysis of voided urine or bladder washing. Among the total of 1,570 tests, 484 consisted of primary cytoanalysis, 892 were follow-ups of positive cases, and 194 were follow-ups of negative cases. Surgical biopsies were taken in all cases with a positive cytology except for 7 cases that were excluded for clinical reasons.

Biopsy specimens were classified as carcinoma grades I, II, III, and IV. The primary cytoanalysis for the 484 patients was performed on 433 samples of voided urine, 5 bladder washings, and 46 catheterized specimens from the kidney. The cytologic results are summarized in Table 3 according to sex and method of collection.

A total of 372 negative, 26 suspicious, and 86 positive cases were recorded. In this study of urothelial tumors, positive cases were about three times as common in males as in females. The frequency of occurrence was greatest in males in the age group of 60 to 70 years, and in females in the age group of 65 to 75. Histopathologic diagnoses were confirmed in 79 of the 86 positive cases, and the results are summarized in Table 4.

At the first cytologic testing, 7 cases were negative; however, on repeat cytologic tests, 4 of the 7 missed cases were correctly diagnosed. The other negative

TABLE 3. Cytologic Results in 484 Patients with Urinary Tract Complaints

Sample	Result	Total	Male	Female
Voided urine	Negative	332	210	122
	Suspicious	24	19	5
	Positive	77	59	18
Bladder washings	Positive	5	5	—
Renal pelvis	Negative	40	20	20
	Suspicious	2	1	1
	Positive	4	1	3
Total		484	315	169

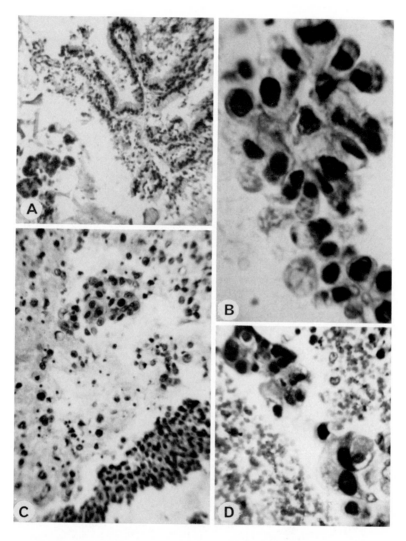

Fig. 10A. PTCB of voided urine. Notice, in the lower left corner, clusters with scalloped distribution of the outside layer. The right upper corner shows a fragment of columnar epithelium that was mucin-positive. Multiple biopsies confirmed our cytologic diagnosis of cystitis cystica with papillary transitional cell carcinoma, grade II. Pap stain. × 110. **B.** PTCB of voided urine. Nuclear hyperchromasia, irregular cell distribution with peripheral scalloping of the cytoplasm as is seen in transitional cell carcinoma, grade II. Pap stain. × 465. **C.** PTCB of voided urine. Notice clusters and scattered isolated malignant cells, a feature characteristic of transitional cell carcinoma, grade III. Pap stain. × 95. **D.** PTCB of voided urine. Marked nuclear hyperplasia with irregular polarity and loose cellular cohesion as seen in transitional cell carcinoma, grade III. Pap stain. × 365.

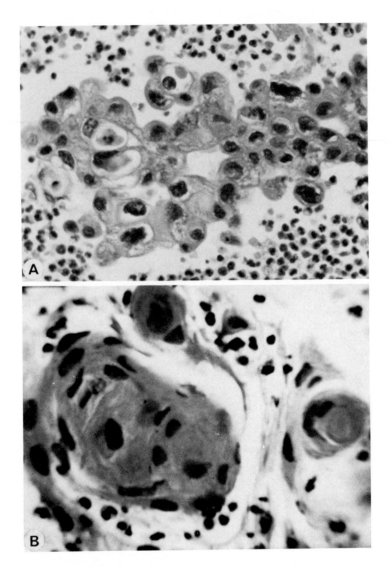

Fig. 11A. PTCB of voided urine. Sheets of cells with eosinophilic cytoplasm, hyperchromatic irregular nuclei and loose cellular cohesion, as can be seen in transitional cell carcinoma of bladder, grade IV. Pap stain. × 365. **B.** PTCB of voided urine. Malignant pearl and tadpole cells in transitional cell carcinoma of bladder, grade IV. Pap stain. × 465.

TABLE 4. Histopathologic Diagnoses of Cytologic Positive Cases

Diagnosis	Urine	Bladder Washings	Kidney
Transitional cell Ca,* grade I	8	2	—
Transitional cell Ca, grade II	21	2	
Transitional cell Ca, grade III	30	—	2
Transitional cell Ca, grade IV	6	—	2
Adenocarcinoma of bladder	1		—
Ureter: Transitional cell—Ca, grade II	2		
Urethra: Squamous cell carcinoma	1		
Kidney: Adenocarcinoma	2		
Total	71	4	4

* Ca: Carcinoma.

cases were nonurothelial tumors that are notoriously difficult to diagnose by urinary cytology. Often when cystoscopy was negative, the cell block preparation showed the presence of malignant cells. Because of these highly significant repeat positive cases, the urologists were alerted to keep these patients under constant observation. In fact, 44 repeat biopsies were reported as follows: 7, grade I carcinoma; 15, grade II; 12, grade III; 6, grade IV; 1, radiation changes; and 3, negative.

In conclusion, the application of the plasma–thrombin cell block technique to urine samples is very reliable for the primary diagnosis of urothelial tumors. This procedure becomes even more important when used as a routine method to follow the course of patients with previous positive biopsies.

Acknowledgments

The author is very grateful to Mrs. Anita C. Day, Debra A. Grabauskas, and Jean MacLauchlan Carvalho for their help during the many years they have worked in cytopathology preparing and reading cell block material; to Mrs. Irene O'Connor, my secretary, for the preparation of the manuscript; to Mr. Aben De Almar for the diagrams; and to Doctor Umberto De Girolami, my son, for his patient cooperation in reviewing the manuscript.

References

1. De Girolami E, Gahres EE, Nelson RB: Instrument and method: Histo-brush technic for endometrial tissue study. Obstet Gynecol 28:861, 1966
2. Bahrenburg LPH: On the diagnostic results of the microscopical examination of ascitic fluid in two cases of carcinoma involving the peritoneum. Cleveland Med Gaz 11:274, 1896
3. Mandlebaum FS: The diagnosis of malignant tumors by paraffin sections of centrifuged exudates. J Lab Clin Med 2:580, 1917
4. Chapman CB, Whalen EJ: The examination of serous fluids by the cell-block technic. N Engl J Med 237:215, 1947

5. Sirtori C: Personal communication, 1948
6. Tonelli L, Alati E: Tenniche e criteri classici ed originali nella citodiagnostica del carcinoma polmonare. Recenti progressi in medicina. Pensiero Scientifico 12:3, 1952 (reprint)
7. Weinberg T: The use of glass fiber paper as an absorbent in the tissue laboratory, a preliminary report. J Mt Sinai Hosp 24:1342, 1957
8. Harris MJ, Keebler CM, Schwinn CP: Cytopreparatory techniques in urinary cytology. Am Soc Clin Pathol, Continuing Education Program No. C31, 1976
9. Shackelford RI, Jones JL: An embedding medium for permanent sections of exudative material and fragments of tissue removed for biopsy. Am J Clin Pathol 32:397, 1959
10. Ayre JE: Rotating endometrial brush: New technic for the diagnosis of fundal carcinoma: Obstet Gynecol 5:137, 1955
11. Boutselis J, Ullery JC: Cannula for obtaining endometrial material for cytologic study. Obstet Gynecol 20:265, 1962
12. Gravlee LC: Jet-irrigation method for the diagnosis of endometrial adenocarcinoma: Its principle and accuracy. Obstet Gynecol 34:168, 1969
13. Jensen JG: Vacuum curettage: Out-patient currettage without anaesthesia. A report of 350 cases. Dan Med Bull 17:199, 1970
14. Abate SD, Edwards CL, Vellios F: A comparative study of the endometrial jet-washing technic and endometrial biopsy. Am J Clin Pathol 58:118, 1972
15. Bibbo M, Shanklin DR, Wied GL: Endometrial cytology on jet wash material. J Reprod Med 8:90, 1972
16. Dowling EA, Gravlee LC, Hutchins KE: A new technique for the detection of adenocarcinoma of the endometrium. Acta Cytol 13:496, 1969
17. Harris M, Bibbo M, Rao C, Wied GL: Cytopreparatory techniques for the endometrial jet wash specimens. Acta Cytol 16:508, 1972
18. So-Bosita J, Lebherz T, Blair O: Endometrial jet washer. Obstet Gynecol 36:287, 1970
19. Barnett JM: Suction curettage on unanesthetized outpatients. Obstet Gynecol 42:672, 1973
20. Bjerre BA, Gardmark SA, Sjoberg NJA: Aspiration curettage: A new diagnostic method. Reprod Med 7:221, 1971.
21. Cohen CJ, Gusberg SB, Koffler D: Histologic screening for endometrial cancer. Gynecol Oncol 2:279, 1974
22. Denis R, Barnett JM, Forbes SE: Diagnostic suction curettage. Obstet Gynecol 42:301, 1973
23. Hamilton JV, Knab DR: Suction curettage: Therapeutic effectiveness in dysfunctional uterine bleeding. Obstet Gynecol 45:47, 1975
24. Holt EM: Outpatient diagnostic curettage. J Obstet Gynaecol Br Commonw 77:1043, 1970
25. Jensen JG: Three years experience of vacuum curettage. Acta Obstet Gynecol Scand 50, 1971 (reprint)
26. Walters D, Robinson D, Park RC, Patow WE: Diagnostic outpatient aspiration curettage. Obstet Gynecol 46:160, 1975
27. Abramson D, Driscoll S: Endometrial aspiration biopsy. Obstet Gynecol 27:381, 1966
28. Gondos B: Recent developments in the cytologic diagnosis of vaginal, endometrial and ovarian cancer. Ann Clin Lab Sci 4:420, 1974
29. Hammond DO, Seckinger DL, LeDrew L: Endometrial cellular study: A new method using membrane filtration. Acta Cytol 11:181, 1967
30. Jimenez-Ayala M, Vilaplana E, Becerro C, et al: Endometrial and endocervical brushing techniques with a Medosa cannula. Acta Cytol 19:557, 1975
31. Papanicolaou GN, Marshall VF: Urine sediment smears as diagnostic procedure in cancers of urinary tract. Science 101:519, 1945

32. Nieburgs HE: Cytologic Technics for Office and Clinic. New York, Grune, 1956, p 233

33. Sagi ES, MacKenzie LL: An improved procedure for the cytological examination of urinary sediment. Cancer Cytol 1:24, 1958

34. Solomon CR: Amelar RD, Hyman RM, Chaiban R, Europa DL: Exfoliated cytology of the urinary tract: A new approach with reference to the isolation of cancer cells and the preparation of slides for study. J Urol 80:374, 1958

35. Seal SH: A method for concentrating cancer cells suspended in large quantities of fluid. Cancer 9:866, 1956

36. Cullen TH, Popham RR, Voss HJ: An evaluation of routine cytological examination of the urine. Br J Urol 39:615, 1967

37. Faide M, Eckert WG, Patterson JN: A comparison of a simple centrifuge method and the millipore filter technique in urinary cytology. Acta Cytol 7:199, 1963

38. Harpst HC, Ware RE, Eisenberg RB, O'Dell JB: Exfoliative cytology of the urinary tract: Evaluation of the millipore technic. Acta Cytol 5:195, 1961

39. Kern WH: The cytology of transitional cell carcinoma of the urinary bladder. Acta Cytol 19:420, 1975

40. Kern WH, Bales CE, Webster WW: Cytologic evaluation of transitional cell carcinoma of the bladder. J Urol 100:616, 1968

41. Merritt JW, Enderson WB, Slate TA: A simplified filter technic for cytologic detection of urinary malignancies. J Urol 82:396, 1959

42. Taft PD, Arizaga-Cruz JM: A comparison of the cell block, Papanicolaou and millipore filter technics for the cytologic examination of serous fluids. Am J Clin Pathol 34:561, 1960

43. Taylor JN, MacFarlane EWE, Ceelen GH, Doolittle K: Cytological studies of urine by millipore filtration technique: Preliminary report. J Urol 88:704, 1962

44. Taylor JN, MacFarlane EWE, Ceelen GH: Cytological studies of urine by millipore filtration technique: Second annual report. J Urol 90:113, 1963

45. Trott PA: Cytological examination of urine using a membrane filter. Br J Urol 39:610, 1967

46. Umiker W: Accuracy of cytologic diagnosis of cancer of the urinary tract. Acta Cytol 8:186, 1964

47. Levy E, Jerusalem K: Experience with cytologic examination of urines with the assistance of multiple parallel methods with and without clinical indication of tumor. Acta Cytol 17:121, 1973

48. Allegra SR, Fanning JP, Streker JF, Corvese NM: Cytologic diagnosis of occult and "in-situ" carcinoma of the urinary system. Acta Cytol 10:340, 1966

49. Chierego F, Fabris P, Pizzetti F: La Citologia dell'Apparato Urogenitale. Milan, Ambrosiana, 1957, p 130

50. Esposti PL, Zajicek J: Grading of transitional cell neoplasms of the urinary bladder from smears of bladder washings. Acta Cytol 16:529, 1972

51. Harris MJ, Schwinn CP, Marrow JW, Gray RL, Brownell BM: Exfoliative cytology of urinary bladder irrigation specimens. Acta Cytol 15:385, 1971

52. Gill WB, Lu CT, Thomsen D: Retrograde brushing: A new technique for obtaining histologic and cytologic material from ureteral and renal pelvic and renal calyceal lesions. J Urol 109:573, 1973

53. Bibbo M, Gill WB, Harris MJ, et al: Retrograde brushing as a diagnostic procedure of ureteral, renal pelvic and renal calyceal lesions. A preliminary report. Acta Cytol 18:137, 1974

54. Constantian H, De Girolami E: Urothelial tumors detected by cytology: A new cell block technique. J Urol 109:304, 1973

55. De Girolami E: Cell block technic for urinary cytology. Bull Pathol 10:127, 1969

CAT-SCRATCH DISEASE

J.A.H. CAMPBELL

Cat-scratch disease (CSD) is an infectious process characterized by mild constitutional symptoms and a prominent lymphadenopathy in the drainage area of a visible or presumed cat scratch. The disease was given this name by Debre et al [1] because he found it almost always followed close contact with cats; but the alternative view that the scratch was more important than the cat led Mollaret et al [2] to suggest the name benign lymphoreticulosis of inoculation.

The clinical and pathologic similarity between CSD and lymphogranuloma venereum has led many people to believe that a virus or chlamydia is the causative agent; yet the use of routine and special bacteriologic media, embryonated eggs, tissue culture, and inoculation of a wide variety of animals have not resulted in an isolation. [3-7]

The discovery of CSD was a rather leisurely process, for although its existence had been suspected by French and North American workers since 1931, the first published descriptions of the disease did not appear until 1950. [1] In reading its romantic history as told by Carithers, [8] one can only marvel at the civilized manners of yesteryear's pathologists who gave discoverer's honors to Lee Foshay of Cincinnati, though he did not write about the subject, as he was of the school that believed one should not publish observations on a disease until the pathologic agent had been identified. In his work on tularemia, however, Foshay had recognized a group of atypical cases with negative bacteriologic and serologic results. It was these cases that became the first to be diagnosed as cat fever after Dr. H. Rose and F. Hanger of New York had supplied Foshay with the antigen for skin testing that now bears their name.

The disease these pioneers discovered proved to be a common one, and it is the experience of many people by now that a first encounter with the disease and the relevant literature [9] soon leads one to observe many more cases. Epidemics of CSD are documented [6] and occur both in minor forms in families and as major outbreaks in the community, particularly in the autumn and winter months of temperate zones.

Clinical Features

Clinically, the disease is encountered most commonly in children and young adults who in playing or sleeping with a boisterous kitten get scratched for their misplaced affection on the arms, head and neck, or legs. The offending cat remains healthy and gives a negative skin test with the Rose–Hanger antigen. About 90 percent of patients report close contact with cats and three-quarters or more begin with a cat scratch.[5, 6, 9, 10] Among the remainder, there has been mention of scratching by other sharp objects, such as thorns, wood splinters, bones, pins, fish hooks, rabbit, dog, and monkey claws, and even such exotic items as porcupine quills.[3-5, 9]

Within a week to 10 days of injury, the skin becomes inflamed and presents as a red macule or papule, sometimes with a central vesicle, pustule, or scab. Persistent ulcers at the scratch site are apparently not common, and the lesion does not itch like an insect bite.[10] Then one to four weeks after appearance of the primary skin lesion, a regional adenopathy develops, involving usually only one node and without a lymphangitis between scratch and the node. It is this lymphadenopathy that generally draws attention to the disease because the primary skin lesion is often insignificant and constitutional symptoms such as headache, fever, and malaise are generally mild in CSD. Rare severe complications such as encephalitis,[11, 12] thrombocytopenic purpura,[13] and Parinaud's oculoglandular syndrome [14, 15] have been recorded, but even the lymphadenopathy disappears in many cases without more distress to the patient than a little local tenderness. In this common clinical situation of a transient mild illness with adenopathy, a diagnosis may be impossible unless the antigen for skin testing is available. On the other hand, in up to half the cases of published series,[3, 5, 9, 10] the nodes remain enlarged and painful, and a small percentage discharge pus. It is this group of nodes that become the object of histologic examination, in the hope of establishing a diagnosis and excluding more serious causes of lymphadenopathy, such as tuberculosis or lymphoma. Sometimes, the clinician will aspirate pus from a fluctuant node which proves sterile by all bacteriologic, mycologic, and virologic methods, and it is an unfortunate fact that too many laboratories discard this sterile material without attempting manufacture of the scarce Rose–Hanger antigen.[5-7] If 0.1 ml of the antigen is injected intracutaneously, it produces induration with surrounding redness in 48 hours in about 90 percent of recorded cases of CSD, with some 4 percent of the false-positives in controls.[5, 10, 16] Warwick and Good [16] and Marshall [7] record an immediate as well as a delayed reaction to the antigen.

Laboratory Tests

No laboratory test yet devised can confirm or exclude the diagnosis of CSD, though many may have to be done to eliminate those conditions with which CSD is confused.

Culture of material is necessary in consideration of pyogenic lymphadenitis, tularemia, brucellosis, tuberculosis, infections with anonymous mycobacteria, and sporotrichosis. Agglutination tests assist in excluding P. tularensis, B. abortus, and S. moniliformis as well as the heterophile antibody of infectious mononucleosis.

Complement fixation with Lygranum, and the Frei test may be done if lymphogranuloma venereum is suspected; serologic tests in secondary syphilis; the Sabin–Feldman dye test in toxoplasmosis; and animal inoculations in rat-bite fever, sporotrichosis, and toxoplasmosis.

Immunoglobulin analysis may be necessary, with immunologic rarities causing persistent adenopathy such as chronic familial granulomatosis.[17]

Comprehensive laboratory services of this order are, however, not always available, and diagnostic criteria on simpler grounds have been devised. The minimum would seem to be a lymphadenopathy following contact with a cat, a positive Rose–Hanger skin test and a negative Frei test.[7] Aspiration of sterile material from the node and histologic nodal changes compatible with CSD add greater certainty to the diagnosis.[5]

Pathologic Examination

Skin Lesion

The microscopic features of the primary skin lesion have been described by Johnson and Helwig [18] and Winship.[19] They found small areas of dermal necrosis surrounded by a larger zone of acellular necrobiosis around which, in turn, is a palisade of finely vacuolated epithelioid histiocytes and giant cells, with an outer mantle of small lymphocytes. Polymorphs and plasma cells may be found in perivascular distribution, and eosinophils can be prominent in the early phases.

Lymph Node Lesions

The lymph nodes most commonly affected in the larger series of published cases have been, in descending order of frequency, the axillary, head and neck, and inguinal groups.[4, 6, 10] Curiously, lymph nodes that are seldom involved by infections or neoplasms may be enlarged in CSD, causing confusion with submental abscess, thyroglossal cyst, and even a breast lump of the axillary tail. The lymph node enlargement is generally only moderate in degree. In a group of 14 cases seen personally, the nodes ranged from 0.7 to 3.5 cm in diameter. One must be prepared for a variety of gross appearances, and it is a good rule to suspect CSD whenever one encounters an unexplained lymph node enlargement. Some nodes are firm in consistency and well defined though possibly with a thickened capsule and adherent to surrounding adipose tissue. Generally, the cut surface is tan colored and homogeneous, but bulging small yellow foci should alert one to possible microabscess (Fig. 1), and even hemorrhagic areas may be a clue to the diagnosis, as indicated by Winship.[19]

Apart from the Rose–Hanger skin test, histologic examination of a lymph node is the only other source of positive supporting evidence for a clinical diagnosis of CSD.

The lymph nodes have customarily been described as showing an early phase of lymphoid hyperplasia, an intermediate phase of granuloma formation, and

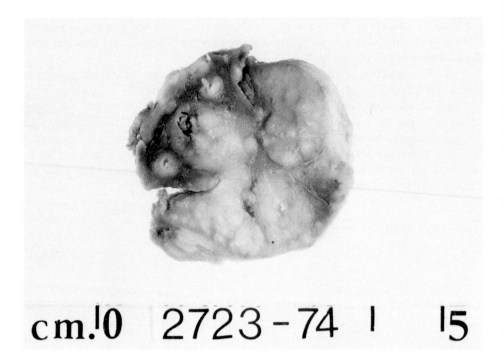

cm.⁰0   2723-74   l   l5

Fig. 1. Axillary lymph node from a boy of 15 years with adenopathy of 1 month's duration. The capsule is thickened and numerous pale microabscesses can be seen in all areas. × 2.2.

a final stage of suppuration. It is, however, uncommon for a surgically removed node to show only one phase histologically, and usually all three are present together. This is a fortunate and distinctive feature of most cases of CSD, which distinguishes them from almost all the common persistent lymphadenopathies with which confusion is possible. Infectious mononucleosis for instance shows hyperplasia, but neither granulomas nor suppuration, and toxoplasmosis has hyperplasia and granulomas, but lacks suppuration.

The list of all persistent lymphadenopathies in the differential diagnosis of CSD is long and includes nodular lymphoma and Hodgkin's disease, infectious mononucleosis, rheumatoid arthritis, dermatopathic, postvaccinial, and drug-induced lymphadenopathies, secondary syphilis, tuberculosis, sarcoid reactions, tularemia, brucellosis, sporotrichosis, lymphogranuloma venereum, toxoplasmosis, pyogenic lymphadenitis, and many others of lesser frequency. The more important members of this group have been discussed in the *Pathology Annual 1970* by Sieracki and Fisher,[20] by Ackerman and Rosai,[21] and Dorfman and Warnke.[22] For a long time, lymphogranuloma venereum and tularemia have been regarded as the only conditions showing nodal histology identical to CSD, but the references just quoted indicate that one must pay more attention to immunologic rarities and to infections with Yersinia or anonymous mycobacteria.

The detailed morphology of the lymph node lesion has been described by Winship [19] and by Naji et al.[23] Both papers describe the earliest change as areas of reticulum cell hyperplasia at the site of entrance of afferent lymphatics in the periphery of the node. These foci, which in our material were interpreted as hyperactive germinal centers, may be so prominent as to simulate nodular lymphoma (Fig. 2). However, these often assume the bizarre shapes and show the cytologic variety of reactive lymphoid tissue, with tingible histiocytes and large hyperchromatic, mitotically active lymphocytes in the germinal centers (Fig. 3), together with a peripheral rim of small lymphocytes. Confusion may arise when sheets of large lymphocytes form in the interfollicular or medullary tissues, giving a monomorphic lymphomalike picture (Fig. 4), but this transformation is a local change and never completely effaces the nodal architecture (Fig. 5).

Cells with characteristics that have variously been described as those of immunoblasts or reticular lymphoblasts can be found in CSD, predominantly in and around the cortical germinal centers (Fig. 6), but they seldom occur in large numbers or diffusely. One feels instead that the germinal centers of nodes in CSD retain their tingible histiocytes until abscesses develop and that the picture they present is one of multiple nodules with starry-sky appearance rather than the

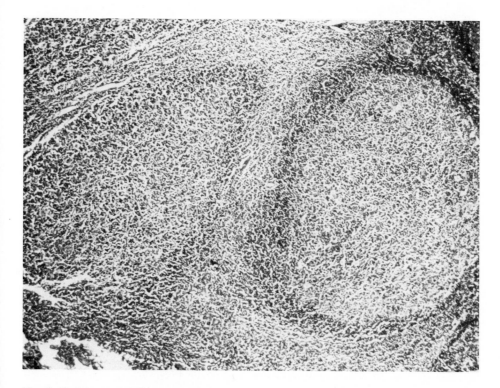

Fig. 2. Nodular and diffuse lymphoid hyperplasia of a degree that might cause confusion with lymphoma. Signs of subsiding abscess were present elsewhere in the node. Submental lymph node from female aged 25 years, removed May, 1970, and patient in excellent health June, 1976. × 40.

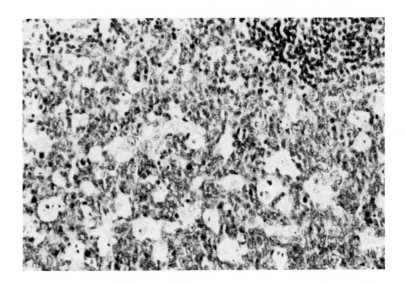

Fig. 3. The more usual appearances of lymphoid hyperplasia in CSD with many tingible histiocytes in the germinal centers. × 400.

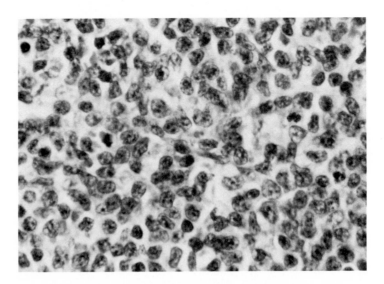

Fig. 4. Monomorphic lymphocyte proliferation which might cause confusion with lymphoma. × 800.

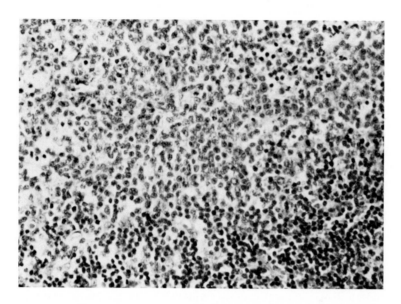

Fig. 5. Lower-power view of Figure 4 showing merging of normal and abnormal areas. × 250.

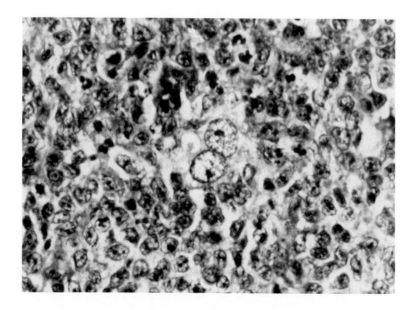

Fig. 6. Immunoblasts in a germinal center. × 800.

diffuse mottling described in postvaccinial lymphadenitis [24] and infectious mono-nucleosis.[25] This phase of lymphoid hyperplasia must represent antigenic stimulation of the so-called B system of lymphocytes and results finally in the plasma cells one finds later. These changes are presumably the maximum lesion occurring in those patients who clinically have only a transient lymphadenopathy and a positive skin test.

Winship also described the stages of microabscess formation in these areas of what he called reticulum cell hyperplasia, and he illustrated how, when well established, the lesions acquire a palisade of epithelioid histiocytes, giving a stellate abscess.

In the developing microabscess (Fig. 7), which in our material is often near or within a germinal center, one finds at first simply necrotic cells with karyorrhectic nuclei, acidophilic debris, and fibrin exudate centrally. More peripherally, there are dilated capillary channels that may proceed later to capillary thrombosis (Fig. 8). Polymorphs appear early in the central areas (Fig. 9), while plasma cells and epithelioid histiocytes are found later on the periphery of the microabscess (Fig. 10). Caseous necrosis does not occur, but giant cells do form and may be numerous in some cases (Fig. 11). The peripheral lymph sinuses are dilated and filled with cells (Fig. 12), and by the time abscesses are established, there is a prominent pericapsular inflammation outside the node with edema, capillary granulations, and fibroblastic tissue (Fig. 13). This perinodal inflammation may be impressive in bulk and is characteristic of CSD, being caused at least partly, no doubt, by back pressure effects following blockage of the filtering network and lymphatic channels within the node.

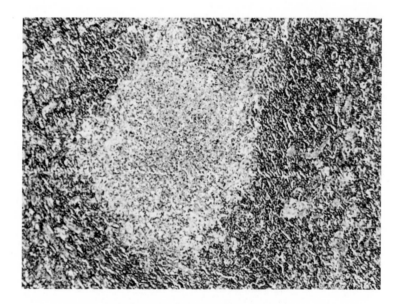

Fig. 7. Early microabscess composed principally of necrotic debris. The lesion appears to be within a vaguely defined lymphoid follicle also containing scanty epithelioid histiocytes. × 100.

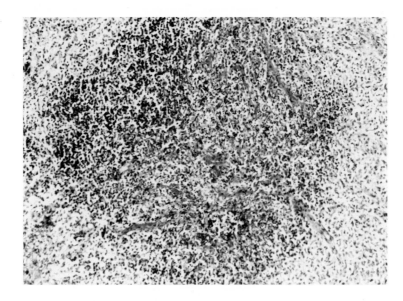

Fig. 8. Capillary thrombi in a microabscess. Large numbers of plasma cells are present in the surrounding tissues. × 100.

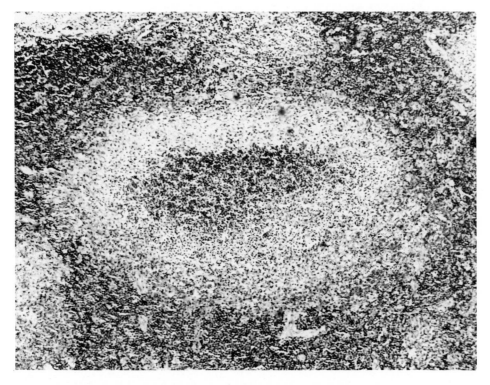

Fig. 9. Microabscess with numerous polymorphs centrally. × 100.

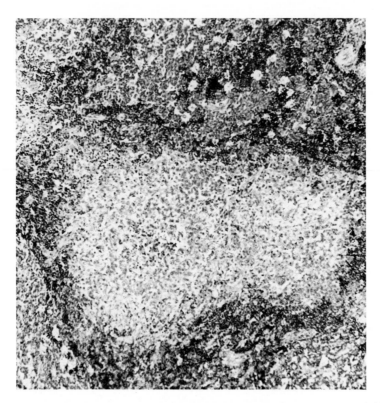

Fig. 10. Microabscess formed predominantly of epithelioid histiocytes. × 100.

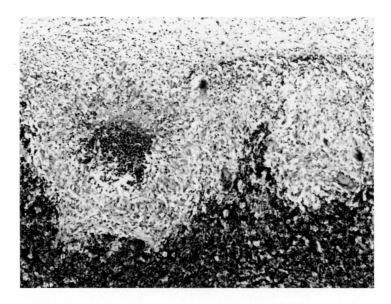

Fig. 11. Microabscess with central polymorphs surrounded by epithelioid histiocytes and several giant cells. × 100.

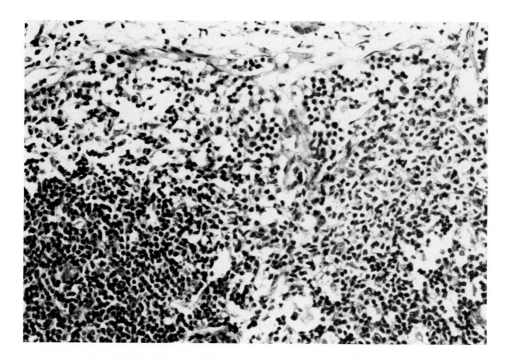

Fig. 12. Peripheral sinus dilated and filled with cells. × 250.

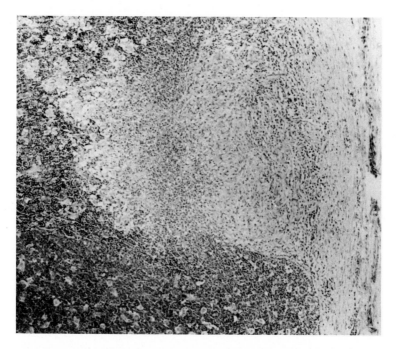

Fig. 13. Cortical microabscess and capsular fibroblastic response. × 40.

Microabscesses form in both cortical and deep parts of the node and may coalesce to replace large areas, with the production of a painful suppurating node requiring aspiration or surgical removal. Alternatively, the microabscesses may remain small or scanty and yet induce widespread plasma cell formation, while other cases are characterized by a prominent epithelioid cell response and giant cells. Some authors refer to a typical stellate microabscess, but one doubts if there is such an entity, because all of the following microabscesses can be found in CSD, all star shaped, and each in its own way bringing the possibility of CSD to mind:

Necrosis and cell debris (Fig. 7).
Necrosis and numerous polymorphs (Fig. 9).
Necrosis and numerous epithelioid histiocytes, with or without polymorphs (Fig. 10).
Necrosis, polymorphs, palisaded epithelioid histiocytes and giant cells (Fig. 11).

The last type of abscess can certainly occur in tuberculosis and Yersinia infections, causing confusion to the histologist. In the majority of cases, epithelioid histiocytes and giant cells are confined to the periphery of the microabscess within the node, but they may be found also in the perinodal inflammatory reaction (Fig. 14) or in the peripheral sinus. Exceptionally, epithelioid cells occur diffusely in the node in small clusters, as in toxoplasmosis, though not without suppuration in some part (Fig. 15).

The frequency of giant cell formation is variable in CSD, Winship having found them in 25 of 29 cases, but Naji et al in only 1 of 3 and Marshall in only 1 of

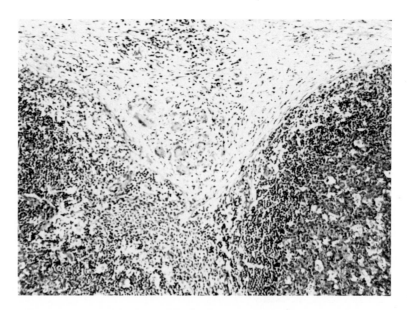

Fig. 14. Epithelioid histiocytes and giant cells in perinodal inflammatory reaction. × 100.

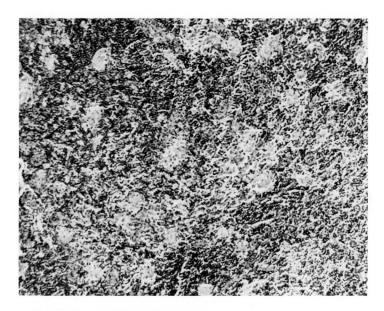

Fig. 15. Small clusters of epithelioid histiocytes in a germinal center not unlike toxoplasmosis. × 100.

11 cases. In 14 nodes seen personally, giant cells were present with varying frequency in 13 cases. One will also find that epithelioid and giant cells can be present around one microabscess and absent around another close by. This suggests that their formation is influenced more by local than by systemic factors, such as the level of circulating humoral antibody or the state of delayed hypersensitivity in the patient as a whole. The wide variations in the frequency of giant cell formation reported by the different authors just quoted also incline one to think that differences in local strains of the causative agent, or a possible inert adjuvant introduced on the cat's claws, may operate in different patients or in different communities.

A detailed account of the immunologic processes that take place in CSD cannot be given at the present time, because no organism or specific antigen is available for study. One can, therefore, only speculate on the basis of what occurs in lymphadenopathies of known causation to which CSD bears clinical and pathologic similarities.

The phase of lymphoid hyperplasia in CSD is similar, for instance, to that which occurs after smallpox vaccination; the microabscesses are regarded as identical to those of lymphogranuloma venereum, and the epithelioid and giant cell granulomas are the same as one may find in mycobacterial or Yersinia infections. One can, therefore, by analogy picture the foreign antigen, infectious or otherwise, introduced on the cat's claws as being transported, possibly with an adjuvant, from the primary lesion to the regional lymph node and initiating there both humoral and cell-mediated responses, the former resulting in stimulation of germinal centers and plasma cell formation, the latter in epithelioid granulomas and the specifically sensitized lymphocytes responsible for the delayed tuberculin-type skin test responses. Both the intervals between the scratch, the primary lesion, and the lymphadenopathy, as well as the nature of the response to intradermal injection of the Rose–Hanger antigen, are consistent with the long-held view that a cell-mediated hypersensitivity develops in CSD.

The possibility of a local Arthus reaction in the skin or lymph nodes has apparently not been considered, but an observation in our material (Figs. 16 and 17) that acute arteritis can occur in cat-scratch lymphadenitis makes one wonder whether so-called immune complex reactions between antigen, antibody, and complement may not be involved in these sites. The cell necrosis and polymorph response in CSD lymph nodes has always tacitly been ascribed to a viral or chlamydial toxin, but the discovery [26, 27] that immune complexes are chemotactic to polymorphs and cause capillary thrombosis offers at least a theoretical alternative to direct toxic action. Presumably, the presence of plasma cells in the nodes of CSD indicates that humoral antibody is available locally for the formation of antibody complexes. Normally, such complexes are easily cleared by phagocytosis, but as lymph nodes are filtering organs, they may be peculiarly susceptible to the effects of these complexes, as is known to be the case with the renal glomerulus.[28] These immune complexes are also claimed to cause local release of substances such as histamine and serotonin, and these might be responsible for the extranodal inflammatory changes that form so prominent a part of CSD.

All such conjectures remain theoretical, however, until a causative organism is isolated, but one would be interested to know if other unpublished observations of arteritis in the nodes of CSD have been made.

If detailed ultrastructural studies have been done in CSD, they have not yet received prominence in the literature. Limited observations on our material have

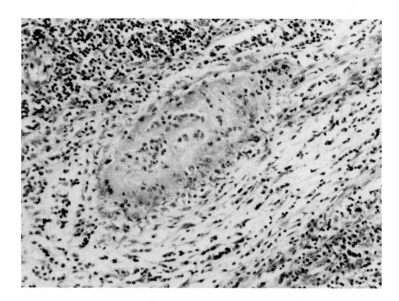

Fig. 16. Acute arteritis within the substances of a lymph node that contained numerous microabscesses in other areas. × 250.

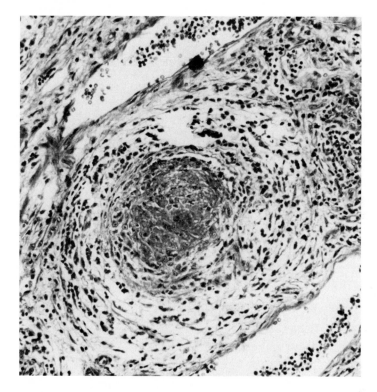

Fig. 17. Same vessel as Figure 16 at different levels of section. $\times$ 400.

not shown any specific features in transformed lymphocytes or epithelioid cells, nor have acceptable viral particles been discovered.

In trying to summarize the subject of CSD, one is left with the impression that little has been added since the disease was last reviewed.[9] With its low morbidity and homely name, CSD has never been taken seriously by patient or physician. This good-natured contempt has been shared, one suspects, by the research worker too, who has allowed it to remain an old-fashioned mystery in an age of immunologic marvels.

References

1. Debre R, Lamy M, Jammet ML, Costil L, Mozziconacci P: La maladie des griffes de chat. Bull Mem Soc Med Hôp Paris 66:76, 1950
2. Mollaret P, Reilly J, Bastin R, Tournier P: La decouverte du virus de la lympho-reticulose benigne d' inoculation. Presse Med 59:681, 1951
3. Daniels WB, MacMurray FG: Cat scratch disease. Arch Intern Med 88:736, 1951
4. Daniels WB, MacMurray FG: Cat scratch disease: Non-bacterial regional adenitis. Ann Intern Med 37:697, 1952
5. Margileth AM: Cat scratch disease: Non-bacterial regional adenitis. Pediatrics 42:803, 1968

6. Warwick WJ, Good RA: Cat scratch disease in Minnesota. (I) Evidence for its epidemic occurrence. (II) Family epidemic. Am J Dis Child 100:228, 1960
7. Marshall CE: Cat scratch fever. Can Med Assoc J 75:724, 1956
8. Carithers HA: Cat scratch disease. Notes on its history. Am J Dis Child 119:200, 1970
9. Warwick WJ: Cat scratch syndrome. Many diseases or one disease? Prog Med Virol 9:256, 1967
10. Carithers HA, Carithers CM, Edwards RO, Jr: Cat scratch disease. JAMA 207:312, 1969
11. Stevens H: Cat scratch fever encephalitis. Am J Dis Child 84:218, 1952
12. Thompson TE, Jr, Miller KF: Cat scratch encephalitis. Ann Intern Med 39:146, 1953
13. Jim RTS: Thrombocytopenic purpura in cat scratch disease. JAMA 176:1036, 1961
14. Levitt JM: The oculoglandular form of cat scratch disease. JAMA 165:1955, 1957
15. Margileth AM: Cat scratch disease as a cause of the oculoglandular syndrome of Parinaud. Pediatrics 20:1000, 1957
16. Warwick WJ, Good RA: Cat scratch disease in Minnesota. (III) Evaluation of the intradermal skin test to cat scratch disease antigen. Am J Dis Child 100:241, 1960
17. Johnston RB, McMurray JS: Chronic familial granulomatosis. Am J Dis Child 114:370, 1967
18. Johnson WT, Helwig EB: Cat scratch disease: Histopathologic changes in the skin. Arch Dermatol 100:148, 1969
19. Winship T: Pathological changes in so-called cat scratch fever. Am J Clin Pathol 23:1012, 1953
20. Sieracki JC, Fisher ER: Diagnostic problems involving nodal lymphomas. Pathol Annu 5:91, 1970
21. Ackerman LV, Rosai J: Surgical Pathology. St. Louis, Mosby, 1974
22. Dorfman RF, Warnke R: Lymphadenopathy simulating the malignant lymphomas. Hum Pathol 5:519, 1974
23. Naji AF, Carbonell F, Barker HJ: Cat scratch disease. Am J Clin Pathol 38:513, 1962
24. Hartsock RJ: Postvaccinial lymphadenitis. Cancer 21:632, 1968
25. Salvador AH, Harrison EG, Kyle RA: Lymphadenopathy due to infectious mononucleosis: Its confusion with malignant lymphoma. Cancer 27:1029, 1971
26. Cochrane CG, Dixon FJ: Cell and tissue damage through antigen antibody complexes. Calif Med 111:99, 1969
27. Dixon FJ, Cochrane CG: The pathogenicity of antigen–antibody complexes. Pathol Annu 5:355, 1970
28. Gell PGH, Coombs RRA, Lachman PJ: Clinical Aspects of Immunology. London, Blackwell, 1975

HEPATIC TUMORS AND ORAL CONTRACEPTIVES

ROBERT E. FECHNER

Introduction

In 1973 Baum et al [1] reported seven women with benign hepatic tumors who were taking oral contraceptive hormones (OCH). The cluster of cases was considered significant because three of the patients were from a single hospital where no other benign hepatic tumors could be found in a search going back to 1913. The common denominator of OCH therapy suggested that the hormones might be causal. In the subsequent two and a half years, a flurry of additional reports of hepatic tumors in women taking OCH has ensued totaling nearly 100 cases. Seven have been diagnosed as either hepatoma [2-4] or hepatoblastoma,[5] but the vast majority of liver lesions has been considered benign (ie, nonmetastasizing), with diagnostic labels including focal nodular hyperplasia, hamartoma, adenoma, benign hepatoma, and minimal deviation hepatoma. In studying the descriptions and illustrations of the benign lesions, it is obvious that several diagnostic terms are being applied to two pathologically distinct lesions, to wit, focal nodular hyperplasia and liver cell adenoma. Many authors have not made the distinction, which has impeded the understanding of the possible relation (or lack of relation) of OCH to these two different entities.

The fundamental problem of inaccurate classification is unnecessary because Edmondson separated and defined focal nodular hyperplasia (FNH) and liver cell adenoma (LCA) in the late 1950s.[6, 7] The histologic criteria are clear and recently have been reaffirmed by others.[8-11] A lesion is classified as liver cell adenoma when the tumor is (a) composed of liver cells with nuclear variation no greater than that of normal liver and (b) lacks bile ducts or ductules (Figs. 1 and 2). Focal nodular hyperplasia requires (a) one or more grossly visible localized nodules in an otherwise normal liver, (b) a predominance of normal hepatic cells, but with some bile ducts or ductules, and (c) fibrous septa in the nodule which usually radiate from a central stellate fibrous area (Figs. 3 and 4). These criteria exclude nodules in cirrhotic livers, nodular regenerative hyperplasia, hepatocellular

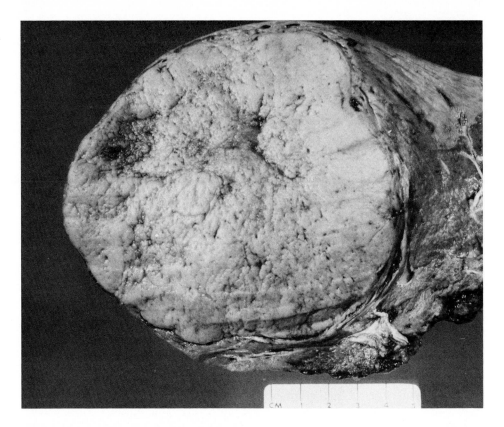

Fig. 1. Liver cell adenoma lacks central scar and is pale yellow in color, probably due to glycogen abundance. Note irregular, finely nodular appearance. Normal liver on right. Patient had taken oral contraceptives for 5 years.

adenomatosis, and partial nodular transformation, although all of them share some microscopic features with FNH, eg, hepatic cell hyperplasia and the presence of bile ducts within nodules. The differentiations are made readily because the grossly detectable masses of partial nodular regenerative hyperplasia and hepatocellular adenomatosis involve the liver diffusely.[12]

Personal Experience

The benign hepatic lesions in the surgical pathology files between 1968 and 1976 at The Methodist Hospital yielded seven cases of LCA and six cases of FNH; all in women. Six of the seven women with LCA were taking OCH at the time the lesion was diagnosed, as were two of the six women with FNH. The negative histories were confirmed by specific interview with the women. The details of these cases will be published elsewhere. The clinical and pathologic features paralleled those to be discussed in this review and will be alluded to when appropriate.

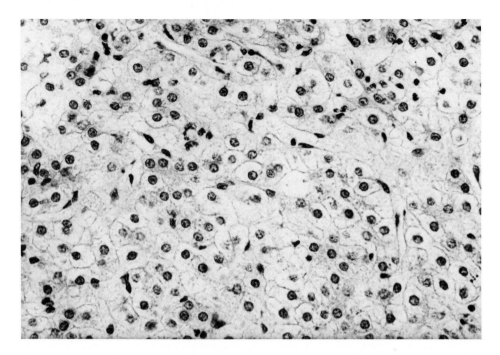

Fig. 2. Liver cell adenoma consists of liver cells and sinusoids without bile ducts or ductules. × 220.

Summary of Literature

The Anglo-American literature on benign hepatic tumors has been reviewed from 1940 to the present in an effort to place the recent reports in perspective. In this paper, the phrases "before 1960" and "after 1960" will be repeatedly used, since 1960 was the year that hormones were approved by the Federal Drug Administration for use as oral contraceptives. The literature prior to 1960 serves as one type of control because patients reported before then were not taking oral contraceptives. The literature between 1960 and 1973 is also valuable as another control since hepatic lesions reported in those years were *not* selected for publication because of the history of OCH therapy, although in retrospect, some patients were taking OCH. This is important because papers on benign hepatic lesions going to press after late 1973 have dealt almost exclusively with lesions from women taking oral contraceptives. The first criterion for publication is that the patient is taking hormones, which results in selected case reports with a positive association between OCH and liver tumors, rather than series of consecutive patients unselected as to hormone history. Anecdotal literature of this sort can be important and may detect a genuinely new trend. However, it also tends to be self-fulfilling and becomes weighted toward an apparently positive association between the two events under consideration.

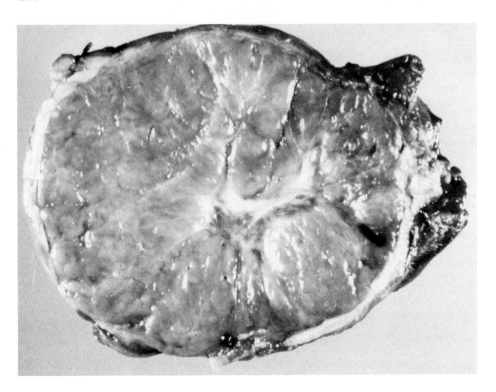

Fig. 3. Focal nodular hyperplasia has a centrally located fibrous scar with a coarse nodular arrangement of the tumor around it. The color and consistency is that of normal liver. Patient had taken oral contraceptives for 4 years.

Turning first to the literature between 1940 and 1960, one finds 37 surgically treated benign hepatic masses excluding mesenchymal hamartomas and hemangiomas.[13-35] Of these, 24 were felt to be clearcut examples of FNH,[13-27] and eight were accepted as unequivocal cases of liver cell adenoma.[17, 28-32]

Since 1960 there have been 125 cases of benign liver lesions diagnosed during life which were reported individually or in small series,[36-82] plus the pathologic study of Phillips et al [80] and two large groups of patients reported by Edmondson et al [84] and by Ishak and Rabin.[83] The latter was a brief preliminary survey. It will not be included in the tabulations of this paper, since it spans the pre- and post-hormone eras and includes cases from surgical and autopsy material without designating the exact source.

There was a positive history of OCH usage in 59 of the 125 cases in the numerous small series and in 29 of 36 of the cases of Edmondson et al.[84] (These figures have been corrected for the multiple reporting of several patients. Six of the 42 adenomas reported by Edmondson et al were previously reported.[53, 66, 67] Four of the 8 cases of Americks et al [73] were previously reported by Baum et al [1] and partly duplicated by Goldstein et al.[75] Four of the 13 cases reported by Mays et al [4] in 1976 were previously published by Mays et al [43] in 1974.) Nine were

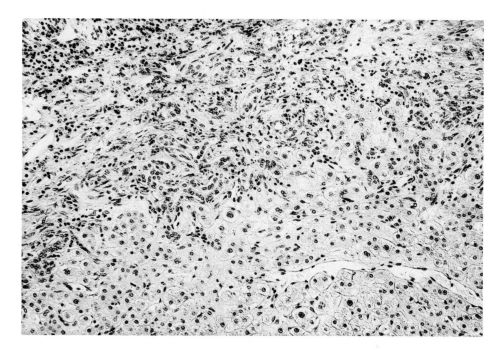

Fig. 4. Numerous bile ductules are formed at the periphery of the nodules in focal nodular hyperplasia. × 80.

identifiable as cases of FNH, 48 as LCA, and 31 are of uncertain pathologic types since pathologic descriptions were not given or were too vague to be certain as to the nature of the tumor.

Since focal nodular hyperplasia and liver cell adenomas are morphologically distinct lesions, they will be discussed separately.

Focal Nodular Hyperplasia

The 24 cases of FNH diagnosed during life reported between 1940 and 1960 included 11 in children and 13 in adults: 10 were women and 3 men.[14, 20, 23, 24, 26] The women were 23, 28, 28, 28, 32, 38, 39, 46, 47, and 63 years old. Since 1960, 37 cases of FNH diagnosed during life have been published, of which 26 were older than 19 years. Twenty-three were women between 21 and 51 years old, 13 of whom were between 21 and 29 years of age.

When comparing the adults surgically treated for FNH before 1960 and after 1960, there were many similarities and only a single difference which may be related to OCH. Both groups had a similar age range: 23 to 64 years before 1960 and 21 to 51 years after 1960. Approximately half of the female patients in both groups were in the third decade, indicating that FNH in adults was a tumor detected predominantly in young women even when they were not taking oral contraceptives.

The lesions in adults have been evenly distributed between the left and right lobes both before and after 1960, which was also borne out in the subgroup known to be taking OCH. The frequency of multiple lesions in adults was virtually identical before 1960 (two of 13) and after 1960 (three of 24). Moreover, five of 34 cases of FNH had multiple nodules in an autopsy series studied before the hormone era,[85] which was a similar proportion to the surgical groups. Against this background, the fact that two of the three patients with multiple lesions reported since 1960 were taking OCH is unimpressive and can be considered coincidental.

No gross or microscopic differences could be discerned in the lesions of FNH from women taking OCH, compared with women having a negative history with the possible exception of alterations in the vasculature. Mays et al [43] discussed a variety of abnormalities, including arterial medial hypertrophy with varying degrees of occlusion, phlebitis, fresh organizing thrombi, and intimal proliferation in small vessels. The authors thought the changes might have caused hemorrhagic necrosis, but were aware that they might be merely secondary to such necrosis. Similar changes were described in two other lesions of FNH from women taking OCH in whom hemorrhage was absent.[46, 47] Therefore, vascular changes did exist without producing bleeding and were not secondary to hemorrhage in these particular instances. Furthermore, arterial and venous hypertrophy were described by Edmondson [7] in 1958 and by Benz and Baggenstoss [85] who found "occasional venous thrombi" in their lesions of noninfarcted FNH in autopsy material before OCH were available. For these reasons, one should not too quickly attribute to OCH the rare thrombi or changes in the vessel walls. However, even though there were no qualitative differences in the vascular changes in FNH lesions from women taking OCH, there may be a quantitative difference in a few lesions which might be secondary to hormones.

The one clinical difference that stands out since 1960 has been the dramatic complication of acute life-threatening hemorrhage. Prior to 1960, no one with FNH had presented with bleeding, although occasional small foci of old or recent hemorrhage were found in resected lesions.[14] In 1967 a 25-year-old woman was described who had hemorrhage from FNH, but there was no information regarding the use of oral contraceptives.[41] Among the nine women with FNH known to be taking OCH, two presented with intrahepatic or intraperitoneal bleeding.[43] It is possible that a woman taking OCH might be more susceptible to hemorrhage than a nonuser of OCH, in view of the increased frequency of thrombotic episodes in other organs during OCH usage. In hepatic lesions, this complication may be a direct consequence of OCH therapy and could occur even if the underlying lesion itself was not caused by hormone administration.

The incidence of FNH is not known and an accurate statistical assessment of the influence of OCH cannot be made. The problem can be approached indirectly if one analyzes the years 1960 through 1973 before the rush of selected cases begins. There were 26 surgical cases, 15 of whom were adults (58 percent). This percentage is not far removed from the 24 patients before 1960, which included 13 adults (53 percent). The frequency of FNH in childhood is unrelated to OCH and serves as a constant before and after 1960. Since the proportion of adults and childhood cases has stayed about the same, this can be interpreted as evidence against an increased frequency of lesions in adults.

Proof of an association between FNH and OCH requires consecutive cases unselected by sex and unselected by hormone history in which the sex ratio overwhelmingly favors women and the vast majority are taking OCH. Only our small group of six consecutive cases of FNH seen since 1968 is available. Although all were women, only two had a positive history of OCH usage which was comparable to the 20 percent of premenopausal women in our hospital population known to be taking OCH during these years.[86] Another bit of information regarding frequency is provided by the survey at the Armed Forces Institute of Pathology. As of 1975, exactly half of the cases of FNH on file occurred before the induction of OCH, and there has not been a conspicuous increase in recent years.[83] At the moment, we must conclude that convincing evidence is lacking for a cause and effect relationship between OCH and FNH.[10, 83] Nevertheless, the lesion of FNH is of special significance to the user of OCH since it appears to be at risk for hemorrhage. It would seem prudent to eliminate the use of OCH in a woman found to have FNH, especially if the lesion is not resectable and is only biopsied.

Liver Cell Adenomas

Liver cell adenomas were rarely reported before 1960. Henson et al [22] encountered no liver cell adenomas at surgery at the Mayo Clinic between 1907 and 1954. They listed four lesions diagnosed as "hepatoadenomas," but their detailed histologic description is classic for FNH. Only two adenomas measuring less than 0.5 cm were found in autopsies at the Mayo Clinic between 1922 and 1951.[85] There are eight adequately documented surgical cases of LCA before 1960.[17, 28-32]

Since 1960, there have been reports of two women with LCA diagnosed at autopsy. One was 70 years old [42] and the other was 37. The latter had taken OCH for "many years" and died at home due to hemorrhage from an adenoma.[56] The literature on LCA diagnosed during life includes 42 cases reported by Edmondson et al and 36 cases in several smaller series. There is duplication in these numbers since six of the cases of Edmondson et al [84] are previously reported.[53, 66, 67] (These figures also have been corrected for the repetitive reporting of some of the cases of Baum et al [1] in two later papers.[73, 75]) The 36 cases reported individually and the series of Edmondson will be kept separate for the purposes of this discussion.

Of the 36 cases, four were children, all girls, ages 1, 2, 3, and 15 years.[45, 57, 71] The 32 adults spanned 20 to 67 years of age with a preponderance of 18 patients between 20 and 29 years of age, and 13 more between 30 and 40 years old. With the sole exception of a 20-year-old man,[42] all were women. The 31 women can be divided into three groups: 19 known to be taking oral contraceptives, seven who never used oral contraceptives, and five in whom no history of OCH usage is available.

The age distribution for the women taking OCH included eight in their twenties, ten in their thirties, and one who was 40 years old. The single most common presenting symptom was acute pain and collapse due to intrahepatic or intraperitoneal hemorrhage. This occurred in nine women. Five others had vague pain leading to discovery of a mass, and three had an asymptomatic mass, one of which was found incidentally at the time of cholecystectomy. In one patient the presenting symptoms were not known.[61]

Cessation of OCH therapy did not eliminate the risk of future hemorrhage from an adenoma. Two women who had stopped OCH and completed a subsequent pregnancy ruptured an adenoma 3 and 5 weeks postpartum, respectively.[55, 66] A third woman who had stopped OCH but did not become pregnant went into shock from hemorrhage 9 months later.[76]

There were seven women with adenomas who did not have a history of oral contraceptive medication (cases 1, 3, and 4 of Galloway et al,[58] case 3 of Hilliard et al,[59] case 2 of Davis et al,[87] and cases 1 and 3 of Albritton et al [88]). The women were 22, 24, 25, 26, 34, 35, and 67 years old. Case 3 of Albritton et al [88] and case 2 of Davis et al [87] presented with massive hemorrhage.

The five women reported before 1960 who could not have used OCH and the seven female patients just mentioned include two elderly women. However, it is of interest that nine of the ten remaining females were less than 40 years old, and seven of them were between 19 and 27. As with FNH, young women were the ones most likely to develop liver cell adenomas even when they were not taking OCH.

The presenting signs or symptoms in users of OCH were not particularly different from nonusers, with the exception that acute massive hemorrhage was more often seen in women taking OCH (eight of 18 users [44 percent] as opposed to two of 12 nonusers [17 percent]). Edmondson et al [84] noted that four of the ten women with ruptured adenomas were menstruating at the time of rupture, and they hypothesized that spasm of arteries in the adenoma leading to ischemic necrosis might occur at the same time as spasm of the endometrial spiral arterioles.

The size of the lesions from women who did not use OCH ranged from 5 to 16 cm, with a median of 10 cm. In women using OCH, there was a tendency to slightly larger tumors, ranging from 8 to 25 cm with a median of 13 cm.

All adenomas reported before 1960 were solitary, while nine of 36 since 1960 were multiple. Three of the cases of multiple adenomas were in women using OCH, but four of seven women with a definitely negative history for oral contraceptives also had multiple lesions.

The probability of an increased incidence of LCA since 1960 seems likely. We are cognizant of the extreme limitations of trying to judge the incidence of a lesion by the frequency with which it appears in the literature, but the following observations seem pertinent. There are eight acceptable surgical cases of LCA reported between 1940 and 1960, and 36 cases since 1960, plus the 36 new cases of Edmondson et al.[84] The brief reports of Baum et al [1] and Berg et al [74] indicated that their sources of material contained no liver cell adenomas until after 1960. As stated before, there were apparently no adenomas as defined by Emondson's criteria in the surgical files of the Mayo Clinic between 1907 and 1954, and only two tiny lesions were diagnosed at autopsy between 1922 and 1951.

Only one study provided figures on the frequency of adenomas removed at one institution before and after 1960. Albritton et al [53] reported one adenoma removed at the UCLA Health Center in 1948. Four tumors found between 1965 and 1973 were diagnosed as adenomas.* Two of the latter patients were taking OCH and two were not.[88]

If there was an increase in LCA since 1960, can it be attributed at least in part to OCH therapy? There were 20 adults (19 women) in papers published or in press before 1973, when the positive selection factor of OCH and liver cell tumors took hold. Through the courtesy of several authors, we have been able to obtain histories of OCH medication in 12 of their patients.[87-91] Nine women were taking OCH, and three were not. In addition, the report in 1972 by Horvath et al [60] included a history of OCH, but this was not the primary reason the case was published. Therefore, ten of the 13 women for whom information was available prior to 1973 were taking OCH. This is suggestive of a relation, since only about 16 percent of American women were taking OCH between 1964 and 1972.[92] Furthermore, the group of three cases of LCA reported by Hilliard et al [59] and our seven cases provided ten additional consecutive patients with adenomas unselected for OCH therapy. Eight of these ten had a positive history of OCH.

Edmondson et al [84] found that 29 of 34 women with adenomas were taking OCH. Interestingly, a similar proportion of controls (24 of 34) without liver tumors were taking OCH. A significant difference did exist between the two groups in that the mean duration of usage was 80 months in the patients with adenomas, but only 38 months in the women without neoplasms.

Edmondson et al [84] noted that the OCH in women with adenomas was heavily weighted by preparations containing mestranol. (All OCH contain either mestranol or ethinyl estradiol as the estrogenic component.) They found that over 90 percent of women with adenomas were taking OCH containing mestranol, whereas only 55 percent of the control users of OCH were taking mestranol compounds.† There are 5 cases in the literature with well-documented LCA in which the exact hormone is given, and four of five were mestranol. In all six of our cases of LCA, the OCH contained mestranol and not estradiol. We interpret these observations as strongly suggestive of an association between LCA and oral contraceptives, especially those that contain mestranol.

Seven cases diagnosed as hepatoma have been reported in young women taking OCH. In two of these, the patients were well 3 and 6 years after resection.[3] The histologic slides have been reviewed and are now felt to be compatible with adenomas.[91] Davis et al [2] have illustrated an hepatic cell tumor with bizarre nuclei, but the follow-up is too short to judge the biologic potential. Mays et al [4]

---

* On review, case 4 of this series has been diagnosed as focal nodular hyperplasia and reported again along with a new case of liver cell adenoma from a woman with a 7-year history of oral contraceptive usage. (McAvoy JM, Tompkins RK, Longmire WP: Benign hepatic tumors and their association with oral contraceptives. Case reports and survey of the literature. Arch Surg 111:761, 1976)

† Several aspects of the experimental design of the study by Edmondson et al [84] have been criticized, especially the analysis that concluded that users of mestranol are at greater risk compared to users of ethinyl estradiol. Edmondson's group has expanded and reanalyzed part of their data and find no reason to alter their original conclusions. (Correspondence. N Engl J Med 294:1061, 1976; N Engl J Med 295:51, 1976)

listed four cases of hepatoma with vein invasion. Two of the patients had unresectable tumors and have died, although details were not given. One of the other two is alive 2 months after right lobectomy, and the fourth died during surgery. It is of interest that three of the four patients had used OCH for one year or less, which contrasts sharply with the adenomas that are in women who usually have taken OCH for 3 to 5 years or longer.

Ultrastructural Studies

Ultrastructural studies on the livers of women taking OCH have shown alterations of ergastoplasm and mitochondria. Nonneoplastic liver cells from women taking OCH have shown dilatation and vesicle formation in both the smooth and rough profiles of ergastoplasm (ER).[93] This could reflect an induction or activation of microsomal drug-metabolizing enzymes which are responsible for the metabolism of at least some synthetic and endogenous sex steroids.

By contrast, Kay [90] and Kay and Schatzki [61] found no conspicuous alterations in the ergastoplasm of a liver cell adenoma from a woman taking OCH, and Horvath et al [60] specifically noted that the ER in their adenoma did not differ from normal hepatocytes "in any way." On the other hand, in one extensive study of liver cell adenomas, smooth ER was consistently decreased, but no drug histories were given.[80] The decrease of ER in these lesions may be analogous to experimentally induced minimal deviation hepatomas which have a decreased activity of microsomal enzymes when compared to normal.[94]

The mitochondrial alterations in both nonneoplastic and neoplastic hepatocytes consist of mitochondriomegaly with formation of intramitochondrial crystalloid inclusions (Fig. 5). The inclusions have been the focus of considerable attention, but their pathogenesis and chemical structure remain obscure. They have been seen in livers injured by such diverse agents as obstructive jaundice, alcohol, viral hepatitis, obesity, and toxic hepatitis.[95] Gonzales-Angulo et al [93] found inclusions in livers during pregnancy, but not in women whose pregnancy had terminated 5 to 12 months before the biopsy and they suggested that the inclusions were a reflection of increased metabolic demand. Perez et al [96] found inclusions in eight of 13 women who received OCH for more than a year. There was no correlation with the duration of therapy, since one patient taking OCH for 30 months had no inclusions, but they were numerous in two women after only 1 year of treatment. The presence of inclusions did not correlate with abnormal liver function tests. After discontinuing OCH for 6 months, repeat biopsies in six women contained diminished numbers of persistent inclusions.[116] Identical inclusions have also been illustrated in the 2 liver cell adenomas mentioned previously,[60, 90] but the significance of the inclusions in both neoplastic and nonneoplastic liver cells was difficult to assess because of the inconsistency of ultrastructural studies on apparently normal liver. Bhagwat et al [97] examined livers from five persons (one female) defined as normal by the absence of a history for liver diseases, normal hepatic function tests, and a grossly and microscopically normal liver. None contained inclusions. Using similar criteria of normalcy, others have found inclusions in a total of 15 of 18 livers, but neither the sex nor a statement regarding OCH

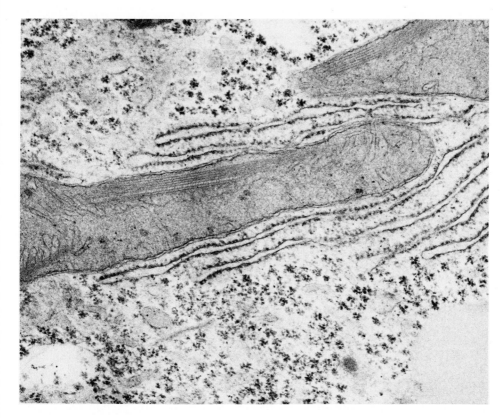

Fig. 5. Intramitochondrial crystalloid formation in a cell from liver cell adenoma. Glycogen is abundant within the cytoplasm. Patient had taken oral contraceptives for 5 years. × 32,000.

or other drug therapy is given in these reports.[98-100] Whatever the mechanism for their formation, the inclusions in patients taking OCH seem to be, at best, a quantitative and not a qualitative difference when compared with normal liver or livers damaged by other agents.

Experimental Studies

When turning to the experimental production of hepatic tumors in animals treated with OCH, one finds variable results. For example, increased numbers of liver cell tumors were produced in both male and female rats given megestrol compounds (progestins), but only male rats developed tumors when given the progestins norethynodrel, norethisterone, or norethisterone plus the estrogen mestranol.[101] The same compounds failed to produce an excess number of liver cell tumors in three strains of mice. Furthermore, female mice in one hepatoma-susceptible strain actually developed fewer neoplasms than expected when given the combination of norethynodrel and mestranol (Enovid).[102] Dogs and Rhesus monkeys have not developed hepatic tumors during six years of OCH administration.[103] Such inconsistencies have not contributed to understanding the possible relationship of these hormones to hepatic tumors in humans.

The mechanism by which sex hormones might promote or inhibit the growth of experimental liver cell neoplasms is unclear. Progestins are mildly cholestatic, and this might increase the intrahepatic concentration of carcinogenic substances normally excreted in the bile.[104] Another mechanism may be related to the fact that sex hormones share the same or similar metabolic enzymes with some well-recognized nonhormonal chemical carcinogens.[105] Because progestins are capable of enzyme induction, they might enhance the tumorogenicity of nonsteroidal compounds by increasing the intracellular concentration of these compounds. Specific evidence to prove enzyme induction by OCH was provided in one experimental model. Utilizing chick embryos, several progestin components of oral contraceptives induced higher than normal levels of hepatic aminolevulinic acid synthetase. The estrogen components, when administered alone, failed to be inductive, nor did they have an enhancing effect when injected along with the progestins.[106] In addition to demonstrating enzyme induction, these experiments were of interest because some women taking OCH excreted this particular enzyme in abnormally elevated quantities.[107]

Vascular Alterations

Two women taking OCH have suffered hepatic rupture in the absence of trauma or a recognizable tumor. Case 3 of Stauffer et al [70] is a 29-year-old woman taking OCH for six years who had the onset of acute pain. At laparotomy, an intrahepatic hematoma was drained, and a biopsy from the edge of the lesion yielded only necrotic tissue. This, of course, did not fully rule out an underlying neoplasm, since some adenomas with hemorrhage have a rim of neoplasm no more than a few millimeters wide as the only remnant. This could easily go undetected unless a well-oriented intact specimen were examined. Nonetheless, this patient recovered, and on scan three months later, there was diminution of the filling defect at the site of the original hematoma. More convincing proof of hemorrhage from a tumor-free liver is found in the 28-year-old patient of Frederick et al [108] who described a large intrahepatic hematoma with bleeding into the peritoneal cavity treated by lobectomy. Examination of the resected tissue failed to show tumor, and the only abnormalities were hepatic vein thrombi that presumably precipitated the infarct. Parenthetically, several cases of extrahepatic hepatic vein thrombosis have been reported in women taking OCH, but none have been accompanied by hepatic rupture.[109]

Sinusoidal dilatation is another morphologic abnormality of the vasculature which might predispose to hemorrhage. Winkler and Poulsen [110] reported four women taking OCH who had liver biopsies showing conspicuous dilatation of sinusoids and attenuation of adjacent liver plates in the periportal area. Three of the women had clinically enlarged livers. Stauffer et al [70] described dilated sinusoids in the liver adjacent to nodules of FNH which could have been secondary to outflow obstruction by the masses.

The term peliosis hepatis has been applied rather loosely to adenomas containing focal hemorrhage and thrombi, although peliosis is not described in the adjacent liver.[56, 63] Mays et al [43] also described "small blood-filled lakes" within nodular hyperplasia while specifically noting their absence in the adjacent normal liver. We are unaware of an example of diffuse peliosis hepatis in a woman using OCH. Such an event would not be totally unexpected in view of the several cases of peliosis reported in patients taking male sex steroids, one of whom died of fatal intraperitoneal bleeding.[111] The most frequently used progestin components of OCH are C-17 substituted testosterone derivatives, which are weak androgens.

Androgens and Hepatic Tumors

Another group of hepatic neoplasms is pertinent to this discussion. Twelve men and women taking androgens have been diagnosed as having hepatocellular carcinoma. Several were patients with Fanconi's anemia, which seems to predispose to a variety of hematopoietic and epithelial neoplasms, including one 24-year-old man who developed a hepatoma and had never taken androgens.[112] A peculiarity of the patients with hepatomas who have received androgens is the long survival and the absence of metastases in those coming to autopsy. Since the lesions are usually histologically well differentiated, one suspects that they might have been adenomas. Indeed, Farrell et al [113] made the diagnosis of adenoma in one patient taking androgens. One patient with androgen-associated hepatoma probably has had distant metastases.[114] Another interesting feature in this group is the regression in tumor size when androgen therapy ceases. This phenomenon has been documented in three patients,[113, 114] and strongly suggests that the androgens caused these neoplasms or that their enlargement or growth was dependent on the hormones.

Conclusions

In an age of proliferating environmental carcinogens, the firm identification of any single one as a causative agent becomes progressively more difficult. It is easy to ask for a history of hormone therapy, and having obtained an affirmative statement, to assume that it is a contributing factor. Thus far, the finding of clinically detectable hepatic tumors in women taking OCH is a rare event among the more than 20 million women who have used or are using oral contraceptives.[115] Every disease can be expected by chance alone within such a large population, especially when the peak years for the spontaneous occurrence of liver cell adenomas and focal nodular hyperplasia are the same as the peak years for oral contraceptive usage. Because there are no qualitative differences between the hepatic tumors from users and nonusers of OCH, one can only rely on statistical data and so far the data are meager.

Our analysis of the literature before and after the start of the hormone era discloses nothing to suggest that focal nodular hyperplasia has increased in frequency or is associated with oral contraceptives, with the possible exception that the lesion may be more prone to hemorrhage in women taking oral contraceptives.

Conversely, there is an unequivocal increase in liver cell adenomas reported since 1960. The tumors have been almost exclusively in young women, the majority of whom have been using oral contraceptives for at least three years. This provides indirect support, but certainly not proof, of an association. The cases of hepatoma in women taking oral contraceptives are too few to warrant even a tentative judgment at this time.

References

1. Baum JK, Holtz F, Bookstein JJ, et al: Possible association between benign hepatomas and oral contraceptives. Lancet 2:926, 1973
2. Davis M, Portmann B, Searle M, et al: Histological evidence of carcinoma in a hepatic tumor associated with oral contraceptives. Br Med J 4:496, 1975
3. Hermann RE, David TE: Spontaneous rupture of the liver caused by hepatomas. Surgery 74:715, 1973
4. Mays ET, Christopherson WM, Mahr MM, et al: Hepatic changes in young women ingesting contraceptive steroids. Hepatic hemorrhage and primary hepatic tumors. JAMA 235:730, 1976
5. Meyer P, Livolsi VA, Cornog JL: Hepatoblastoma associated with an oral contraceptive. Lancet 2:1387, 1974
6. Edmondson HA: Differential diagnosis of tumors and tumor-like lesions of liver in infancy and childhood. Am J Dis Child 91:168, 1956
7. Edmondson HA: Tumors of the Liver and Intrahepatic Bile Ducts. Atlas of Tumor Pathology. Section VII, Fascicle 25. Armed Forces Institute of Pathology, Washington, DC, 1958
8. Ackerman LV, Rosai J: Surgical Pathology, 5th ed. St. Louis, Mosby, 1974, p 533
9. Knowles DM, Wolff M, Casarella WJ: Hepatic cell adenomas. Arch Surg 110:1154 (Letter), 1975
10. Knowles DM, Wolff M: Systemic contraceptives and the liver. Ann Intern Med 83:907 (Letter), 1975
11. Sorensen TIA, Baden H: Benign hepatocellular tumors. Scand J Gastroenterol 10:113, 1975
12. Knowles DM, II, Kaye GI, Goodman GC: Nodular regenerative hyperplasia of the liver. Gastroenterology 69:746, 1975
13. Bartlett WC, Shellito JG: Hamartoma of the liver. Surgery 29:593, 1951
14. Begg CF, Berry WH: Isolated nodules of regenerative hyperplasia of the liver. Am J Clin Pathol 23:447, 1953
15. Benson CD, Penberthy GC: Surgical excision of primary tumor of the liver (hamartoma) in infant seven months old with recovery. Surgery 12:881, 1942
16. Branch A, Tonning DJ, Skinner GF: Adenoma of the liver. Can Med Assoc J 53:53, 1945
17. Christopherson WM, Collier HS: Primary benign liver-cell tumors in infancy and childhood. Cancer 6:853, 1953
18. Clay RC, Finney GG: Lobectomy of the liver for benign conditions. Ann Surg 147:827, 1958
19. Cleland RS: Benign and malignant tumors of the liver. Pediatr Clin North Am 6:427, 1959
20. Franklin RG, Downing CF: Primary liver tumors. Am J Surg 73:390, 1947
21. Gerding WJ, Popp MF, Martineau PC: Hamartomatous cholangiohepatoma. Report of a case. JAMA 145:821, 1951
22. Henson SW, Gray HK, Dockerty MB: Benign tumors of the liver. I. Adenomas. Surg Gynecol Obstet 103:23, 1956

23. Hoffman HS: Benign hepatoma: Review of the literature and report of a case. Ann Intern Med 17:139, 1942
24. Hunter WR: A case of benign hepatoma. Br J Surg 36:425, 1949
25. Kay S, Talbert PC: Adenoma of the liver, mixed type (hamartoma). Report of two cases. Cancer 3:307, 1950
26. McBurney RP, Woolner LB, Wollaeger EE: Solitary hyperplastic nodule of the liver simulating a neoplasm: Report of a case. Proc Staff Meet Mayo Clin 25: 606, 1950
27. Packard GB, Stevenson AW: Hepatoma in infancy and childhood; discussion and report of patient treated by operation. Surgery 15:292, 1944
28. Berkheiser SW: Recurrent liver cell adenoma. Gastroenterology 37:760, 1959
29. Jager BV, Nugent CA: Solitary benign adenoma of the liver associated with progressive hepatic insufficiency. Report of a case with autopsy findings. Arch Intern Med 101:645, 1958
30. Longmire WP, Scott HW: Benign adenoma of the liver; successful surgical resection of tumor involving both right and left lobes. Surgery 24:983, 1948
31. Wallace RH: Resection of the liver for hepatoma. Arch Surg 43:14, 1941
32. Warvi WN: Primary tumors of the liver. Surg Gynecol Obstet 80:643, 1945
33. Duckett JW, Montgomery HG: Resection of primary liver tumors. Surgery 21:455, 1947
34. Hershey CD: Partial hepatectomy in certain primary tumors of the liver. South Surg 12:245, 1946
35. Levenson RM, Mason DG: Mixed adenoma (hamartoma) of the liver: Report of a case. Ann Intern Med 38:136, 1953
36. Aronsen KF, Ericsson B, Lunderquist A, et al: A case of operated focal nodular cirrhosis of the liver. Scand J Gastroenterol 3:58, 1968
37. Crispin HA: A case of hepatic adenoma. Acta Chir Belg 70:91, 1971
38. Field CA: Hamartoma of the liver in a pregnant woman. Minn Med 52:639, 1969
39. Garancis JC, Tang T, Panares R, et al: Hepatic adenoma. Biochemical and electron microscopic study. Cancer 24:560, 1969
40. Hertzer NR, Hawk WA, Hermann RE: Inflammatory lesions of the liver which simulate tumor: Report of two cases in children. Surgery 69:839, 1971
41. Kwittken J: Hamartoma of the liver. NY State J Med 67:3254, 1967
42. Malt RA, Hershberg RA, Miller WL: Experience with benign tumors of the liver. Surg Gynecol Obstet 130:285, 1970
43. Mays ET, Christopherson WM, Barrows GH: Focal nodular hyperplasia of the liver. Possible relationship to oral contraceptives. Am J Clin Pathol 61:735, 1974
44. McLoughlin MJ, Colapinto RF, Gilday GL, et al: Focal nodular hyperplasia of the liver. Angiography and radioisotope scanning. Radiology 107:257, 1973
45. Nikaido H, Boggs J, Swenson O: Liver tumors in infants and children. Clinical and pathological analysis of 22 cases. Arch Surg 101:245, 1970
46. Nissen ED, Kent DR: Liver tumors and oral contraceptives. Obstet Gynecol 46:460, 1975
47. O'Sullivan JP, Wilding RP: Liver hamartomas in patients on oral contraceptives. Br Med J 2:7, 1974
48. Ramchand S, Suh HS, Gonzalez-Crussi F: Focal nodular hyperplasia of the liver. Can J Surg 13:22, 1970
49. Thomas PA, McCusker JJ, Merrigan EH, Conte NF: Lobar cirrhosis with nodular hyperplasia (hamartoma) of the liver treated by left hepatic lobectomy. Am J Surg 112:831, 1966
50. Westbrook RI, Raines M: Hamartoma: Case report. Nebr Med J 54:588, 1969
51. Whelan TJ, Baugh JH, Chandor S: Focal nodular hyperplasia of the liver. Ann Surg 177:150, 1973

52. Wilson TS, MacGregor JW: Focal nodular hyperplasia of the liver: The solitary cirrhotic liver nodule. Can Med Assoc J 100:567, 1969
53. Albritton DR, Tompkins RK, Longmire WP: Hepatic cell adenoma: A report of four cases. Ann Surg 180:14, 1974
54. Antoniades K, Campbell WN, Hecksher RH, et al: Liver cell adenoma and oral contraceptives. Double tumor development. JAMA 234:628, 1975
55. Antoniades K, Brooks CE, Jr: Hemoperitoneum from liver cell adenoma in a patient on oral contraceptives. Surgery 77:137, 1975
56. Contostavlos DL: Benign hepatomas and oral contraceptives. Lancet 2:1200, 1973
57. Davis JB, Schenken JR, Zimmerman O: Massive hemoperitoneum from rupture of benign hepatocellular adenoma. Surgery 73:181, 1973
58. Galloway SJ, Casarella WJ, Lattes R, et al: Minimal deviation hepatoma. Am J Roentgenol 125:184, 1975
59. Hilliard JL, Graham DY, Spjut HJ: Hepatic adenoma: A possible complication of oral contraceptive therapy. South Med J 69:683, 1976
60. Horvath E, Kovacs K, Ross RC: Ultrastructural findings in a well-differentiated hepatoma. Digestion 7:74, 1972
61. Kay S, Schatzki PF: Ultrastructure of a benign liver cell adenoma. Cancer 28:755, 1971
62. Kelso DR: Benign hepatomas and oral contraceptives. Lancet 1:315, 1974
63. Knapp WA, Ruebner BH: Hepatomas and oral contraceptives. Lancet 1:270, 1974
64. Minow RA, Tompkins RK, Gitnick GL: Diarrhea syndrome in hepatic adenoma. Am J Dig Dis 20:182, 1975
65. Monaco AP, Hallgrimsson J, McDermott WV: Multiple adenoma (hamartoma) of the liver treated by subtotal (90%) resection: Morphological and functional studies of regeneration. Ann Surg 159:513, 1964
66. Motsay GJ, Gamble WG: Clinical experience with hepatic adenomas. Surg Gynecol Obstet 134:415, 1972
67. Palubinskas AJ, Baldwin J, McCormack KR: Liver-cell adenoma. Angiographic findings and report of a case. Radiology 89:444, 1967
68. Sackett JF, Mosenthal WT, House RK, et al: Scintillation scanning of liver cell adenoma. Am J Roentgenol 113:56, 1971
69. Scorer CG: Spontaneous rupture of a hepatic adenoma: A possible hazard of flying. Br J Surg 56:633, 1969
70. Stauffer JQ, Lapinski MW, Honold DJ, et al: Focal nodular hyperplasia of the liver and intrahepatic hemorrhage in young women on oral contraceptives. Ann Intern Med 83:301, 1975
71. Tate RC, Chacko MV, Singh S, et al: Parenchymal hamartoma of the liver in infants and children. Am J Surg 123:346, 1972
72. Tountas C, Paraskevas G, Deligeorgi H: Benign hepatoma and oral contraceptives. Lancet 1:1351 (Letter), 1974
73. Ameriks JA, Thompson NW, Frey CF, et al: Hepatic cell adenomas, spontaneous liver rupture, and oral contraceptives. Arch Surg 110:548, 1975
74. Berg JW, Ketalaar RJ, Rose EF, et al: Hepatomas and oral contraceptives. Lancet 2:349 (Letter), 1974
75. Goldstein HM, Neiman HL, Mena E, et al: Angiographic findings in benign liver cell tumors. Radiology 110:339, 1974
76. Model DG, Fox JA, Jones RW: Multiple hepatic adenomas associated with an oral contraceptive. Lancet 1:865, 1975
77. Mosonyi L: Multiple benign hepatomas and virilization by ovarian tumor. Lancet 2:1263, 1973
78. O'Reilly K: Focal nodular hyperplasia of the liver. Aust NZ J Surg 44:142, 1974

79. O'Reilly K: Focal nodular hyperplasia of the liver: A further contribution. Aust NZ J Surg 45:76, 1975
80. Phillips MJ, Langer B, Stone R, et al: Benign liver cell tumors. Classification and ultrastructural pathology. Cancer 32:463, 1973
81. Pollice L: Primary hepatic tumors in infancy and childhood. Am J Clin Pathol 60:512, 1973
82. Vosnides G, O'Keefe B, Brander W, et al: Liver hamartomas in patients on oral contraceptives. Br Med J 5:580, 1974
83. Ishak KG, Rabin L: Benign tumors of the liver. Med Clin North Am 59:995, 1975
84. Edmondson HA, Henderson B, Benton R: Liver-cell adenomas associated with use of oral contraceptives. N Engl J Med 294:470, 1976
85. Benz EJ, Baggenstoss AH: Focal cirrhosis of the liver: Its relation to the so-called hamartoma (adenoma, benign hepatoma). Cancer 6:743, 1953
86. Fechner RE: Fibroadenomas in patients receiving oral contraceptives. A clinical and pathologic study. Am J Clin Pathol 53:857, 1970
87. Schenken JR: Personal communication, 1975
88. Albritton DR: Personal communication, 1975
89. Gamble WG: Personal communication, 1975
90. Kay S: Personal communication, 1975
91. Hermann RE: Personal communication, 1976
92. Tyler ET: International aspects of the use of norgestrel. In Fairweather DVI (ed): International Norgestrel Symposium. New York, Elsevier, 1974, pp 1–8
93. Gonzales-Angulo A, Aznar-Ramos R, Marquez-Monter H, et al: The ultra-structure of liver cells in women under steroid therapy. I. Normal pregnancy and trophoblastic growths. Acta Endocrinol (Kbh) 65:193, 1970
94. Rogers LA, Morris HP, Fouts JR: The effect of phenobarbital on drug metabolic enzyme activity, ultrastructure, and growth of a "minimal deviation" hepatoma (Morris 7800). J Pharm Exp Ther 157:227, 1967
95. Bhagwat AG, Ross RC: Hepatic intramitochondrial crystalloids. Arch Pathol 91:70, 1971
96. Perez V, Gorosdisch S, DeMartire J, et al: Oral contraceptives: Long-term use produces fine structural changes in liver mitochondria. Science 165:805, 1969
97. Bhagwat AG, Ross RC, Currie DJ: Ultrastructure of normal human liver. Arch Pathol 93:227, 1972
98. Lynn JA: Hepatic ultrastructural variations in apparently "normal" humans. Lab Invest 20:594 (Abstract), 1969
99. Roth GJ, Trump BF, Smuckler EA: Occurrence and nature of mitochondrial matrix striations. J Cell Biol 23:79A (Abstract), 1964
100. Wills EJ: Crystalline structures in the mitochondria of normal human liver parenchymal cells. J Cell Biol 24:511, 1965
101. Committee on Safety of Medicines. Carcinogenicity test of oral contraceptives. HMSO, London, 1972
102. Heston WE, Vlahakis G, Desmukes B: Effects of the antifertility drug Enovid in five strains of mice, with particular regard to carcinogenesis. J Natl Cancer Inst 51:209, 1973
103. Lancaster MC: Long-term results of toxicological studies with norgestrel combinations. In Fairweather DVI (ed): International Norgestrel Symposium. New York, Elsevier, 1974, pp 16–27
104. Sherlock S: Hepatic adenomas and oral contraceptives. Gut 16:753, 1975
105. Conney AH, Burns JJ: Metabolic interactions among environmental chemicals and drugs. Science 178:576, 1972
106. Rifkind AB, Gillette PN, Song CS, et al: Induction of hepatic aminolevulinic acid synthetase by oral contraceptive steroids. J Clin Endocrinol Metab 30:330, 1970

107. Koskelo P, Eisalo A, Toivonen I: Urinary excretion of porphyrin precursors and coproporphyrin in healthy females on oral contraceptives. Br Med J 1:652, 1966
108. Frederick WC, Howard RG, Spatola S: Spontaneous rupture of the liver in patients using contraceptive pills. Arch Surg 108:93, 1974
109. Hoyumpa AM, Schiff L, Helfman EL: Budd-Chiari syndrome in women taking oral contraceptives. Am J Med 50:137, 1971
110. Winkler K, Poulsen H: Liver disease with periportal sinusoidal dilatation: A possible complication of contraceptive steroids. Scand J Gastroenterol 10:699, 1975
111. Bagheri SA, Boyer JL: Peliosis hepatis associated with androgenic-anabolic steroid therapy. Ann Int Med 81:610, 1974
112. Cattan D, Vesin P, Wautier J, et al: Liver tumors and steroid hormones. Lancet 1:878, 1974
113. Farrell GC, Uren RF, Perkins KW, et al: Androgen-induced hepatoma. Lancet 1:430, 1975
114. Johnson FL, Feagler JR, Lerner KG, et al: Association of androgenic-anabolic steroid therapy with development of hepatocellular carcinoma. Lancet 2:1273, 1972
115. Lehfeldt H: Current status of oral contraceptives. Obstet Gynecol Annu 2:261, 1973
116. Martinez-Manautou J, Aznar-Ramos R, Bautista-O'Farrill J, et al: The ultrastructure of liver cells in women under steroid therapy. II. Contraceptive therapy. Acta Endocrinol (Kbh) 65:207, 1970

Addendum

Since completion of this paper, several relevant communications have appeared.

Andersen PH, Packer JT: Hepatic adenoma. Observations after estrogen withdrawal. Arch Surg 111:898, 1976

Baek S, Sloane CE, Futterman SC: Benign liver cell adenoma associated with use of oral contraceptive agents. Ann Surg 183:239, 1976

Brander WL, Vosnides G, Ogg CS, et al: Multiple hepatocellular tumours in a patient treated with oral contraceptives. Virchows Archiv [Pathol Anat] 370:69, 1976

Christopherson WM, Mays ET: Liver tumours and oral contraceptives. Lancet 1:1076, 1976

Fechner RE: Bleeding from adenoma of the liver. Arch Surg 112:100, 1977

Glassberg AB, Rosenbaum EH: Oral contraceptives and malignant hepatoma. Lancet 1:479, 1976

Henderson BE, Benton B, Edmondson HA: Hepatocellular carcinoma and oral contraceptives, JAMA 236:560, 1976

Kalra TMS, Mangla JC, DePapp EW: Benign hepatic tumors and oral contraceptive pills. Am J Med 61:871, 1976

Knowles II DM, Wolff M: Focal nodular hyperplasia of the liver. A clinicopathologic study and review of the literature. Hum Pathol 7:533, 1976

O'Sullivan JP, Rosswick RP: Oral contraceptives and malignant hepatic tumours. Lancet 1:1124, 1976

Ross D, Pina J, Mirza M, et al: Regression of focal nodular hyperplasia after discontinuation of oral contraceptives. Ann Intern Med 85:203, 1976

Schenken JR: Hepatocellular adenoma; Relationship to oral contraceptives? JAMA 236:559, 1976

Sears HF, Smith G, Powell Jr RD: Hepatic adenoma associated with oral contraceptive use. An unusual clinical presentation. Arch Surg 111:1399, 1976

Stauffer JQ, Hill RB: Systemic contraceptives and liver tumors. Ann Intern Med 85:122, 1976

THE ROLE OF ELECTRON MICROSCOPY IN THE IDENTIFICATION OF VIRUSES IN HUMAN DISEASE

EDUARDO J. YUNIS, YOSHIE HASHIDA, AND JOEL E. HAAS

The value of electron microscopy in the study of many human diseases has been well documented.[1-4] Its contributions to diagnostic pathology and to our understanding of the pathogenesis of both common and rare disorders are underscored by the large volume of published reports of studies utilizing the electron microscope. Electron microscopy has been widely used experimentally and clinically in the study of glomerulonephritis, thus improving our capabilities to diagnose human disease, and giving us considerable insight into its pathogenesis. In the study of certain human tumors, electron microscopy has contributed to the solutions of basic problems in differential diagnosis and histogenesis.[5] Electron microscopy has also been of aid in providing specific diagnostic and confirmatory information in the study of congenital and metabolic myopathies and neuropathies.[1] A new category of diseases, the "lysosomal diseases," [6] has been established, aided by electron microscopic study of morphologic changes associated with many inherited metabolic disorders, such as the various mucopolysaccharidoses, glycogen storage diseases, Tay-Sachs disease, Gaucher's disease, and many others.

Our knowledge of the structure and biology of viruses has been immensely enhanced by electron microscopy.[7] Experience gained from the ultrastructural study of viruses in culture and diseased tissues has been of paramount importance in the elucidation of the pathogenesis of many viral diseases. The extreme importance of electron microscopy in suggesting a role for specific viruses as causative agents in such entities as subacute sclerosing panencephalitis and progressive multifocal leukoencephalopathy is well known.[8, 9] But the usefulness of electron microscopy in the diagnosis of viral infections has not been fully realized.[10-12] This may be due to widely held views that meaningful information may only be obtained from fresh and optimally fixed tissue samples. It is the purpose of this chapter to emphasize that a number of available techniques allow electron microscopic detection of virus or virus products not only in ideally prepared material from body fluids, exudates, biopsy material, and fresh or fixed autopsy material, but also in tissue processed and embedded in paraffin for routine histologic examination, and even in hematoxylin and eosin-stained slides. Although the electron microscopic images derived from some of these sources may not be comparable to those obtained in the experimental situation, useful diagnostic information can be obtained from such a variety of material using appropriate precautions.

Crystalline arrays of replicating virions and groups of large viruses may be identified with certainty in suboptimally fixed material. On the other hand, the identification of naked nucleocapsid should be approached with extreme caution in such material, since even in well-fixed material, it has been confused with native nucleoprotein. Individual small virus particles (enteroviruses), not in orderly arranged groups, are difficult to distinguish from cytoplasmic components such as glycogen and ribosomes, even in optimally fixed tissue sections. Thus, images obtained from suboptimally fixed materials must be critically appraised, especially in light of a thorough knowledge of the structure and morphology (their size, site of replication, appearance, capsid symmetry) of various groups of viruses, and knowledge of ultrastructural tissue changes. Even though the electron microscopic images of viruses withstand poor fixation, the danger of mistaking altered or poorly fixed cellular structures for viral particles is inversely proportional to the status of tissue preservation and fixation. However, optimal fixation does not preclude erroneous interpretation. Examples abound in the literature of particles claimed to resemble viruses for which there is as yet no proof. Information concerning virus morphology is available elsewhere.[7]

Identification of Viruses in Negatively Stained Preparations

Negatively stained preparations of fluid from viral skin vesicles and extracts of sonicated crusts of healed vesicles were used as early as 1964 to yield images of a diagnostic character.[13] A small drop of the vesicle fluid can be readily mixed with an equal volume of phosphotungstic acid, placed on a carbon-coated electron microscopic grid, and immediately examined in the electron microscope. The negatively stained viral images allow ready differentiation between such viruses as vaccinia and herpes based on their general architecture and size (Fig. 1). Utilization of such simple techniques in the differential diagnosis of vesicular skin lesions may be of great epidemiologic value, since few have had first-hand experience with smallpox.[14] It may be difficult to distinguish clinically between the skin lesions of vaccinia and herpesviruses, especially in patients with spontaneous or iatrogenic disorders of the immune system.[12] The potential value of chemotherapeutic agents in the treatment of herpes infections may make an early and definitive diagnosis important.[12, 15] Myxoviruses have been demonstrated by the negative stain technique in nasal secretions and cerebrospinal fluid.[16]

Immune electron microscopy [17] has contributed to the elucidation of the etiology of nonbacterial gastroenteritis and hepatitis A and B. In this technique, the immune complexes formed by mixing the virus suspension and the antiserum are pelleted by ultracentrifugation, stained negatively with phosphotungstic acid, and examined by electron microscopy. This is one of the most sensitive methods for establishing the presence of an immune reaction and allows the direct visualiza-

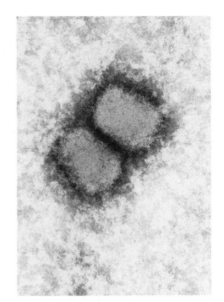

Fig. 1. These vaccinia virions negatively stained with phosphotungstic acid were obtained from a dermal vesicle of an 11-month-old girl. Their size and rectangular outline allow differentiation from herpes virions. × 79,000.

tion of viral particles aggregated by specific antisera. It is particularly of great value to detect small viruses present in low titers.

The agent of infantile epidemic gastroenteritis was originally thought to be a reoviruslike agent. More recently it has been termed rotavirus and duovirus, and it has been demonstrated in a high proportion of the stools of patients with infantile epidemic gastroenteritis in a number of reports from all over the world.[18] It has been demonstrated in stool extracts and in electron microscopic sections of duodenal mucosa to be a distinctive particle 600 to 650 Å in diameter, similar to viruses known to cause diarrhea in infant mice, calves, and pigs.[19] Rapid type-specific identification of enteroviruses is also possible by immune electron microscopy using a serum-in-agar diffusion method.[20]

The inability to demonstrate a virus in tissue culture or by biochemical methods in viral hepatitis has underscored the importance of electron microscopy in the study of this disease.[21, 22] A variety of electron microscopic techniques utilized during the past five years has contributed significantly to our understanding of the morphology, antigenicity, and sites of assembly of a hepatitis virus. Negative staining and routine sections have elucidated the nature of the 42-nm diameter Dane particle and established the relationship of its envelope to the smaller spherical and tubular particles (20 to 22 nm diameter) seen in hepatitis B surface antigen-rich plasma (Fig. 2). Immune electron microscopy [23] established the existence of an antibody to the core of the same particle, opening the way for demonstration of core antigen in nuclei of infected cells. The core is presumably extruded into the cytoplasm where it obtains its HBsAg-containing envelope, thus forming the Dane particle, the complete virion.[22] Immune electron microscopy has also demonstrated a 27-nm viruslike particle in the stool of patients with type A hepatitis.[24]

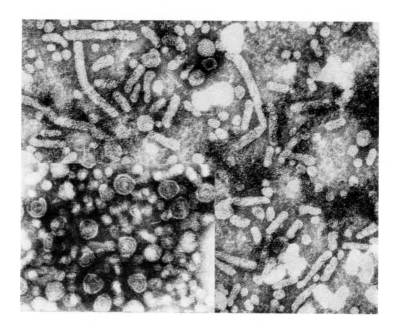

Fig. 2. The filamentous and spherical 20 to 22 nm particles and the 42 nm (Dane) particles (insert) are seen in this negative stain of hepatitis B surface antigen-rich plasma. × 170,000. (Courtesy of Robert Atchison, Ph.D. and Bruce Merrell, Graduate School of Public Health, The University of Pittsburgh.)

The disease has been induced in marmosets [25] and chimpanzees [26] inoculated with human hepatitis A virus, and viral particles have been visualized in the livers of experimentally infected marmoset monkeys.[25]

In this laboratory and others,[11] the simple technique of negative staining of fluids has been extended to the viral diagnostic laboratory. When it is important to establish a diagnosis before a recognizable pattern of cytopathic effect occurs, or when different viruses give a similar cytopathic effect, or it is undesirable to await definitive neutralizing antibody studies, it is possible to examine the nutrient fluid of infected tissue cultures with the negative stain technique. In this manner, one can determine whether or not a virus is present and perhaps make a definitive identification of that virus. If complete virologic diagnostic methods such as a battery of identifying, neutralizing antisera are not available, a standard electron microscopic tissue section of the centrifuged tissue culture pellet may be made, revealing the characteristic morphology of a given virus in tissue culture. Thus, it is possible to identify and distinguish a virus of the herpes group (Fig. 3) from the myxoviruses, enteroviruses, poxviruses (Fig. 4), or adenovirus group (Fig. 5).

The Use of Formalin-Fixed Material

Electron microscopy is useful in the diagnosis of viral infections when facilities for culturing and identifying viruses by routine methods are not available. Appropriately chosen fresh tissues may be obtained at surgical biopsy or even at

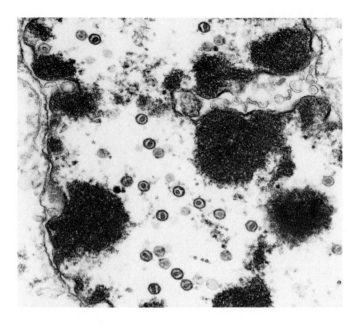

Fig. 3. Naked virions of herpesvirus grown in tissue culture of throat washing are seen within the nucleus. × 43,000.

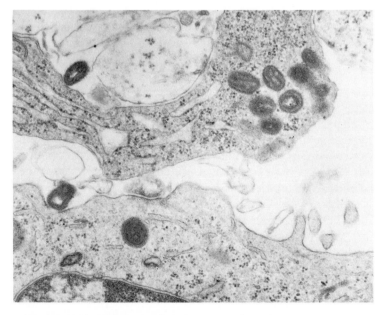

Fig. 4. Section of pellet of tissue culture of the vesicle fluid from the same patient as Figure 1, showing the complex coating of poxviruses. × 46,000.

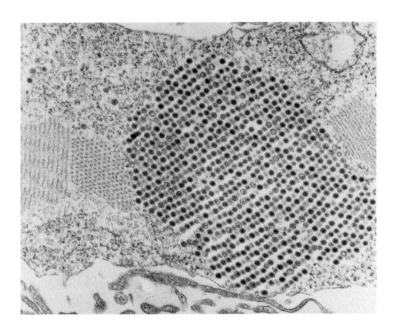

Fig. 5. Adenovirus grown in tissue culture of the liver obtained at postmortem examination of an infant. $\times$ 32,000.

autopsy to establish and corroborate light microscopic diagnoses of viral infections, such as herpetic encephalitis or hepatitis (Fig. 6), adenovirus pneumonia, and disseminated measles. When fresh tissue is not available, it is not impossible to establish such diagnoses with the electron microscope using formalin-fixed tissues stored for varying periods of time. Following the initial reports of the viral nucleocapsid nature of the nuclear inclusions of subacute sclerosing panencephalitis (Fig. 7A), we retrieved formalin-fixed autopsy tissue from eight patients in whom the diagnosis of encephalitis had been made previously by light microscopy. The now widely recognized characteristic nucleocapsidlike detail of the nuclear inclusions was readily recognizable in three of these (Fig. 7B), including one that had been shown previously to contain herpesvirus antigen by immunofluorescence. In the remainder, the diagnosis of herpes was corroborated, the characteristic outline of the individual herpesvirus particles being easily recognized in this tissue that had been formalin-fixed for a period of years.[27] Thus, the electron microscopic examination of formalin-fixed tissue makes possible the differential diagnosis of nuclear inclusions seen in subacute sclerosing panencephalitis, herpes, progressive multifocal leukoencephalopathy,[9] and adenovirus.[28] More recently, togavirus particles were demonstrated for the first time with the electron microscope in the brain of a patient with eastern encephalomyelitis.[29]

The diagnosis of adenovirus pneumonia may be suspected from the examination of lung sections obtained at autopsy. However, the smudged nature of the nuclear changes in routine histopathologic sections often makes it difficult to establish that diagnosis if appropriate viral cultures have not been taken. In this

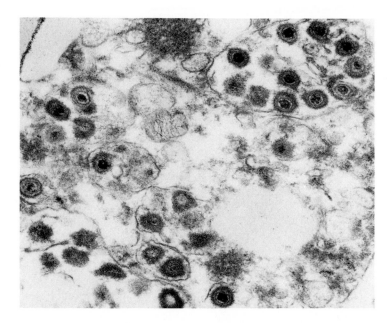

Fig. 6. Enveloped herpesvirus particles are demonstrated in the cytoplasm of a liver cell. Material obtained from a case of neonatal disseminated herpes infection, 7 hours post-mortem. × 54,000.

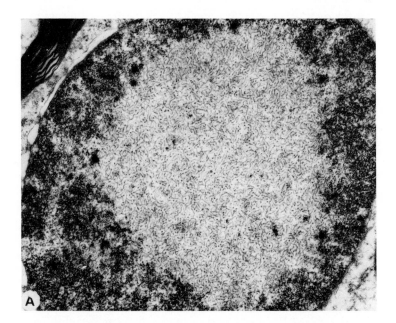

Fig. 7. A. Low-power electron micrograph of oligodendroglial nucleus with typical subacute sclerosing panencephalitis inclusion characterized by margination of the chromatin and a central body composed of tubular structures. Glutaraldehyde-osmium. × 32,000.

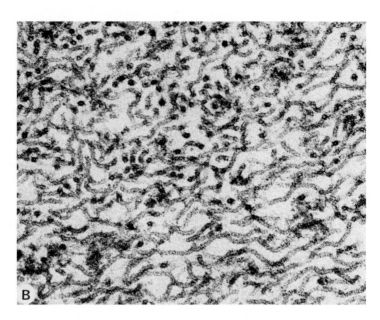

Fig. 7. B. High magnification of tubular structures composing subacute sclerosing pan-encephalitis inclusion to show the cross-sectional hollow profiles and the suggestion of cross-hatching in longitudinal profiles. Material fixed in formalin for 2 weeks. × 143,000.

laboratory, we have been successful in going back to formalin-fixed stock tissue, processing it for electron microscopy, finding similar smudged nuclei in preliminary thick sections, and demonstrating with the electron microscope that such smudged nuclei contain replicating adenovirus (Fig. 8).

Electron microscopy has also demonstrated and confirmed the role of measles virus in the intranuclear inclusions present in cells of tissue biopsies of Koplik spots.[30] We have been able to demonstrate the widespread changes caused by disseminated measles virus in three cases of atypical measles in patients receiving immunosuppressive therapy. The study of measles giant cells in formalin-fixed lungs, liver, kidney, and adrenal gland resulted in the demonstration of intranuclear measles nucleocapsid similar to that seen in subacute sclerosing panencephalitis.[31] This demonstrates that measles nucleocapsid propagates in other tissues just as it does in central nervous system (CNS) tissues in subacute sclerosing panencephalitis, apparently without forming intact virions.

The difficulties in distinguishing viral particles from cytoplasmic components are illustrated in the search for coxsackievirus particles in diseased human tissues. The difficulties are due to the similarities in size, morphology, and staining characteristics that individual virions share with both ribosomes and glycogen. In an extensive search for such configurations in a case of culture documented coxsackievirus B2 encephalomyocarditis, we were successful in demonstrating crystalline arrays within the endothelial cytoplasm of myocardial capillaries.[32] The tissue from which these sections were prepared for electron microscopy had been stored in Jores' autopsy fixative for approximately one month. The fact that a tissue has not

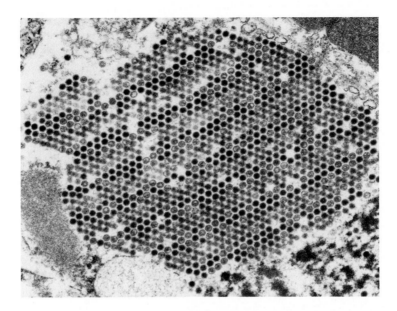

Fig. 8. Crystalline array of virions from a 3-month-old infant with adenovirus pneumonia. The lung had been stored in 10 percent formaldehyde for 3 weeks before embedding in Epon-araldite. × 35,000.

been optimally fixed should not prohibit the application of electron microscopic methods to the diagnosis of viral infections. More recently, crystalline arrays of replicating coxsackievirus A9 have been demonstrated in sections of skeletal muscle from which virus could be identified in tissue culture only after multiple passages.[33] Electron microscopy may reveal viral infection to be more widespread than routine cultures would indicate. Picornaviruslike crystals have also been reported in two culture-negative cases of polymyositis [34] and in skeletal muscle of Reye's syndrome,[35] but their viral nature has been questioned.[36]

The Use of Routine Hematoxylin and Eosin-Stained Slides

Other useful sources of material for the application of electron microscopy to viral diagnosis are paraffin-embedded material [2] and, better yet, routine hematoxylin and eosin-stained paraffin tissue sections. To be able to select a precise area from a hematoxylin and eosin-stained slide for electron microscopic examination has obvious advantages. After demonstrating the remarkably well-preserved appearance of various DNA viruses such as adenovirus, herpes simplex, and cytomegalovirus in routine histologic stained sections, Blank et al [37] extended their observations to the study of viral skin lesions. Using hematoxylin and eosin-stained histologic sections of formalin-fixed paraffin-embedded tissues, they demonstrated the electron microscopic appearance of poxviruses (molluscum contagiosum, vaccinia, smallpox), herpes simplex, and a human papillomavirus. In this technique, the cover slip is removed and the slide rinsed in mixtures of xylol and propylene oxide. The tissue is covered with a thin layer of Epon-araldite and placed in the oven. Upon hardening, the tissue becomes attached to the sheet of Epon-araldite and is removed from the slide by prying with a razor blade. The desired area is cut out under the dissecting microscope, attached to the tip of a Beem capsule block of Epon-araldite, and sectioned for electron microscopy. Using this technique, typical crystalline arrays of adenovirus particles have been demonstrated in the distinctive and smudged nuclear inclusions of 10-year-old histologic sections of lung of infants who died of adenovirus pneumonia.[38] We have extended these observations in our laboratory, utilizing such techniques to rule out or demonstrate the presence of viruses in questionable inclusions or smudged nuclei in cases of suspected viral infection where cultures have not been obtained. Further, in this fashion, we have established the frequent occurrence of adenovirus in nuclei of intestinal and appendiceal mucosa of children with ileocolic intussusception (Fig. 9).[39] Similarly, we have demonstrated intranuclear cytomegalovirus in histologic sections of a case of healing neonatal necrotizing enterocolitis (Fig. 10). In each of these instances, light microscopic slides with suggestive or definite intranuclear inclusions in hematoxylin and eosin-stained sections served as the source of individual cells to be examined with the electron microscope. Similar techniques have been applied to cytology preparations for examination of nuclear and cytoplasmic inclusions.[37] In this laboratory, intranuclear papovaviruslike particles have been demonstrated in the urinary sediment of a child with acute hemorrhagic cystitis (Fig. 11).[40] Only adenovirus had been previously known to be associated with acute hemorrhagic

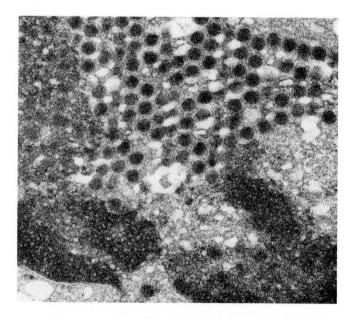

Fig. 9. Intranuclear 58 nm particles from an H&E slide with inclusions within epithelial cells of the appendix, from a case of ileocecal intussusception. × 105,000.

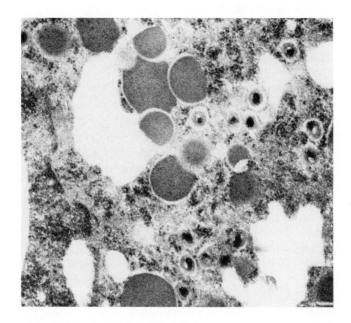

Fig. 10. Herpes-group virions were demonstrated using the H&E-stained slide of material from the surgically resected terminal ileum from a 2.5-month-old infant with healing infantile necrotizing enterocolitis. × 43,000.

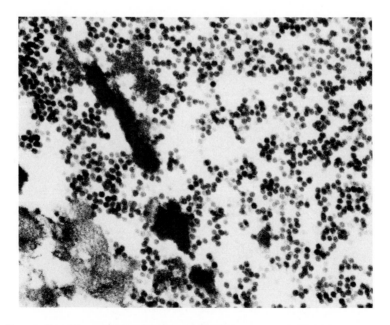

Fig. 11. Papovavirus-like particles demonstrated in the urinary epithelial cells using H&E-stained cytology preparation from a child with acute hemorrhagic cystitis. × 72,000.

cystitis.[41] With this technique, we have also demonstrated pox virions in smears made from lesions suspected to be molluscum contagiosum (Fig. 12).

Nonviral Nuclear Inclusions and Pseudoinclusions

Electron microscopy has also helped in the elucidation of the nature of nuclear pseudoinclusions such as those found in neoplasms,[42] in paraproteinemias, and in pancreatic cells of patients dying with Reye's syndrome (Fig. 13),[43] and of nonviral nuclear inclusions such as those seen in hepatic and renal tubular cells in lead poisoning. The latter inclusions have been shown to be heavy metal protein complexes by histochemical, electron microscopic, and x-ray diffraction studies.[44] Electron microscopy of pseudoinclusions revealed these structures to be cytoplasmic components surrounded by invaginated nuclear membrane or accumulation of material in dilated perinuclear cisterna.

Virus-Like Particles

As discussed earlier, electron microscopy may be of use in establishing the presence of pathogenic viruses when other methods have failed. There are multiple instances, however, when the use of electron microscopy in attempts to demonstrate virus particles may have created more heat than light.

The intense activity in the electron microscopic examination of fresh biopsy

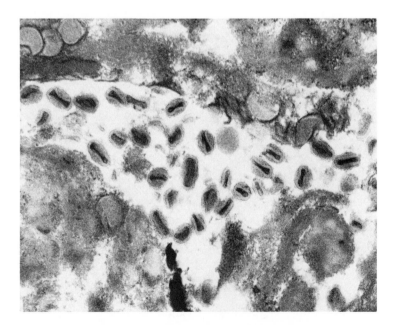

Fig. 12. The complex coating and dumbbell-shaped inner core of pox virions are seen in this preparation made from a cytology smear containing the cytoplasmic inclusion of molluscum contagiosum. × 56,000.

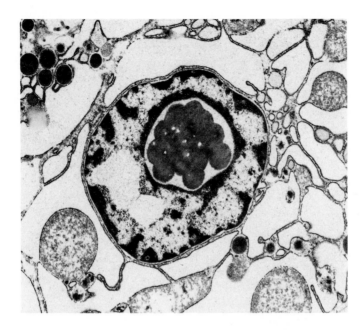

Fig. 13. This pseudoinclusion body in a pancreatic acinar cell nucleus bordered by condensed chromatin material was obtained at autopsy of a 4.5-year-old boy who died of Reye's syndrome. The tissue had been stored in 10 percent formaldehyde for 3 weeks. × 14,000.

material and the search for a human tumor virus or viruses has resulted in a deluge of reports of viral particles or viruslike structures associated with a variety of lesions. These are intracytoplasmic, intranuclear, or extracellular nucleocapsidlike structures; and intranuclear, intracytoplasmic, or extracellular, naked or enveloped, round, viruslike particles.

Widely recognized are the myxoviruslike inclusions in the endothelial cytoplasm of patients with systemic lupus erythematosus, first reported in 1969.[45] These tubuloreticular structures occur within endoplasmic reticulum and were cited to be similar to nucleocapsid of paramyxovirus in both dimensions and appearance (Fig. 14). However, since the initial report, a spate of subsequent papers have pointed out a number of discrepancies, casting great doubts onto their alleged viral nature. These include the lack of previously known intracisternal viral products,[46] size discrepancies (a diameter of 200 to 300 Å versus 180 Å of paramyxovirus nucleocapsid), their near ubiquity,[47] nonspecies specificity (their occurrence in equine viral arteritis and rhesus monkey endothelium as well as in human tissues [46]), their reproducibility in lymphoid cell cultures stimulated with 5-bromo-deoxyuridine,[48] the repeated failure to yield a culturable virus, their glycoprotein nature,[48] and lack of cytochemically identifiable nucleic acid.[49] They may somehow be related to viral replication in other regions of a cell,[50] but are most likely nonspecific alterations in the structure of endoplasmic reticulum.[51] These and other viruslike structures associated with systemic lupus erythematosus have been discussed by Andres et al.[52]

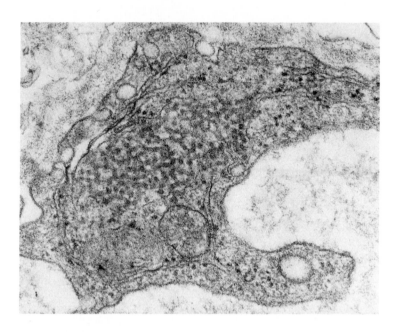

Fig. 14. Myxovirus-like inclusion in the cytoplasm of an endothelial cell found in a brain biopsy specimen obtained from a 6-month-old infant with spongy degeneration of the brain (Canavan's disease). × 80,000.

Intranuclear nucleocapsidlike structures have been reported in muscle nuclei of patients with polymyositis.[53] These inclusions, while similar to myxovirus in external diameter of 180 Å, are likewise similar in diameter to myofilaments and have been seen in nuclei of other diseased muscle (Fig. 15).[54]

Structures said to be similar to the nucleocapsid seen in subacute sclerosing panencephalitis have been illustrated in three cases of Goodpasture's syndrome.[55] However, the illustration is not unlike the appearance of native nucleoprotein in suboptimally fixed nuclei or nuclei in tissue primarily fixed in osmium tetroxide. Similar images of native nucleoprotein may be dependent upon the stage of the cell cycle and probably represent altered chromatin images in severely injured cells. Thus, in a glomerular lesion that is characterized by epithelial proliferation and often necrosis, such images must be judged with caution. Similarly, images illustrated as viral, alleged to represent measles nucleocapsid occurring in alveolar lining cells of patients with leukemia,[56] and paramyxoviruslike particles seen in mononuclear cells of patients with multiple sclerosis,[57] most likely represent altered nuclear chromatin.[58]

Extracellular nucleocapsidlike particles have been seen in both glomerular and skin lesions [59, 60] in deposits of lupus erythematosus. These coiled and straight aggregates of material with distinct periodicity are much larger in diameter (600 Å) than known viral nucleocapsids and are now thought to be crystalline, physicochemically altered proteins. As such, they seem to be specific for systemic lupus erythematosus.[60]

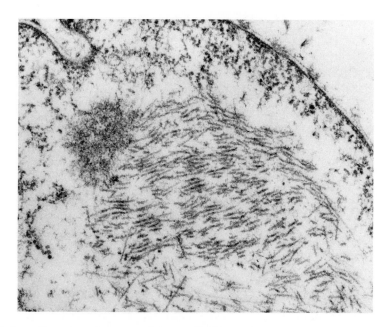

Fig. 15. A portion of nucleus containing a fibrillar nucleocapsidlike inclusion body from muscle biopsy material of a case of inclusion body myositis. The specimen had been stored in formaldehyde for 2 weeks. × 46,000.

Particles said to resemble intact virus have been reported in nuclei of patients with serum hepatitis.[61] Their resemblance to perichromatinic granules and dissimilarity to noncoated particles seen in hepatocytic nuclei and cytoplasm of patients with type B hepatitis [23] renders their vital nature doubtful.

Originally seen in nuclei of virus-infected tissues, nuclear bodies have since been recognized in a variety of conditions including a number of tumors (Fig. 16). Their exact nature remains unclear, but they do not resemble images of known viruses, and they are considered to be a manifestation of cellular reactivity.[62]

Enveloped viruslike particles have been described within the glomerular basement membrane of a renal biopsy from a patient with proteinuria who had serologic evidence of mumps infection.[63] These particles were thought to be mumps virus due to morphologic similarities. However, virus could not be cultured from the urine, and the structures lacked distinct nucleocapsid. Thus, such inclusions within the glomerular basement membrane may alternatively be interpreted as tangentially sectioned extensions of glomerular cells.

In the search for human tumor viruses, the technique of negative staining has given rise to premature claims for recognition of virus particles. Although negative staining of concentrated samples of viruses has been of obvious value, negatively stained cell debris can easily be confused with individual particles.[64] There have also been reports of standard electron microscopic images of isolated particles resembling the murine B- (Fig. 17) and C-type particles in mammary carcinoma, other human tumors, human milk, and cultures of various human tissues

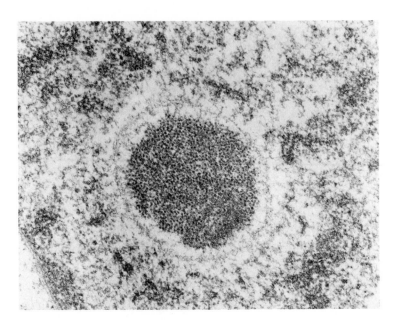

Fig. 16. A portion of a nucleus with a nucleolar body from a mesenchymal sarcoma of the neck of a 6.5-year-old boy. × 47,500.

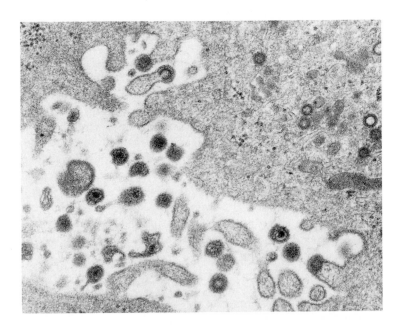

Fig. 17. Intracytoplasmic A, budding and mature B particles from mouse mammary carcinoma. × 63,000.

and tumors. However, these particles have not occurred in the same numbers with which they occur in the murine tumors. They have been mostly isolated particles, showed variable morphology, and have not been corroborated by other investigators. Additionally, there has not been consistent biochemical evidence for the presence of viral components analogous to that which occurs in the animal tumors.[64] Small vesicles and other cellular structures can resemble isolated virus particles. These include tangentially sectioned nuclear pores, annulate lamellae, pinocytotic vesicles, and altered organelle membranes.[65] Hence, the appearance of isolated intracellular and budding particles said to be similar to those occurring in animal tumor systems must be interpreted with great caution and with the same rigorous criteria used to judge the identity of such particles in the experimental tumor systems.

Particles said to resemble C-type animal viruses have been seen in sections of a wide variety of tissues, including many renal lesions. These should be particularly acknowledged because of the widespread use of electron microscopy in evaluating renal biopsies. Variously termed round extracellular particles,[66] extracellular granular material,[66] and spherical microparticles,[67] they have appeared within dense deposits, within the glomerular basement membrane, mesangium, and associated with but not within all three varieties of glomerular cells. At least two classes of these materials, based on size and appearance, may be associated with membrane fragments and are usually present in clusters that have the appearance of fibrinoid deposits by light microscopy. There is a tendency for these particles to occur' in proliferative lesions or injured glomeruli with cellular destruction, and their resemblance to contents of injured nuclei has been cited. The associated membrane fragments may also be nuclear in origin.[66] Round extracellular particles range from 400 to 1200 Å in diameter, and may have a dense core with an adjacent clear halo and a single limiting membrane. Spherical microparticles are pleomorphic and average 500 to 580 Å in diameter. These particles are most frequently seen adjacent to cytoplasmic processes of epithelial and mesangial cells and to glomerular lesions where sclerosis and electron-dense deposits predominate. Despite their resemblance to herpesviruses, C-type particles, or particles seen in cultured lymphocytes from patients with infectious mononucleosis, their location, variation in size, and their frequent association with cellular debris suggest their origin from damaged cells.[66] They have been considered cytoplasmic microvesicles or crystalline lipoprotein bodies released from damaged cells.[67] The virallike particles recently reported in cases of Reye's syndrome [68] as representing herpes and myxovirus/paramyxovirus, resemble secretory granules and coated vesicles. Absence of nuclear replication is against herpes.

Whether or not any of these structures should prove to be viral in origin, the contributions of electron microscopy to their discovery and initial steps in elucidation of their nature and potential pathogenesis are self-evident. Such was the case with subacute sclerosing panencephalitis and progressive multifocal leuko-encephalopathy. However, caution should prevail, and the rigorous criteria used for acceptance of a given image as virus or virus-related should be strictly applied now and in the future as it was in the past. Conclusions must be reached in light of knowledge of the structure and site of replication of the alleged virus, the source of the material in which the images are seen, fixation methods, and most importantly, the wide variety of documented ultrastructural images of normal cell components and changes occurring in diseased tissues, not known to be due to virus replication or to virus-mediated cell damage.

References

1. Haust MD: The clinical value of electron microscopy. Bull Int Acad Pathol 12:21 (Autumn), 1972
2. Zimmerman LE, Font RL, Ts'o M, Fine BS: Application of electron microscopy to histopathologic diagnoses. Trans Am Acad Ophthalmol Otolaryngol 76:101 (January–February), 1972
3. Neustein HB: Electron microscopy in diagnostic pathology. Perspect Pediatr Pathol 1:369, 1973
4. Bloodworth JMB, Azar HA, Yodaiken RE (eds): Symposium on electron microscopy. Hum Pathol 6:403, 1975
5. Rosai J, Rodriguez HA: Application of electron microscopy to the differential diagnosis of tumors. Am J Clin Pathol 50:555, 1968
6. Hers HG, Van Hoof F (eds): Lysosomes and Storage Diseases. New York, Academic Press, 1973
7. Dalton AJ, Haguenau F (eds): Ultrastructure of Animal Viruses and Bacteriophages: An Atlas. Ultrastructure in Biological Systems, vol. 5. New York, Academic Press, 1973
8. Bouteille M, Fontaine C, Vedrenne C, Delarue J: Sur un cas d'encéphalite subaiguë à inclusions. Etude anatomo-clinique et ultrastructurale. Rev Neurol (Paris) 113:454, 1965
9. ZuRhein GM, Chou SM: Particles resembling papova viruses in human cerebral demyelinating disease. Science 148:1477, 1965
10. Rapid diagnosis of virus diseases. Lancet 1:1411 (Editorial), 1975
11. Pennington TH, Follett EAC, Timbury MC: Rapid diagnosis of virus infections. Lancet 2:182 (Letter), 1975
12. Banatvala JE, Chrystie JL, Flower AJE: Rapid diagnosis of virus infections. Lancet 2:79 (Letter), 1975
13. Nagington J: Electron microscopy in differential diagnosis of poxvirus infections. Br Med J 2:1499, 1964
14. Confinement of the poxvirus. Lancet 2:561 (Editorial), 1974
15. Ch'ien LT, Whitley RJ, Nahmias AJ, et al: Antiviral chemotherapy and neonatal herpes simplex virus infection: A pilot study-experience with adenine arabinoside (ARA-A). Pediatrics 55:678, 1975
16. Doane FW, Anderson N, Chatiyanonda K, et al: Rapid laboratory diagnosis of paramyxovirus infections by electron microscopy. Lancet 2:751, 1967
17. Almeida JD, Waterson AD: The morphology of virus-antibody interaction. In Smith KM, Lauffer MA, Bang FB (eds): Adv Virus Res, vol 15. New York, Academic Press, 1969, pp 307–38
18. Almeida JD: Visualization of fecal viruses. N Engl J Med 292:1403, 1975
19. Rotaviruses of man and animals. Lancet 1:257 (Editorial), 1975
20. Anderson N, Doane FW: Specific identification of enteroviruses by immuno-electron microscopy using a serum-in-agar diffusion method. Can J Microbiol 19:585, 1973
21. Alter HJ, Holland PV, Purcell RH: Commentary: Viral hepatitis. Light at the end of the tunnel. JAMA 229:293, 1974
22. Virus hepatitis updated. Lancet 1:1365 (Editorial), 1975
23. Huang SN, Groh V: Immunoagglutination electron microscopic study of virus-like particles and Australia antigen in liver tissue. Lab Invest 29:353, 1973
24. Feinstone SM, Kapikian AZ, Purcell RH: Hepatitis A: Detection by immune electron microscopy of a virus-like antigen associated with acute illness. Science 182:1026, 1973

25. Provost PJ, Wolanski BS, Miller WJ, et al: Biophysical and biochemical properties of CR326 human hepatitis A virus. Am J Med Sci 270:87, 1975
26. Maynard JE: Hepatitis A. Perspectives and recent advances. Am J Pathol 81:683, 1975
27. Hashida Y, Yunis EJ: Re-examination of encephalitic brains known to contain intranuclear inclusion bodies: Electron microscopic observations following prolonged fixation in formalin. Am J Clin Pathol 53:537, 1970
28. Chou SJ, Burrell R, Harley J, Gutmann L, Roos R: Subacute focal adenovirus encephalitis. J Neuropathol Exp Neurol 31:173 (Abstract), 1972
29. Bastian FO, Wende RO, Singer DB, Zeller RS: Eastern equine encephalomyelitis. Histopathologic and ultrastructural changes with isolation of the virus in a human case. Am J Clin Pathol 64:10, 1975
30. Suringa DWR, Bank LJ, Ackerman AB: Role of measles virus in skin lesions and Koplik's spots. N Engl J Med 283:1139, 1970
31. Breitfeld V, Hashida Y, Sherman FE, Odagiri K, Yunis EJ: Fatal measles infection in children with leukemia. Lab Invest 28:279, 1973
32. Haas JE, Yunis EJ: Viral crystalline arrays in human Coxsackie myocarditis. Lab Invest 23:442, 1970
33. Tang TT, Sedmak GV, Siegesmund DA, McCreadie SR: Chronic myopathy associated with coxsackievirus type A9: A combined electron microscopical and viral isolation study. N Engl J Med 292:608, 1975
34. Chou SM, Gutmann L: Picornavirus-like crystals in subacute polymyositis. Neurology 20:205, 1970
35. Alvira MM, Mendoza M: Reye's syndrome: A viral myopathy? N Engl J Med 292:1297 (Letter), 1975
36. Hanson PA, Urizar RE: Reye's syndrome—virus or artifact in muscle? N Engl J Med 293:505 (Letter), 1975
37. Blank H, Davis C, Collins C: Electron microscopy for the diagnosis of cutaneous viral infections. Br J Dermatol 83:69, 1970
38. Pinkerton H, Carroll S: Fatal adenovirus pneumonia in infants. Correlation of histologic and electron microscopic observations. Am J Pathol 65:543, 1971
39. Yunis EJ, Atchison RW, Michaels RH, DeCicco FA: Adenovirus and ileocecal intussusception. Lab Invest 33:347, 1975
40. Hashida Y, Gaffney PG, Yunis EJ: Acute hemorrhagic cystitis of childhood and papovavirus-like particles. J Pediatr (in press)
41. Numazaki Y, Kumasaka T, Yano N, et al: Further study on acute hemorrhagic cystitis due to adenovirus type 11. N Engl J Med 289:344, 1973
42. Sobel HJ, Schwarz R, Marquet E: Nonviral nuclear inclusions. I. Cytoplasmic invaginations. Arch Pathol 87:179, 1969
43. Collins DN: Ultrastructural study of intranuclear inclusions in the exocrine pancreas in Reye's syndrome. Lab Invest 30:333, 1974
44. Goyer RA, May P, Cates MM, Krigman MR: Lead and protein content of isolated intranuclear inclusion bodies from kidneys of lead-poisoned rats. Lab Invest 22:245, 1970
45. Györkey E, Min KW, Sinkovics JG, Györkey P: Systemic lupus erythematosus and myxovirus. N Engl J Med 280:333 (Letter), 1969
46. Haas JE, Yunis EJ: Tubular inclusions of systemic lupus erythematosus. Ultrastructural observations regarding their possible viral nature. Exp Mol Pathol 12:257, 1970
47. Uzman BG, Saito H, Kasac M: Tubular arrays in the endoplasmic reticulum in human tumor cells. Lab Invest 24:492, 1971
48. Schaff Z, Barry DW, Grimley PM: Cytochemistry of tuboreticular structures in lymphocytes from patients with systemic lupus erythematosus and in cultured human lymphoid cells. Comparison to a paramyxovirus. Lab Invest 29:577, 1973
49. Schaff Z, Heine U, Dalton AJ: Ultramorphological and ultracytochemical studies on tuboreticular structures in lymphoid cells. Cancer Res 32:2696, 1972

50. Barringer JR, Swoveland P: Tubular aggregates in endoplasmic reticulum: Evidence against their viral nature. J Ultrastruct Res 41:270, 1972
51. Chandra S: Undulating tubules associated with endoplasmic reticulum in pathologic tissues. Lab Invest 18:422, 1968
52. Andres GA, Speile H, McCluskey RT: Virus-like structures in systemic lupus erythematosus. In Schwartz RS (ed): Progress in Clinical Immunology, vol 1. New York, Grune, 1972, pp 23–44
53. Chou SM: Myxovirus-like structures in a case of human chronic polymyositis. Science 158:1453, 1967
54. Yunis EJ, Samaha FJ: Inclusion body myositis. Lab Invest 25:240, 1971
55. Tsai CC, Kissane JM, Germuth FG, Jr: Paramyxovirus-like structures in Goodpasture's syndrome. Lancet 2:601, 1974
56. Akhtar M, Young I: Measles giant cell pneumonia in an adult following longterm chemotherapy. Arch Pathol 96:145, 1973
57. Prineas J: Paramyxovirus-like particles associated with acute demyelination in chronic relapsing multiple sclerosis. Science 178:760, 1972
58. Hayano M, Sung JH, Mastri AE: "Paramyxovirus-like particles" occurring in various tissues in diverse unrelated conditions. Presented at 51st meeting, American Association of Neuropathologists, New York, May 30, 1975
59. Fresco R: Virus-like particles in systemic lupus erythematosus. N Engl J Med 283:1231 (Letter), 1970
60. Grishman E, Porush JC, Rosen SM, Churg J: Lupus nephritis with organized deposits in the kidneys. Lab Invest 16:717, 1967
61. Skikne MI, Talbot JH: The identification and structural analysis of viral particles in serum hepatitis. Lab Invest 31:246, 1974
62. Dupuy-Coin AM, Lazar P, Kalifat SR, Bouteille M: A method of quantitation of nuclear bodies in electron microscopy. J Ultrastruct Res 27:244, 1969
63. Smith RD, Northrop RL: Paramyxovirus-like structures in the nephrotic syndrome. Am J Clin Pathol 56:97, 1971
64. de Harven E: Remarks on the ultrastructure of type A, B, and C virus particles. In Lauffer MA, Bang FB, Maramorosch K, Smith KM (eds): Adv Virus Res, vol 19. New York, Academic Press, 1974, pp 221–64
65. Haguenau F: "Virus-like" particles as observed with the electron microscope. In Dalton AJ, Haguenau F (eds): Ultrastructure of Animal Viruses and Bacteriophages: An Atlas. New York, Academic Press, 1973, pp 391–97
66. Bariety J, Callard P, Appay MD, Grossetete J, Mandel C: Ultrastructural study of some frequent and poorly known intraglomerular structures. In Hamburger J, Crosnier J, Maxwell MH (eds): Advances in Nephrology from the Necker Hospital, vol 3. Chicago, Yearbook, 1974, pp 153–172
67. Burkholder PM, Hyman LR, Barber TA: Extracellular clusters of spherical microparticles in glomeruli in human renal glomerular diseases. Lab Invest 28:415, 1973
68. Tang TT, Siegesmund KA, Segmak GV, et al: Reye syndrome. A correlated electron-microscopic, viral, and biochemical observation. JAMA 232:1339, 1975

ANATOMIC PATHOLOGY AND PATHOGENESIS OF THE LESIONS OF SMALL ARTERIES AND ARTERIOLES OF THE KIDNEY IN ESSENTIAL HYPERTENSION

ANIL K. MANDAL, RICHARD D. BELL, JOHN A. NORDQUIST, AND ROBERT D. LINDEMAN

The renal pathology associated with essential hypertension has been labeled arteriolar nephrosclerosis.[1] Nephrosclerosis has been considered as benign when the small arteries and arterioles exhibit hyaline (or eosinophilic) thickening of the vessel wall, with little or no change in other component parts of the kidney. In contrast, malignant nephrosclerosis is characterized by necrotic and proliferative changes in the arterioles, necrosis and hyalinization in the glomeruli, loss of tubular mass, and variable interstitial changes.

Many investigators [2-7] have reported on the detailed ultrastructure of the renal arteriole in benign essential and malignant hypertension. These studies failed to delineate the morphogenesis of the vascular and renal lesions and the importance of the blood pressure elevation in the development of the observed changes. Although much of this chapter will deal with the morphologic changes observed in the renal arterial vasculature of patients with benign essential and malignant hypertension and spontaneously hypertensive rats, three additional objectives will be pursued, specifically: to demonstrate a relationship between the extent of renal vascular lesions and both severity and duration of the hypertension; to delineate the mechanism of the renal failure seen to develop in hypertension, ie, is the renal failure due to the lesion of the arterial vessels alone, or is it the result of a more diffuse lesion in the kidney; and to add electron microscopic observations to our understanding of the pathology and morphogenesis of the renal lesions associated with hypertension.

331

Materials and Methods

Human

Twelve kidneys from 10 hypertensive patients were studied. Renal tissues were obtained by either percutaneous or open renal biopsies and after nephrectomies. In 2 patients (patients 5 and 7), two separate studies were performed, at intervals of 43 months and 12 months, respectively, between biopsies and nephrectomies. The clinical features and pertinent laboratory findings in all these patients are listed in Tables 1 and 2. Laboratory studies done to exclude secondary forms of hypertension were all negative, so that all patients were considered to have essential hypertension.

Rat

Kidneys from 40 spontaneously hypertensive rats (SHR) and 38 normotensive Wistar control rats (NR) of similar age distribution (9 to 103 weeks) were studied. Kidneys were removed from these rats after direct recording of their arterial pressures under light anesthesia. Each rat was coded for later identification.

Pieces of cortical renal tissue from whole kidneys of patients and rats and 1 mm pieces from either end of biopsy cores were fixed in 10 percent buffered aqueous formalin and 4 percent iced glutaraldehyde for light microscopy (LM) and electron microscopy (EM) studies, respectively. Cortical renal tissue from

TABLE 1. Clinical Features in Hypertensive Patients

Serial No.	Age, Sex	Presenting Symptoms	Blood Pressure	Known Duration of Hypertension (yr)	Fundoscopic Findings (K-W-B grading)
1	14,M	None	170/100	2	0
2	39,M	Weakness	210/110	6	II
3	22,M	Vomiting	220/130	2	II
4	51,M	Recurrent chest pain	140/110	23	II
5	25,M	Headache	240/140	Unknown	II
6	33,F	Headache and ecchymosis	160/110	6	I
7	23,M	Headache and faintness	240/140	Unknown	IV
8	33,M	Headache	230/130	Unknown	IV
9	32,M	Urinary tract infection	230/130	Unknown	IV
10	19,M	Swelling of tongue	240/140	2	IV

TABLE 2. Laboratory Information in Hypertensive Patients

Serial Number	Urinary Protein	Other Urinary Findings	Serum Urea Nitrogen	Serum Creatinine
1	0	0	12	0.9
2	4+(0.5) *	0	48	2.6
3	4+(0.35) *	0	22	1.6
4	4+(0.12) *	0	26	1.6
5	4+	0	27	2.3
6	4+	Pyuria	84	10
7	4+	0	110	13
8	4+	0	100	12
9	4+	Pyuria	139	21
10	4+(0.6) *	Numerous RBCs	112	13

* Gram per 24 hr.

With kind permission from the Editor, Annals of Clinical and Laboratory Science.

some of these patients also was fixed in ice-cold saline for immunofluorescence microscopy (IM) study.

LM STUDY.   Sections of 3 to 4 μm were cut and stained with hematoxylin and eosin (H&E), periodic acid–Schiff's reagent (PAS), Gomori's trichrome, and Hart and Verhoeff's elastic stain. The findings under the light microscope were photographed on 35-mm films from which 5-×-7-inch prints were made for analysis of the findings.

EM STUDY.   Tissues were postfixed in 1 percent osmium, dehydrated, and embedded in Spurr low-viscosity embedding media (blocks). From the blocks, 0.5 μm (thick) sections were cut, stained with methylene blue and azure II, and examined by LM. When an arterial vessel was found, the block was prepared for thin sectioning. Thin (300 Å) sections were cut and collected on copper and gold grids. The copper grids were stained with uranyl acetate and lead citrate (UA and LC) in the conventional way. The gold grids were stained with 1 percent periodic acid and methenamine silver (PASI) according to the technique described by Olson et al.[8] The gold grids were also stained with silver tetraphenyl porphyrin sulfonate (STPPS), a specific electron-dense stain for elastic tissue according to the technique developed in the authors' laboratory.[9]

All grids were photographed using an EMU (RCA) 3F electron microscope. Findings were photographed on 2-×-2-inch film, from which 8-×-10-inch prints were made for analysis of the findings.

IM STUDY.   Sections of 4 μm were cut in a cryostat and stained with fluorescein isothiocyanate conjugated antibodies against human IgG, IgM, IgA, and C_3 component of complement. The sections were examined by immunofluorescence microscopy.

Detailed Clinical Information and Renal Pathology

PATIENTS 1 THROUGH 4.   The pertinent clinical and laboratory information are shown in Tables 1 and 2.

Renal Pathology.   Kidneys from all four patients demonstrated a normal appearance in most of the glomeruli, in the tubules, and in the interstitium. In one patient (patient 2), about 5 percent of the tubules were dilated. The arterioles showed a normal appearance or thickening of the intima by lightly stained PAS-positive strands (material) and thinning of media due to the presence of excessive amounts of PAS-positive strands. All arterioles were hypocellular (Fig. 1). There was no evidence of necrotic change in any of the component parts of the kidney. By electron microscopy, the arterioles revealed thickening of the basement membranes (BM) between endothelial cells and smooth muscle cells (SMC) and between individual SMC, excessive BM-like material in the SMC layer, and normal or atrophic SMC (Figs. 2 and 3).

PATIENT 5.   A 25-year-old black male had his first admission to the Oklahoma City VA Hospital in November, 1972, for investigation of hypertension. He presented at the general medicine clinic with complaint of persistent headache and was found to have a blood pressure of 240/140 mm Hg and grade II (K-W-B) retinopathy without papilledema. Laboratory investigations failed to demonstrate an underlying cause for hypertension. Serum urea nitrogen and serum creatinine concentrations were 27 mg and 2.3 mg per 100 ml, respectively. A wedge biopsy of the kidney was taken during exploratory laparotomy, and renal tissue was studied using LM, EM, and IM. He was placed on antihypertensive drugs, his

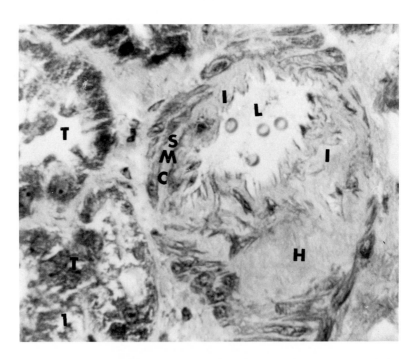

Fig. 1. An arteriole from a patient with benign hypertension (patient 1) in which marked thickening of the intima (I) by PAS-positive (hyaline) material (H) and thinning of smooth muscle cellular (SMC) layer are seen. Lumen of the arteriole (L) is shown. Adjacent tubules (T) appear normal. PAS, × 320.

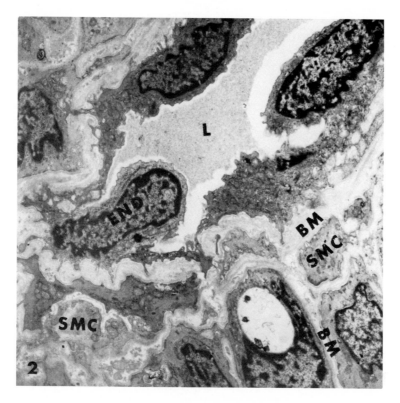

Fig. 2. An electron micrograph of an arteriole from patient 1 shows normal endothelial cell (END), moderate thickening of the basement membrane (BM) between END and smooth muscle cell (SMC), mild thickening of BM between SMC, and atrophy of some SMC. In the lumen (L), proteinaceous material is seen. UA and LC, × 8,750.

headache promptly disappeared, and his serum urea nitrogen and serum creatinine fell to near normal levels. On routine visits to the renal clinic, he experienced elevations of his blood pressures in excess of 240/140 mm Hg, which necessitated numerous hospital admissions for control of the blood pressures. His serum urea nitrogen and serum creatinine concentrations were always below those observed on his first admission. After 36 months, he had the sudden onset of exertional dyspnea and paroxysmal nocturnal dyspnea and was admitted to the hospital. His blood pressures were in the range of 250–260/140–150 mm Hg. He showed grade III (K-W-B) retinopathy. He developed rapid impairment of renal function, with an increase in serum urea nitrogen and creatinine concentrations to 110 and 11.5 mg per 100 ml, respectively. After aggressive treatment with antihypertensive drugs, digitalis, and diuretics, his blood pressure decreased markedly, and his serum urea nitrogen and creatinine concentrations decreased to 80 mg and 8.5 mg per 100 ml, respectively. Eight weeks following this episode, his renal function again began to deteriorate, his blood pressure increased, and he was placed on the maintenance hemodialysis program. Despite hemodialysis and aggressive treat-

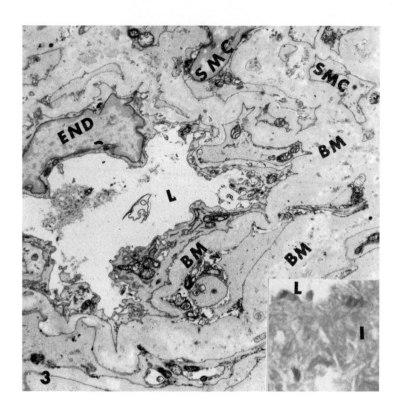

Fig. 3. The electron micrograph of an arteriole from another patient with benign hypertension (patient 2) shows atrophy of endothelial cell (END), moderate thickening of basement membrane (BM) between END and smooth muscle cell (SMC), marked thickening of BM between SMC, and atrophy of SMC. Lumen (L) of the arteriole is shown. PASI, × 6,450. Inset: A part of an arteriole from the same patient as in Figure 3 under light microscopy is shown at the lower right. Lumen (L) and thickening of intima (I) are shown. PAS, × 340.

ment with antihypertensive drugs, his blood pressure continued to increase. He underwent bilateral nephrectomy 43 months after the initial biopsy, and the renal tissue was studied by LM, EM, and IM.

Biopsy Specimen. The renal biopsy specimen showed a loss of 5 to 10 percent of the tubules, a few atrophic tubules, and mild interstitial fibrosis (Fig. 4). Studies of arterioles demonstrated moderate to marked intimal thickening and hyperplasia of SMC in large arterioles and thickening of the intima in the small arterioles (inset for Fig. 4). Thick sections (0.5 μm) stained with methylene blue and azure II and studied by LM revealed marked SMC hyperplasia. Glomeruli showed moderate to marked irregular thickening of the peripheral capillary loops. Ultrastructurally, the arterioles revealed intact endothelial cells, hyperplasia, atrophy or necrosis of SMC, a few fibroblasts, small amounts of collagen fibers, and electron-dense deposits (Fig. 5). There were increased amounts of electron-

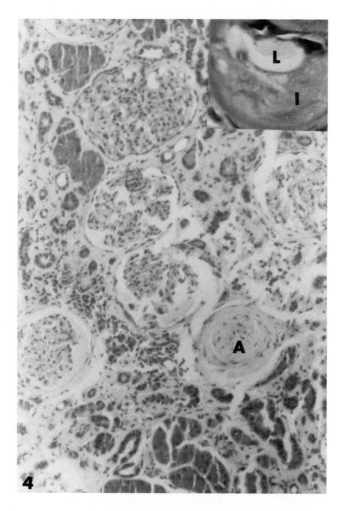

Fig. 4. This light micrograph from the biopsy of patient 5 shows general appearance of all component parts of the kidney. A small arteriole (A) reveals marked thickening of the intima with narrowing of the lumen. Normal glomeruli, mild scarcity of tubules, and mild interstitial fibrosis are seen. H&E, × 80. Inset: An arteriole from the same biopsy as in Figure 4 under higher magnification exhibits marked thickening of the intima (I) by PAS-positive (hyaline) material and thinning of smooth muscle cellular layer. Lumen (L) is shown. PAS, × 320.

dense elastic tissue. Glomeruli showed irregular thickening and tortuosity of basement membranes (GBM), small discrete deposits of electron-dense materials within GBM, and crescent formation (Fig. 6).

    Nephrectomy Specimen. The LM study revealed impressive changes in the arterioles, glomeruli, tubules, and interstitium (Fig. 7). The arterioles demonstrated marked intimal thickening and an excessive amount of intimal fibroblasts and fibrous tissue. A loss of endothelial cells and occlusion of the lumina were

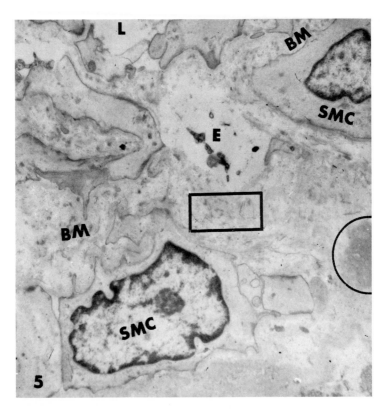

Fig. 5. This electron micrograph of an arteriole from the biopsy of patient 5 reveals atrophy of an endothelial cell. The basement membranes (BM) between endothelial cell and smooth muscle cell (SMC) and between SMC are poorly defined. Electron-dense material (circle) suggestive of necrosis between SMC is shown. Large electron-lucent space suggestive of edema (E) is demonstrated. A small number of collagen fibers (square) are shown. Lumen (L). UA and LC, × 12,000.

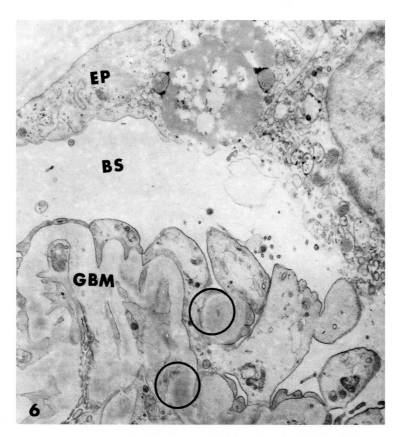

Fig. 6. This electron micrograph of a part of a glomerulus from the biopsy of patient 5 shows proliferating Bowman's epithelial cells (EP), irregular thickening of glomerular basement membrane (GBM), discrete electron-dense deposits within GBM (circles), and collapse of capillaries. Bowman's space (BS) is shown. UA and LC, × 17,500.

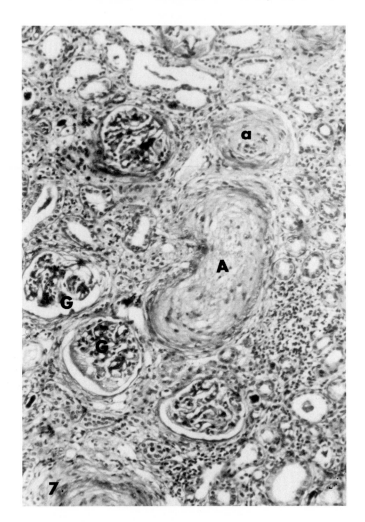

Fig. 7. This light micrograph from nephrectomy specimen of patient 5 shows a small artery (A), an arteriole (a), and several glomeruli. The artery and the arteriole reveal fibroplastic proliferation of the intima with occlusion of the lumina. Two of the 4 glomeruli (G) showed segmental necrosis. Marked disappearance of tubules, dilatation of a few tubules, and small foci of cellular infiltration are seen. H&E, × 80.

found in most arterioles. Intense PAS-positive material suggestive of necrosis in the intima and marked SMC hyperplasia forming concentric layers with occlusion of the lumen were observed in some arterioles. Thrombi occluding arteriolar lumina were sometimes observed. Rarely, aneurysmal dilatation through a disrupted segment of an arteriole produced a conspicuous histologic change. The periphery of this arteriole revealed excessive periadventitial fibrous tissue without inflammatory infiltrates (Fig. 8). About two-thirds of all glomeruli revealed marked, irregular thickening of the basement membrane of the peripheral capillary loops.

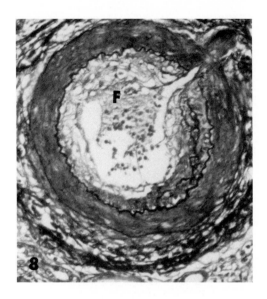

Fig. 8. A small artery from the nephrectomy of patient 5 shows fibroplasia (F) of the intima, disruptive changes through the media with aneurysm formation, and excessive fibrous tissue without inflammatory infiltrates surrounding the peripheral part of the vessel. Trichrome, × 320.

Twenty percent of the glomeruli were hyalinized and revealed fibrotic crescents; an equal number showed necrosis of capillaries and exudation of plasma material into Bowman's space. Few glomeruli appeared normal. The tubular changes were variable with some being normal, some atrophic, and some dilated and filled with casts. Necrotic changes were seen in 10 to 20 percent of the tubules, and a few tubules were filled with red cells.

Ultrastructural studies of two arterioles demonstrated predominantly hyperplasia of SMC in one arteriole (Fig. 9) and necrosis of most SMC in the other (Fig. 10). The hyperplastic SMC were characterized by large, notched nuclei, multiple nuclei, numerous ribosomes, and often dilated endoplasmic reticulum. Along with hyperplasia of SMC, atrophy of a few SMC also was observed. There was a marked increase in collagen fibers in the basement membranes between SMC. The presence of platelets in the subendothelial spaces and electron-dense deposits between necrotic SMC were observed. There were marked increases in fibroblasts (Fig. 10) and electron-dense elastic tissue (Fig. 11). Ultrastructure of glomeruli revealed pronounced but irregular thickening and tortuosity of GBM in most capillary loops, with necrosis of some capillaries, presence of discrete deposits of electron-dense material, atrophy of endothelial and visceral epithelial cells, hyperplasia of parietal (Bowman's) epithelial cells, and the presence of exudation in Bowman's space (Fig. 12). IM studies were negative for all immunoglobulins in both biopsy and nephrectomy specimens. However, fine granular deposits of C_3 component of complement in the walls of small arteries and dense deposits of fibrinogen in occasional small arteries were found. In summary, two separate histologic studies of renal tissue at an interval of 43 months using LM, EM, and IM techniques revealed striking differences in all component parts of the kidney. The differences were characterized by marked increases in hyperplastic

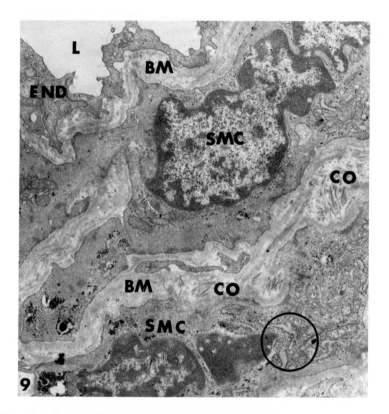

Fig. 9. This arteriole from the nephrectomy specimen of patient 5 shows layers of hyperplastic smooth muscle cells (SMC) evidenced by dilated rough-surfaced endoplasmic reticulum and ribosomes (circle). Basement membrane (BM) is electron dense throughout. Collagen fibers (CO) are seen within the BM between SMC. Lumen (L) and atrophic endothelial cell (END) are shown. UA and LC, $\times$ 18,500.

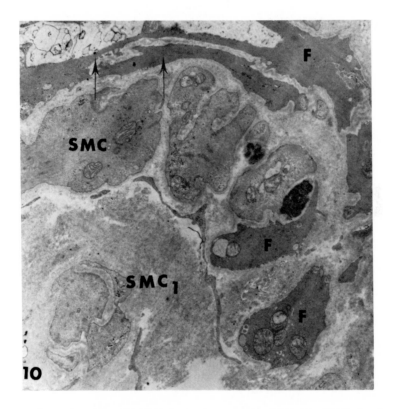

Fig. 10. An excessive number (proliferation) of smooth muscle cells (SMC) is seen in this arteriole. Some smooth muscle cells (SMC₁) are necrotic. Fibroblasts (F) between SMC and in the subendothelial space are conspicuous by their long processes (arrows) that invade between necrotic SMC. UA and LC, × 10,200.

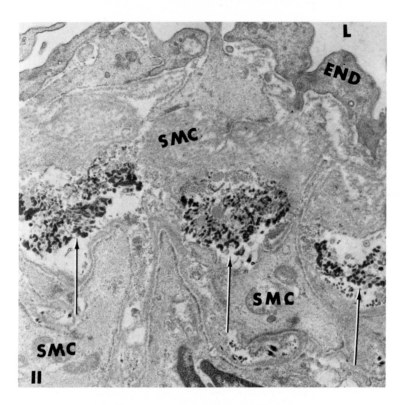

Fig. 11. An electron micrograph of a renal arteriole from the nephrectomy specimen of patient 5 reveals excessive amounts of electron-dense elastic tissue (arrows) between necrotic smooth muscle cells (SMC). Lumen (L) and endothelial cell (END) are shown. STPPS, × 18,750.

SMC and increases in collagen fibers and elastic tissue in most arterioles, necrosis of SMC in a few arterioles, necrosis and hyalinization in one-third of the glomeruli, atrophy and dilatation of most tubules with frank necrosis of 10 to 20 percent of these tubules, and a conspicuous increase in interstitial infiltrates and fibrosis.

PATIENT 6.   A 33-year-old white female was first admitted to the University of Oklahoma Hospitals in January, 1975, with a 6-year history of severe hypertension first appearing during pregnancy and the recent onset of epistaxis and generalized ecchymoses. Antihypertensive therapy was taken intermittently, and her admission blood pressure was 160/100. Her admission laboratory studies included a urinalysis showing numerous white cells with a few red cells. Repeated urine cultures grew no organisms. Her hematocrit was 25 vol percent, and her serum urea nitrogen and serum creatinine concentrations were 84 mg and 10.4 mg per 100 ml, respectively. She began twice weekly hemodialysis beginning February, 1975; and she underwent a bilateral nephrectomy in October, 1975, in preparation for a renal transplant. The renal tissue was studied using LM, EM, and IM.

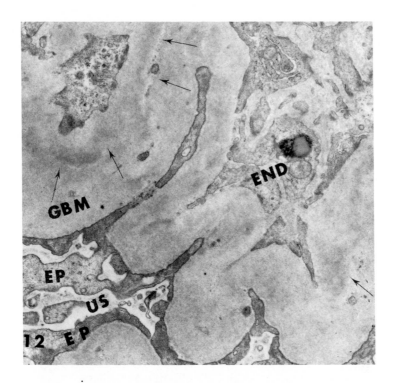

Fig. 12. Glomerular capillaries from the nephrectomy specimen of patient 5 show marked but irregular thickening of basement membranes (GBM), discrete intramembranous deposits (arrows) within GBM, atrophy of epithelial cell (EP), and collapse of capillaries. Urinary space (US) and endothelial cell (END) are shown. UA and LC, × 26,000.

Renal Pathology. LM study of the kidneys showed a variety of changes in the small arteries and arterioles characterized by proliferation of SMC in some arterioles, diffuse necrotic changes in other arterioles, and a combination of proliferation of SMC and necrotic change in the intima in still other arterioles. Complete occlusion of the lumen by homogenous necrotic material was a consistent finding (Fig. 13). Marked widening of the intima by proliferating fibroblasts and fibrous tissue with proliferative changes in the SMC were observed in the small arteries. A total of 60 to 70 percent of the glomeruli were involved. A third of these were totally hyalinized, a third revealed segmental necrosis, and a third were diffusely necrotic. There was a disappearance or atrophy of a vast majority of the tubules and dilatation of most of the remaining tubules with casts filling the lumina. Foci of round cells were seen focally in the interstitium.

By EM study, arterioles revealed diffuse necrosis of all component parts and collections of electron-dense materials that might be necrotic SMC or deposits of immunoglobulins. Fibrin was conspicuous by its absence (Fig. 14 and inset). IM study revealed irregular deposits of IgG, IgM, and C_3 in the GBM, amorphous deposits of IgG and IgA in the tubules, and scattered deposits of fibrinogen in the interstitium.

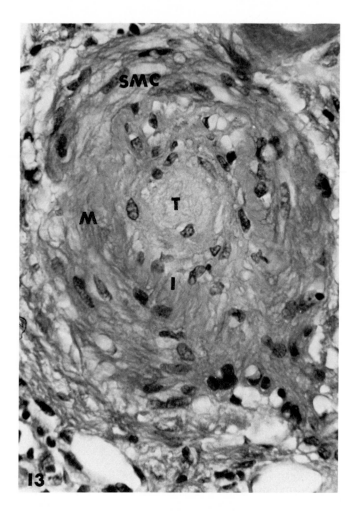

Fig. 13. A large arteriole from the nephrectomy specimen of patient 6 shows necrotic change in the intima (I) and media (M) with thrombotic (T) occlusion of the lumen. Hyperplasia of smooth muscle cells (SMC) is evident. PAS, × 320.

PATIENT 7.   A 25-year-old white male was brought to the emergency room following the sudden onset of severe headache followed by unconsciousness during a football game. On admission, his blood pressure was 240/140 mm Hg, and he showed grade IV (K-W-B) retinopathy with bilateral papilledema. A right percutaneous biopsy was done after his hypertensive crisis was brought under control. Satisfactory reduction of his blood pressure could not be maintained by the aggressive administration of multiple antihypertensive drugs. His renal function rapidly deteriorated, necessitating hemodialysis therapy. One year later, he underwent bilateral nephrectomy in order to achieve control of intractable hypertension.

Renal Pathology.   LM studies of both biopsy and nephrectomy specimens at an interval of 12 months revealed similar findings of concentric hyperplasia of

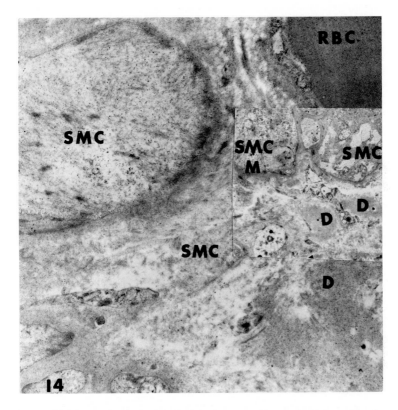

Fig. 14. The electron micrograph of an arteriole from the nephrectomy specimen of patient 6 displays widespread necrosis of smooth muscle cells (SMC), basement membrane, and endothelial cells. Also, collections of electron-dense materials (D) are seen. Red blood cells (RBC) occupy the lumen. UA and LC, × 35,000. Inset: (right center part). Same arteriole as in Figure 14 showing necrotic smooth muscle cells (SMC) and collections of electron-dense material (D). These electron-dense materials (D) may be necrotic material with immunoglobulin deposits. UA and LC, × 7,500.

smooth muscle cells of the arterioles with complete occlusion of the lumina. Necrotic changes were seldom observed. The interlobar arteries revealed a moderate amount of intimal fibroplasia. Most glomeruli were partially or completely hyalinized, a few glomeruli showed segmental necrosis, and a few glomeruli were normal. The vast majority of the tubules had disappeared, with the remaining tubules showing dilatation and hyaline casts within the lumina. A few foci of inflammatory cells were seen.

EM study demonstrated hyperplasia of the outer SMC as well as necrosis of inner SMC, and the presence of disrupted and electron-dense (necrotic) basement membrane between endothelial cells and SMC. Widening of the space between endothelial basement membrane and smooth muscle cell (normally not present) with infiltration of these spaces by fibroblasts, platelets, and lymphocytes was a conspicuous feature (Figs. 15 and 16). Discrete deposits of electron-dense material were found between SMC. Large electron-lucent spaces (appearing to be

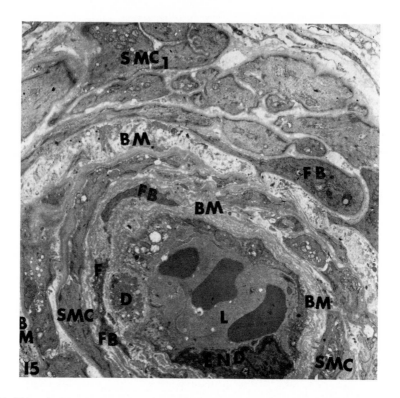

Fig. 15. This whole arteriole from the nephrectomy specimen of patient 7 shows occlusion of the lumen (L) by homogeneous electron-dense material (thrombus), necrosis of the portion of endothelial cell, fibrillar and electron-dense subendothelial basement membrane (BM), fibroblasts (FB) in the subendothelial space and in the smooth muscle cellular layer, necrosis of inner smooth muscle cell (SMC), and necrosis of basement membrane (BM) between inner and outer smooth muscle cell (SMC_1). The outer smooth muscle cells (SMC_1) appear proliferating. Electron-dense deposit (D) in subendothelial space is seen. UA and LC, $\times$ 8,200.

edema) were observed between SMC. The two glomeruli studied revealed necrosis of most of the capillary loops.

PATIENTS 8 AND 9.   Clinical details were unavailable. The renal pathology by LM and EM was similar to that observed in patient 7.

PATIENT 10.   A 19-year-old black male with documented mild hypertension (blood pressure 150/100 mm Hg) for two years was admitted to the University of Oklahoma Hospitals with complaints of dysphagia and fatigue. The admission physical examination revealed pallor, a blood pressure of 240/140 mm Hg, and grade IV (K-W-B) retinopathy. Admission laboratory studies included the urinalysis, which revealed 4+ proteinuria, 6 to 8 white cells, and numerous red cells per high-power field. His serum urea nitrogen and serum creatinine concentrations were 112 mg and 13 mg per 100 ml, respectively. After initiation of maintenance hemodialysis, a percutaneous right renal biopsy was performed, and the tissue was studied by LM, EM, and IM.

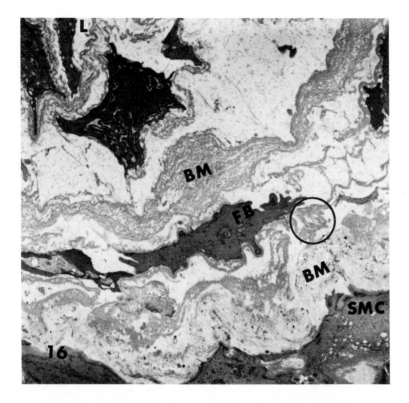

Fig. 16. Part of another arteriole from the same patient as in Figure 15 showing fibrillar basement membrane (BM), fibroblast (FB), fibrin (circle), and necrosis of smooth muscle cell (SMC). Lumen (L) is shown. UA and LC, × 21,000.

Renal Pathology. LM study revealed predominantly hyperplasia of SMC and intimal fibroblastic proliferation with loss of endothelial cells producing luminal occlusion of all caliber vessels (Figs. 17 to 19). Half of the glomeruli were hyalinized. Most of the remaining glomeruli revealed diffuse or segmental necrosis. Tubules had mostly disappeared. The remaining tubules were dilated; a few dilated tubules contained numerous red blood cells (RBCs) within the lumina. A few foci of inflammatory cells were seen throughout the interstitium.

Electron microscopy revealed wide necrotic endothelial basement membranes containing fine granular electron-dense deposits. The SMC were hyperplastic; however, necrosis as well as atrophy of a few SMC also were observed. The BM between individual SMC and in the outer parts of SMC were electron-dense (necrotic) (Fig. 20). Immunofluorescence microscopy revealed no immunoglobulin deposits.

The LM and EM findings of the kidneys in all patients are summarized in Tables 3 and 4. The light microscopic study of renal pathology separates these patients into two groups. Group I consisted of patients 1 through 4 and the first biopsy specimen of patient 5. In patient 5, the study of the biopsy specimen using

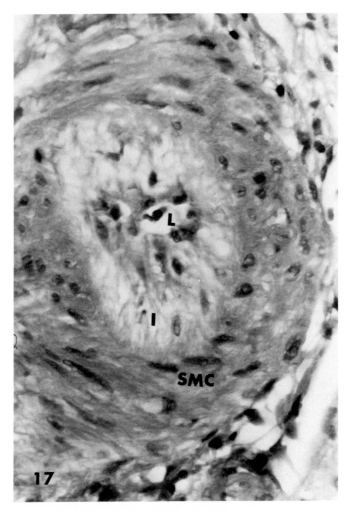

Fig. 17. This large arteriole from patient 10 reveals hyperplasia of smooth muscle cells (SMC) and intimal thickening (I) due to fibroblasts and fibrous tissue. Lumen (L) is occluded. H&E, × 320.

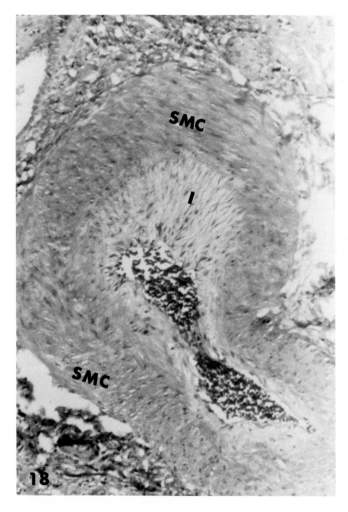

Fig. 18. A small artery from patient 10 shows pronounced thickening of intima (I) due to numerous fibroblastic cells and marked proliferation of smooth muscle cells (SMC). Lumen is occluded by numerous red blood cells. H&E, × 320.

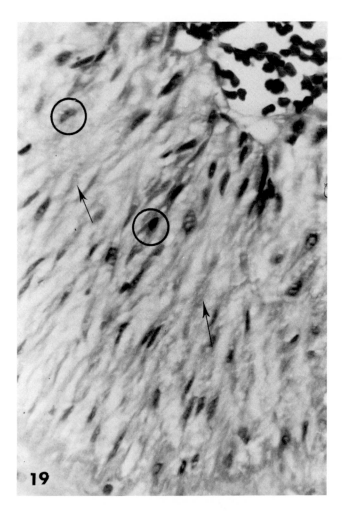

Fig. 19. Higher magnification of the intimal layer from the same artery as in Figure 18 showing fibroblasts (circles) and fibrous tissue (arrows). H&E, × 1,000.

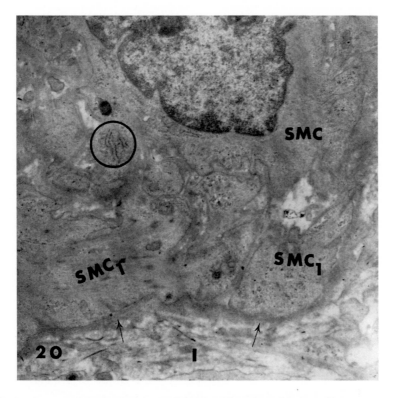

Fig. 20. In this arteriole from the renal biopsy of patient 10, one finds hyperplasia of smooth muscle cells (SMC) evidenced by prominent rough-surfaced endoplasmic reticulum (circle), as well as necrosis of other smooth muscle cells (SMC_1) featured by electron-dense basement membrane (arrows) and absence of normal cytoplasmic constituents. Interstitium (I) is shown. UA and LC, $\times$ 22,500.

TABLE 3. Light Microscopy Study of Renal Tissue

Patient Groups	Glomeruli	Arteriole	Tubule	Interstitium
I: Patients 1–4 Patient 5 (biopsy 1)	Normal to thickened basement membrane of peripheral capillary loops	Normal or thickening of intima and media by PAS-positive strands	Mostly normal, atrophy of 5–10% tubules	Normal or mild fibrosis
II: Patient 5 (nephrectomy) Patients 6–10	Hyalinized, necrotic, normal	Hyperplasia and necrosis of SMC, proliferation of fibroblasts, and excessive amounts of fibrous tissue in the intima	Conspicuous disappearance of most of the tubules, atrophy, and dilatation of 20–25% tubules	Moderate to marked fibrosis and foci of infiltrates

TABLE 4. Summary of the Arteriolar Ultrastructural Findings

	Patients 1–4	Patients 5 *–10
Arteriolar components		
Architecture	N	Distorted
Endothelium	N or atrophic	Mostly lost
BM of endothelial cell	2+–3+ thick	Fibrillar and dark
BM material	2+–3+ increase	None
Smooth muscle cell	N or atrophic	Necrosis in the inner part, hyperplasia and hypertrophy in the outer part
Infiltrations		
Fibrin	0	1+ (infrequent)
Fibroblasts	0	1+–2+
Platelets	0	1+
Inflammatory cells	0	1+–2+
Collagen fibers (PASI)	0	3+
Elastic tissue (STPPS)	Occasional	2+–3+
Electron-dense deposits	0	Infrequent
Edema	0	2+–3+
Glomerular changes	Tortuous irregular thickening of the basement membrane	Thickening of basement membrane, intramembranous and subendothelial electron-dense deposits, and necrosis of capillary loops

0: none; 1+: mild or few; 2+: moderate; 3+: marked; N: normal.
* Changes in the biopsy specimen were milder than in the nephrectomy specimen 43 months later.
With kind permission from the Editor, Annals of Clinical and Laboratory Science.

LM revealed findings that resembled those in group I patients but EM findings in the biopsy were similar to those in group II patients (patients 6 through 10). LM and EM features in the nephrectomy were similar to those in patients 6 through 10.

Studies of the Histology of the Kidney in Spontaneously Hypertensive Rats and Normotensive Wistar Rats

The morphology of the kidney was scored based on the severity of the changes by light microscopy in a manner somewhat similar to that reported by Sommers et al [10] and Heptinstall.[11] The scoring system is shown in Table 5. The histology of the kidney was evaluated and scored without prior knowledge of age, arterial pressure or strain of the rat from which the material was obtained. The histologic scores were then related to age, mean arterial pressure, and rat strains. The renal morphologic changes were graded in order of increasing severity: grade 1 (0 to 2 points, normal); grade II (3 to 7 points, mild); grade III (8 to 19 points, moderate); and grade IV (20 to 39 points, severe). In the 40 SHR, the distributions of morphologic grading were grade I (12.5 percent), grade II (50 percent), grade III (12.5 percent), and grade IV (25 percent). The grade IV lesions were found exclusively in old SHR (average age of 91 weeks). Grade IV lesions were evident

TABLE 5. Scoring of Renal Lesions (Light Microscopy) in Rat Study

Histologic Changes in All Component Parts of the Kidney	*Score*
A. ARTERY AND ARTERIOLE	
1. No change observed	0
2. PAS-positive material	
a. Minimal (+) PAS-positive material in the intima only	1
b. Much (++) PAS-positive material throughout the vessel wall	2
3. Vacuoles	
a. Few vacuoles in media only	1
b. Many vacuoles throughout the vessel wall	2
4. Hyperplasia of smooth muscle cells	
a. Without occlusion of the lumen	3
b. With occlusion of the lumen	5
5. Necrotic changes	
a. Intense PAS-positive homogeneous material in the intima	5
b. Intense PAS-positive homogeneous material throughout the vessel wall	5
c. Infiltration of RBC and inflammatory cells within and outside vascular wall	5
B. GLOMERULI	
1. Increase in mesangial matrix	1
2. Intracapillary thrombi	2
3. Necrosis of tufts	2
4. Crescents (greater than 10%)	2
C. TUBULES AND INTERSTITIUM	
1. Atrophy and dilatation of tubules	2
2. Interstitial infiltrates or fibrosis	1
Total Points	39

in 83 percent (10 of 12) of old SHR. In contrast, more than three-fourths of all NR (79 percent) had normal or near normal renal morphology (grade I); 21 percent demonstrated grade II renal lesions; and no old NR demonstrated grade IV lesions.

Summary of Renal Lesions in Rats

Grade II and grade III lesions were characterized by arteriolar thickening by excessive PAS-positive strands (of material), and many vacuoles, and variable proliferation of smooth muscle cells without and with compromise of arteriolar lumina (Fig. 21). Grade IV (severe or malignant) lesions were featured by necrotic changes in the arterioles and glomeruli, with relative sparing of the tubules and interstitium. Periarteritis and granuloma of the small arteries and granuloma of glomeruli constituted a pronounced feature in grade IV lesions. Large arterioles revealed proliferative and necrotic changes, while small arterioles revealed mainly necrotic changes (Fig. 22). Necrotic changes were revealed in 25 to 75 percent of the glomeruli, and there was a presence of abundant fibrin

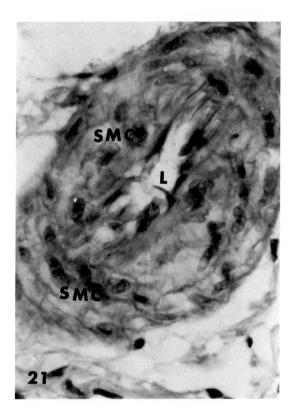

Fig. 21. This light micrograph of a renal arteriole from a 50-week-old SHR showing PAS-positive strands (material) and smooth muscle cell (SMC) hyperplasia. Lumen (L) is shown. PAS, × 320.

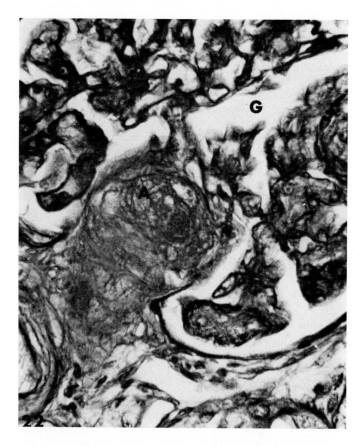

Fig. 22. A necrotic arteriole (A) with necrosis of glomerular capillaries (G) from an 89-week-old SHR. H&E, × 320.

within glomerular capillaries (Fig. 23) (Table 6). It was not uncommon to find several normal glomeruli in the vicinity of a necrotic glomerulus. Ultrastructurally, mild thickening of the basement membrane (BM) between endothelial cells and SMC and between individual SMC were observed. In an occasional rat, marked thickening of the BM giving rise to nodule formation was observed. SMC hyperplasia and atrophy were observed in the arterioles in younger rats. Arterioles from the old SHR exhibited diffuse necrosis of SMC with slight or no fibrin present (Fig. 24). Glomeruli revealed numerous platelets and massive amounts of fibrin in most of the capillary loops (Fig. 25). Some capillary loops were necrotic while others were intact.[12]

Pathophysiologic Correlation Between Mean Arterial Pressure and Age and Severity Index of Renal Lesions in NR and SHR

The mean arterial pressure (MAP) of the NR and SHR population was 125.5 mm Hg ± 2.7 (SEM) and 184 mm Hg ± 4.0 (SEM), respectively. In-

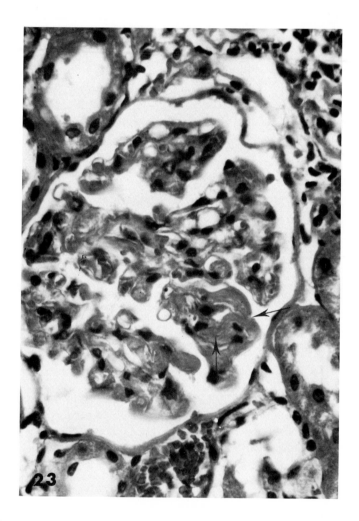

Fig. 23. A necrotic glomerulus from 89-week-old SHR shows abundant fibrin within glomerular capillaries (arrows). Bowman's space is clear. Adjacent tubules are normal. H&E, × 320.

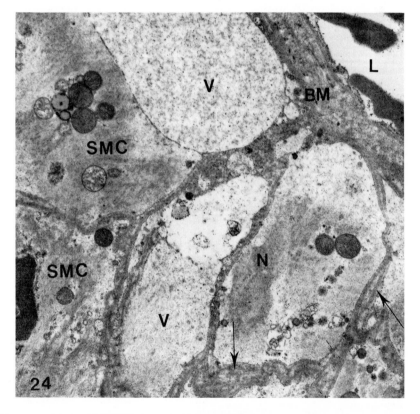

Fig. 24. This electron micrograph of a renal arteriole from an 89-week-old SHR shows necrosis of smooth muscle cell (SMC), marked electron-density (necrosis) of the basement membrane (arrows) between SMC, and occlusion of the lumen by a thrombus (T). UA & LC, × 19,500.

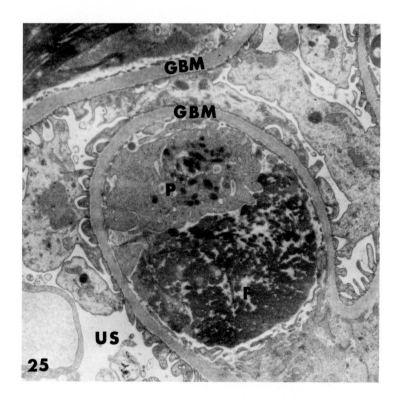

Fig. 25. This electron micrograph of the glomerular capillaries from a 90-week-old SHR rat demonstrates luminal occlusion of a glomerular capillary by a massive amount of fibrin (F) and aggregates of platelets (P). Fibrin (F) is also seen inside the lumen of another capillary at the top. The capillary basement membranes (GBM) are intact. Urinary space (US) is shown. UA and LC, × 10,500.

dividual renal histologic scores of two strains of rats were plotted against MAP. No significant correlation was found between the severity of the renal lesions and the MAP in either the NR or SHR. The mean ages of the NR and SHR populations were 44.1 ± 4.9 (SEM) and 46.4 ± 5.0 (SEM) weeks, respectively. The renal histologic scores were plotted against age. No significant correlation was found between the severity of renal lesions and age in the NR. In contrast, a highly significant correlation (P < .001) was found between age and the severity of renal lesions in SHR (Fig. 26). Thus, severe (or malignant) renal changes were observed in 10 of 12 old SHR (average age 91 weeks). This contrasted with the normal renal histology observed in kidneys of 10 old (average age, 90 weeks) NR.[12] Since SHR had significantly elevated arterial pressure from the earliest age (4 weeks) at which pressure can be measured,[13] age in SHR can be considered equivalent to duration of hypertension. This highly significant association between age (or duration of hypertension) and severity of renal lesions in SHR, therefore, provides evidence to support the concept that the severity of the renal lesions is more dependent on the duration than the severity of the hypertension.[12]

**TABLE 6. Grading of Renal Morphologic Changes in Order of Increasing Severity.
Rat Study**

Grade	Morphologic Changes	Score	Severity
I	No change, minimal PAS-positive material in intima or few vacuoles in media	0–2	Normal
II	Much PAS-positive material throughout and few vacuoles in media, or both throughout and smooth muscle cell (SMC) hyperplasia without occlusion of the lumen. Normal tubules and interstitium	3–7	Mild
III	Any of the above combinations as in grade II plus more marked hyperplasia of SMC with occlusion of the lumen plus any one or all these: increase in mesangial matrix, glomerular crescents, tubular atrophy, and dilatation (5%) and mild interstitial infiltrates	8–19	Moderate
IV	Periarteritis and granuloma of arteries; marked SMC hyperplasia, and intimal necrosis in the larger arterioles, predominant necrosis in the smaller arterioles, diffuse necrosis in the glomeruli; atrophy and dilatation of tubules (10%) and mild interstitial change	20–39	Severe (or malignant)

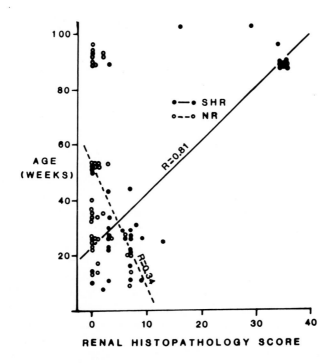

Fig. 26. Displays correlation between renal histopathologic score and age in SHR and NR. (From Ann Clin Lab Sci 7:158, 1977)

Relationship Between Severity of the Renal Lesions and Severity and Duration of Hypertension

Renal Lesions in Essential Hypertension

Although a clear association has been established between the renal lesion of essential hypertension, ie, nephrosclerosis, and the presence of hypertension, the sequence involved in the development of this association remains poorly defined. In other words, it remains unclear whether the hypertension causes the renal lesions or the renal lesion causes the hypertension. There are good reasons why it has been difficult to establish this important cause and effect relationship in essential hypertension. First, it is difficult to obtain renal tissues for serial studies in otherwise asymptomatic hypertensive patients, and single studies from individual hypertensive patients are simply inadequate to provide an understanding of the sequence of development of the renal lesions in hypertensive patients. Furthermore, biopsies obtained percutaneously often are inadequate for study of blood vessels, and a considerable sampling error for the larger vessels (small arteries and arterioles) may exist. Specimens obtained from autopsy show some degree of autolysis and are less than optimum for light microscopic examination and inadequate for electron microscopic examination. Another major problem is that serial biopsies from kidneys of normotensive subjects also are difficult to obtain, so that the effect of aging on vessel pathology cannot be separated from the effect of the hypertension. Interpretation of renal morphology often is biased by a knowledge of the clinical information available on the patients.

Until recently, no experimental animal model closely resembling human essential hypertension has been available. With the availability of the SHR, an animal model closely resembling human essential hypertension, studies of kidneys in SHR of all ages should provide a better understanding of the development of the renal lesions and their relationship to the severity and duration of the hypertension.

The clinicopathologic relationship between the renal lesion of essential hypertension and the development of renal insufficiency or failure also remains poorly defined. One question that remains to be answered is: "Can the renal failure be associated with morphologic changes in one structure in the kidney, ie, arteriole, glomerulus, tubule, or interstitium, or are there parallel changes in all component structures in the kidney?"

One might also question the appropriateness of the current terminology used to define the renal lesions in patients with essential hypertension. In *Stedman's Medical Dictionary* (18th edition), "nephrosclerosis" is defined as "induration of the kidney from overgrowth and contraction of the interstitial connective tissue." Are we then justified in using this general term to describe the renal lesions in essential hypertension? A component of overgrowth is seen in the arterioles either as excessive thickening of basement membrane (BM) or BM-like materials, or as hyperplasia of smooth muscle cells (SMC). Fibrosis of the interstitium is not a pronounced feature, at least not enough to cause shrinkage of the kidney, regardless of the clinical severity of hypertension. In benign hypertension, there is modest reduction in the size of the kidneys, the total weight being over 200 g [14] (normal total weight, 250 to 300 g). In malignant hypertension, the combined weight varied from 130 to 410 g in one series [15] and from 180 to 380 in another series.[16] This reduction in size has been attributed to the severity of the renal failure.[14] Hyalinization of glomeruli and atrophy of tubular cells can cause reduction in weight. The term nephrosclerosis, then, is not a satisfactory one to describe the microscopic picture of the kidney in hypertension; however, it seems appropriate to use the terms *benign* and *malignant* to indicate mild and severe lesions, respectively.

The lack of a universal agreement on the definition of clinical benign and malignant hypertension has complicated evaluation of the literature on the renal pathology of hypertension. Kincaid-Smith et al [16] indicated from their studies, as well as by reviewing studies in other series, papilledema is the hallmark of malignant hypertension. This definition seems to be acceptable by most individuals. Using this definition, we will attempt to define some of the relationships of the renal lesions to essential hypertension. In this series, patients from 1 through 6 appear to have benign hypertension. The renal histology is similar in the first 4 patients, but renal histology, especially using EM, in patients 5 and 6 resembles that observed in patients 7 through 10 (Tables 3 and 4).

The LM studies in the first four patients are characteristic of arteriolar (ie, benign) nephrosclerosis. Ultrastructurally, the changes consist of thickening of basement membrane (BM) and excessive amounts of BM-like material and atrophy of smooth muscle cells (SMC). McGee and Ashworth [2] and Biava et al [3] found similar ultrastructural arteriolar changes in benign or essential hypertensive patients. These changes appear to be nonspecific, since they can be observed in the renal arterioles in patients with chronic renal disease [17] and in diffuse arteriosclerotic conditions without hypertension (Fig. 27). Biava et al [3] and Fisher et al [4] are in agreement with this concept, ie, there is no specific arteriolar change in benign hypertension. These observations suggest the lack of any specific relationship between clinical benign hypertension and the renal pathology that was found in these patients. In other words, benign hypertension and arteriolar (ie, benign) nephrosclerosis may be independent variables.

Recently Fisher and Pirog [18] produced contracted kidneys by selective partial occlusion of the intrarenal arteriolar bed with microspheres in Sprague-Dawley rats without elevation of blood pressure. LM study of the kidney revealed lesions consistent with arteriolar (ie, benign) nephrosclerosis, which led these authors to conclude that such arteriolar lesions are pathogenetically unrelated to hypertension. In contrast, a direct relationship exists between hypertension and the renal lesions characterized by proliferative and necrotic changes in the arterial vessels associated with hyalinization and necrosis of the glomeruli, profound disappearances of tubules, and moderate to marked interstitial changes. This belief is supported by data in three large clinicopathologic studies of malignant hypertension.[15, 16, 19] Controversy exists over which of the two arteriolar lesions, endarteritis proliferans (proliferation of SMC and intimal fibroplasia with occlusion of the lumen) or necrotizing arteriolitis (arteriolar necrosis), is the principal lesion in malignant nephrosclerosis. This issue continues to intrigue the pathologist and

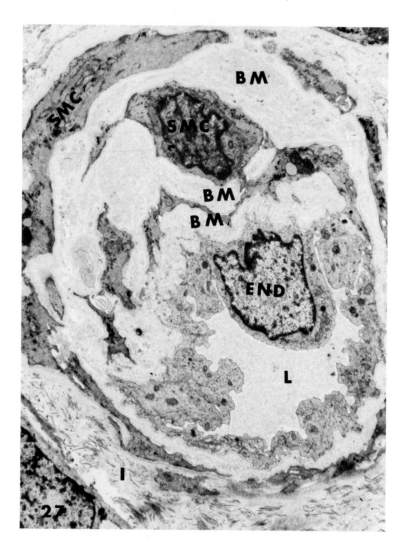

Fig. 27. This electron micrograph of a small arteriole is from the renal biopsy of a 70-year-old woman. She has diffuse arteriosclerotic disease manifested by anginal chest pain, strokes, and renal failure. She gave a history of hypertension. However, admission blood pressure was 140/80 mm Hg. This micrograph shows marked thickening of basement membrane (BM) between endothelial cell (END) and smooth muscle cell (SMC) and between SMC. Atrophy of SMC is seen. Some compromise of the arteriolar lumen (L) is observed. Collagen fibers and fibroblasts are seen in the interstitium (I). UA and LC, × 6,450. (Courtesy of Dr. Robert C. Muehrcke)

practicing physician. A review of the literature indicates there remains a lack of uniform agreement on this question. Kimmelstiel and Wilson [19] and Kincaid-Smith [6] considered diffuse proliferative endarteritis as the characteristic histologic lesion of malignant hypertension, while Heptinstall [14, 15] regarded arteriolar necrosis as the hallmark of malignant hypertension.

Proliferation of smooth muscle cells appears to be the major factor in causing occlusion of the vascular lumen. This is in agreement with observations made in malignant hypertensive patients by Jones [5] and in renovascular hypertensive rats by Spiro et al.[20] When an arteriole with proliferative changes (LM) is examined by EM, it almost always reveals fibrillar or necrotic basement membranes, accompanied by fine discrete electron-dense deposits, necrosis of inner (or intimal) SMC, hyperplasia and hypertrophy of outer SMC, and atrophy of a few scattered SMC. Infiltration with fibroblasts is a constant finding. McCormack and colleagues [21] have found proliferation of fibroblasts and excessive fibrous tissue in the intima (intimal fibroplasia), especially in small arteries in a group of malignant hypertensive patients who received antipressor drugs for 4 to 48 months. Kojima-hara et al [22] found similar changes when malignant hypertensive rats were treated with antipressor drugs. They have suggested this type of change is associated with healing of acute lesions resulting from antihypertensive drug treatment. These vascular changes also were found in the patients studied in this series. Using EM and specific staining techniques, fibroblasts and excessive amounts of collagen fibers and elastic tissue were found in patients 5 through 10, who were receiving drug treatment for variable periods.

Our findings, which are in agreement with those of Jones,[5] suggest that proliferative and necrotic changes may occur simultaneously in the same arteriole, especially if the vessel is studied by EM. Just how these renal lesions (especially arterial vascular lesions) are produced remains unclear. Does hypertension cause these renal (ie, arteriolar) lesions or do the renal lesions produce hypertension? Kimmelstiel and Wilson [19] found a definite correlation between malignant hypertension and malignant nephrosclerosis (severe renal lesions). Heptinstall [15] found vascular necrosis in patients with severe degrees of hypertension (diastolic pressure of 150 mm Hg or over). In contrast, Sommers and colleagues [10] did not find consistency between arteriolar necrosis and any specific level of diastolic pressure. Similarly, Kincaid-Smith and associates [16] found arteriolar necrosis in malignant hypertensive patients with systolic pressures less than 200 mm Hg.

In attempting to answer this question, Wilson and Byrom [23] studied contralateral kidneys from 35 rats between 5 days to 6 months after hypertension was produced by constricting one renal artery. They demonstrated necrotic changes in the arterioles resembling those observed in human malignant nephrosclerosis. Polyarteritis in occasional small arteries was observed. There was no EM study. The authors claimed that severe hypertension caused the renal lesions. Recently Goldby and Beilin [24] studied development and healing of arteriolar lesions using a tracer (carbon particles) and LM and EM techniques in rats made hypertensive by renal artery constriction and contralateral nephrectomy. Three types of lesions were observed. In the first, plasma and carbon particles had entered the media to displace and destroy SMC. In the second, additional intimal deposits containing plasma, fibrin, and macrophages had appeared. In the third, SMC were irregular in outline and surrounded by excessive extracellular material. These authors claimed that the necrotic lesions were the result of the high arterial pressure.

Both groups of authors concluded from their observations that the necrotic arteriolar lesions are caused by severe hypertension. The data in our SHR study are against this concept that the intrarenal arterial vascular lesions are primarily due to the severity of the hypertension alone, and thus in agreement with the conclusions of Sommers and associates [10] and Kincaid-Smith.[6] A significant number of young, severely hypertensive SHR showed normal renal histology or mild renal lesions. Over all ages, severe renal lesions consisting of periarteritis, granulomatous arteritis, and arteriolar and glomerular necrosis appeared in the vast majority of old SHR in contrast to no renal lesions in old NR. Furthermore, one patient (patient 6) with a diastolic pressure of 110 mm Hg showed severe renal lesions. In contrast, another patient (patient 3) with diastolic pressure of 130 mm Hg showed mild (grade II) renal lesions. Progression of the renal lesions over a four-year period was observed in one patient in this series (patient 5). The highly significant association established between the severity of renal lesions and age (ie, duration of hypertension) in SHR led to the conclusion that the development of severe (ie, malignant) renal lesions in hypertension is more dependent on the duration of the hypertension than the severity of the hypertension. This conclusion is supported by Freis,[25] who suggested age, heredity, and environmental influences and not hypertension alone play roles in the severity of the renal lesions.

One hypothesis, then, concerning the mechanism involved in the development of renal vascular lesions in hypertension is that genetic hypertension in the young animal or man is not associated with severe renal lesions, because normal elastic tissue and SMC contents are present in the arterial vascular wall and this structural makeup prevents development of severe lesions until the composition of the vascular elastic tissue and SMC components are altered by age. The demonstration of excessive amounts of elastic tissue by a specific staining technique in the renal arterioles of all SHR,[9] with the most marked increases accompanied by disruptive changes in the renal arteriolar elastic tissue of the vast majority of old SHR, lends support to this hypothesis.[10] It was mentioned in the latter study that degeneration and disappearance of elastic tissue were accompanied by pooling of ground substances and its permeation into adjacent intercellular spaces. These authors were not clear if any hyperplasia of elastic tissue occurred. In the present study, hyperplasia as well as disruptive change in the elastic tissue have been confirmed.

The mechanisms operative in the development of necrotic vascular lesions in the short period of weeks in renovascular hypertensive rats are unlikely to be the same as the ones causing necrotic renal lesions in SHR and hypertensive patients over a period of months or years. The possibility that angiotensin, often elevated in renovascular hypertensive man [14] and assumed to be elevated in these renal-clip hypertensive rats, may produce ischemic (necrotic) renal lesions remains good. This hormone has been found to be normal in most malignant hypertensive patients [14] and is consistently normal in SHR.[13] The cause(s) for proliferation of SMC and overgrowth of collagen fibers and elastic tissue remain to be determined.

Before concluding this chapter, it should be emphasized that there is no single lesion characteristic of malignant nephrosclerosis. A combination of proliferative and necrotic arterial vascular lesions along with obsolescence or necrosis of glomeruli and moderate to marked tubulointerstitial changes constitute the renal lesions of hypertension. This type of massive damage involving all component parts of the kidney is most often found in patients with malignant hypertension (papilledema). However, this renal morphology can be observed in hypertensive patients without papilledema. Thus, the findings in this study support the observations suggesting that the clinical condition of malignant hypertension and the pathologic demonstration of necrotic or proliferative arteriolar lesions in the kidney are related but not necessarily equivalent.

Relationship between Pathology and Functional Failure of the Kidney

Even in the absence of papilledema, hypertensive patients with severe renal lesions tend to develop azotemia. The marked azotemia associated with severe morphologic lesions in hypertensive patients contrasts with the normal or mildly elevated serum urea nitrogen in SHR with similar vascular and glomerular lesions. This raises the question of the mechanism of renal failure in hypertension. Here again, there is no uniform agreement on the impact of the lesions involving individual renal components as the cause of functional failure. Kimmelstiel and Wilson [19] suggested that terminal renal failure was related to the arteriolar necrosis more closely than to the hypertension. McCormack et al [21] stated that intimal cellular proliferation, intimal fibroplasia with marked narrowing of the lumina in small arteries and large arterioles lead to slowly progressive renal failure. Kincaid-Smith [6] found good correlation between the proliferative arteriolar lesion and renal failure. The proliferative arteriolar lesion was more apparent in patients with renal failure than in SHR who did not develop azotemia.

Even though the proliferative arteriolar lesion with intimal fibroplasia is a consistent finding in the kidney of the hypertensive patient with renal failure, it is difficult to confirm this as the cause of the renal failure as the glomeruli also are severely damaged. Furthermore, the effect of widespread loss of tubules and interstitial changes found in severe hypertensive patients must be considered in the pathogenesis of the renal failure. SHR with severe arterial and arteriolar lesions had only slight tubulointerstitial changes and revealed only mild azotemia. Serum urea nitrogen concentrations ranged from 19 to 41 mg per 100 ml with a mean value of 27 mg per 100 ml (normal, 20 to 22 mg per 100 ml). Wilson and Byrom [23] also did not find discernible damage in the tubules and interstitium in rats with experimentally induced hypertension, and their blood urea levels were not different from those observed in control rats.

The diffuse and widespread tubulointerstitial lesions in patients 6 through 10 provided a much different picture from that observed in the SHR where preservation of most tubules and only mild interstitial changes were found. These two studies suggest some relationship between preservation of tubular mass and interstitium and maintenance of normal renal function. In other words, the renal functional impairment seen in severe or malignant hypertensive patients can be associated with a remarkable loss of tubules, damage in the remaining tubules, and moderate to marked interstitial fibrosis and infiltration. This disparity between the morphologic findings and the degree of nitrogen retention observed in hypertensive patients and SHR has previously been described by Risdon et al.[26] They found the best correlation between loss of tubules and changes in the interstitium, and plasma creatinine concentration or creatinine clearance. If this is true, then rapid deterioration of renal function observed in some of the patients with severe or malignant hypertension and with impaired function of the kidneys may be explained by a superimposed ischemic tubular necrosis. This may account for the dramatic deterioration after only mild impairment of renal function, as observed in patient 5. Acute tubular necrosis has been observed by other investigators, also in some patients with accelerated hypertension who developed acute renal failure.[27]

Value of Electron Microscopy in the Study of Kidney Morphology in Hypertension

EM study provides an important technique for evaluating hyaline and necrotic changes, the presence or absence of fibrin, changes in the basement membrane (BM), changes in the amount of elastic tissue and collagen fibers, the presence or absence of fibroblasts and other infiltrative cells, and changes in smooth muscle cells (SMC). This technique proved useful in clarifying hyaline change, fibrinoid necrosis and proliferative changes, and in demonstration of elastic tissue.

Hyaline thickening has been considered as characteristic of arteriolar (ie, benign) nephrosclerosis.[1] This hyaline material is eosinophilic, moderately PAS-positive, and homogeneous. Hyaline material under LM may be under electron microscopy granular deposits, thickened BM between endothelial cells and SMC and between individual SMC and excessive BM-like materials (Fig. 1 versus 2). As proposed by Fisher et al,[4] the term hyaline appears inappropriate.

The LM finding of an eosinophilic and intensely PAS-positive and homogeneous dark material on trichrome staining (fibrinoid necrosis) is considered a hallmark of malignant hypertension.[14] Such an anatomic description also is questionable, since fibrin is seldom found in the arterial vessels in hypertensive patients or in SHR. Diffuse necrosis in the smooth muscle cells appears to provide the light microscopic appearance of intensely PAS- and trichrome-positive material (Fig. 22 versus 24). It is relatively common to find fibrin in the glomeruli in malignant hypertensive patients and in SHR (Fig. 25).

EM distinctively demonstrated hyperplasia and hypertrophy of SMC. Proliferated SMC-formed bundles and the hyperplastic SMC were characterized by a large single or notched nucleus or multiple nuclei, prominent attachment plates, much rough-surfaced endoplasmic reticulum and numerous ribosomes (Fig. 9).

Proliferation of SMC was consistently observed in malignant hypertensive patients. Excessive collagen fibers (PASI) were found in the renal arterioles from malignant hypertensive patients. The presence of collagen fibers, necrosis, and hyperplasia of SMC and electron-dense deposits in the biopsy specimen in patient 5 indicated malignant nephrosclerosis in this patient when LM study revealed changes suggestive of arteriolar (ie, benign) nephrosclerosis. This observation was confirmed by the finding of a marked increase in collagen fibers and elastic tissue, and proliferated SMC in the nephrectomy specimen. Similarly, moderate to marked increases of elastic tissue, especially the presence of elastic tissue around SMC, was consistently observed in the renal arterioles in malignant hypertensive patients and old SHR. Changes observed in the subendothelial elastica were thought by previous authors to be due to separation of its fiber network, resulting in an increased prominence of the mucoprotein PAS-positive matrix.[10] Using a specific staining technique, some of the PAS-positive matrix were found to be elastic tissue.[9]

Infiltration by a variety of cells such as fibroblasts, platelets, lymphocytes, and neutrophils can be identified by EM study. In contrast, intimal SMC can be misinterpreted as fibroblasts and inflammatory cells when the specimen is studied by LM only.

Summary

This section presents data on light (LM) and electron (EM) microscopy studies of kidneys from 10 essential benign (BH) and malignant (MH) hypertensive patients and 40 spontaneously hypertensive rats (SHR).

In BH patients, the hyaline thickening (PAS-positive material or strands) of arterial vessels observed by light microscopy is found to be thickened basement membrane (BM), and excessive BM-like material and atrophic smooth muscle cells (SMC) when the vessel is examined by EM. These arteriolar changes appeared nonspecific and unrelated to hypertension, because similar changes can be found in the ischemic kidney and in chronic renal disease without hypertension.

An array of proliferative and necrotic arterial vascular lesions along with obsolescence and necrosis of glomeruli, marked tubular loss, and interstitial changes are found most commonly in MH patients (with papilledema), but such renal lesions are not uncommon in BH patients (without papilledema). Thus, clinical malignant hypertension and the demonstration of necrotic or proliferative arteriolar lesions in the kidney often are related but not in a clear cause and effect association. In the present study, both hyperplasia and necrosis of arteriolar SMC were found in human malignant hypertension. Both types of arterial changes may coexist in the same arteriole, especially when a vessel is examined by EM.

The cause and effect relationship between hypertension and the associated renal lesions remains undetermined. This study and some previous studies failed to demonstrate any clear correlation between severity of renal lesions (proliferative or necrotic changes) and severity of the hypertension. However, in the SHR study, we found that younger rats had milder lesions. Over all ages, severe lesions resembling those of malignant nephrosclerosis in man appeared in old SHR, and a highly significant association was established between age (ie, duration of hypertension) and pathologic changes ($P < 0.001$). This spectrum of renal lesions and its correlation with duration of hypertension have not been demonstrated previously in experimental hypertension. A relationship between the renal lesions and the duration of hypertension has been demonstrated in at least one patient in this study (patient 5). Thus, it appears that renal lesions in hypertension are more dependent on the duration of the hypertension than the severity of the hypertension.

Azotemia is a consistent finding in hypertensive patients with severe renal lesions. The arterioglomerular changes are similar in man with malignant hypertension and in SHR, but the absence of tubulointerstitial changes and azotemia in

SHR contrast strikingly with the massive tubular loss, interstitial infiltration and fibrosis, and progressive azotemia observed in hypertensive patients. This disparity suggests that renal failure may result more from ischemic loss of tubules and interstitial changes than from merely arterioglomerular lesions.

Fibrin and platelets are inconspicuous in the arterioles, but they are found abundantly in the glomeruli associated with severe renal lesions in both hypertensive man and SHR, especially the latter. The role of fibrin and platelets in the development or acceleration of the renal lesions of hypertension remains to be determined. "Fibrinoid necrosis" appears to be an inappropriate term because this LM appearance in the vessel is, by electron microscopy, electron-dense (necrotic) SMC with slight or no fibrin. Instead, such LM appearance should be described as necrotic change.

EM study can characterize the early stage of severe arteriolar lesions by demonstration of collagen fibers, excessive elastic tissue, and hyperplasia of SMC when LM study reveals intimal thickening or mild SMC hyperplasia. Therefore, the specific renal lesions of hypertension can be distinguished by EM study, even at an early stage, from the nonspecific renal changes of benign hypertension.

Since the SHR has been considered the best animal model thus far developed experimentally for the study of clinical essential hypertension, the studies of the renal pathology in these rats has provided further evidence, underscoring the pertinence of this model for understanding the renal pathology related to essential hypertension in man.

Acknowledgments

The authors would like to express gratitude to Marc A. Pfeffer, M.D., Ph.D., and Janice M. Pfeffer, B.A., of the Department of Medicine, Harvard Medical School (formerly of the University of Oklahoma College of Medicine), for making available kidneys from the rats. The rats were supplied from the SHR and NR colonies of Dr. Edward D. Frohlich, Ochsner Clinic, New Orleans (previously George Lynn Cross Professor of Medicine, University of Oklahoma College of Medicine). The authors are also grateful to Dr. Robert C. Muehrcke, West Suburban Hospital, Oak Park, Illinois, for providing kidneys from his patients (included in this study) and Joseph Uzupick, Electron Microscopy Laboratory, West Suburban Hospital, Oak Park, Illinois, for making available EM prints from studies of kidneys. The authors are grateful to Dr. K. Chrysant, a former fellow in Nephrology (Electron Microscopy), for her participation in part of this study. The authors offer thanks to Mrs. Carolyn Clay for secretarial work in the preparation of this manuscript.

References

1. Papper S, Vaamonde C: Nephrosclerosis. In Strauss MB, Welt LG (eds): Diseases of the Kidney. Boston, Little, Brown, 1971, p. 735
2. McGee WG, Ashworth CT: Fine structure of chronic hypertensive arteriopathy in human kidney. Am J Pathol 43:273, 1963
3. Biava CG, Dyrda I, Genest J, Bencosme SA: Renal hyaline arteriolosclerosis, an electron microscope study. Am J Pathol 44:349, 1964

4. Fisher ED, Perez-Stable E, Pardo V: Ultrastructural studies in hypertension: A comparison of renal vascular and juxtaglomerular cell alterations in essential and renal hypertensions in man. Lab Invest 31:303, 1966
5. Jones DB: Arterial and glomerular lesions associated with severe hypertension. Lab Invest 31:303, 1974
6. Kincaid-Smith P: Participation of intravascular coagulation in the pathogenesis of glomerular and vascular lesions. Kidney Int 7:242, 1975
7. Mandal AK, Frohlich ED, Nordquist J: An ultrastructural analysis of renal arterioles in benign and malignant essential hypertension. Ann Clin Lab Sci 7:158, 1977
8. Olson RL, Nordquist R, Nordquist J, Everett MA: Lysosomes and the skin: XIII Congressus Internationalis Dermatologue. Munchen, 1967. Berlin, Springer-Verlag, 1968, p 1056
9. Mandal AK, Frohlich ED, Bell RD, et al: An electron microscope technique for the study of elastic tissue in small arteries and arterioles of the kidney. Ann Clin Lab Sci 7:42, 1977
10. Sommers SC, Relman AS, Smithwick RH: Histological studies of the kidney biopsy specimens from patients with hypertension. Am J Pathol 34:685, 1958
11. Heptinstall RH: Renal biopsies in hypertension. Br Heart J 16:133, 1954
12. Mandal AK, Bell RD, Nordquist JA, Lindeman RD: Panorama of malignant renal lesions in old spontaneously hypertensive rat. XI Int Cong Int Acad Pathol Book Abs, Oct 17–23, 1976, Washington, D.C., p 173 (abs)
13. Okamoto K, Aoki K, Nosaka S, Kukushima M: Cardiovascular disease in the spontaneously hypertensive rat. Jap Circ J 28:943, 1964
14. Heptinstall RH: Hypertension, Pathology of Kidney. Boston, Little, Brown, 1974, p 121
15. Heptinstall RH: Malignant hypertension: A study of fifty-one cases. J Pathol Bact 65:423, 1953
16. Kincaid-Smith P, McMichael J, Murphy EA: The clinical course and pathology of hypertension with papilledema (malignant hypertension). Q J Med 27:117, 1958
17. Mandal AK, Chrysant K, Nordquist JA, et al: Focal glomerular sclerosis. South Med J 69:997, 1976
18. Fisher ER, Pirog J: Renal arteriolar obstruction without hypertension. Nephron 16:433, 1976
19. Kimmelstiel P, Wilson C: Benign and malignant hypertension and nephrosclerosis. Am J Pathol 12:45, 1936
20. Spiro D, Lattes RG, Wiener J: The cellular pathology of experimental hypertension. I. Hyperplastic arteriolar sclerosis. Am J Pathol 47:19, 1965
21. McCormack LJ, Beland JE, Schneckloth EE, Corcoran AC: Effects of antihypertensive treatment on the evolution of renal lesions in malignant nephrosclerosis. Am J Pathol 34:1011, 1958
22. Kojimahara M, Sekiya K, Ooneda G: Studies on the healing of arterial lesions in experimental hypertension. Virchows Arch [Pathol Anat] 354:150, 1971
23. Wilson C, Byrom FB: Renal changes in malignant hypertensions. Lancet 1:136, 1939
24. Goldby FS, Beilin JJ: The evolution and healing of arteriolar damage in renal-clip hypertension in the rat—an electron microscope study. J Pathol 114:139, 1974
25. Freis ED: Essential hypertension and spontaneous hypertension. In Okamoto K: Spontaneous Hypertension. New York, Springer-Verlag, 1972, p 231
26. Risdon RA, Sloper JC, deWardener HE: Relationship between renal function and histological changes found in renal biopsy specimens. Lancet 2:363, 1968
27. Sevitt LH, Evans DJ, Wrong OM: Acute oliguric renal failure due to accelerated hypertension. Q J Med 40:127, 1971

PAROSTEAL OSTEOMA: A CLINICOPATHOLOGIC APPROACH

LUÍS V. TAMARIT AND JOSÉ PARDO

We present herein a case of parosteal osteoma of the upper third of the femur in a 10-year-old boy. The purpose of this paper is to demonstrate the pathologic and clinical features of this rare tumor that differentiate it from other similar tumorous conditions. We propose to include the tumor within the group of so-called semimalignant new growths, following the general lines of the classification by Uehlinger.[1]

Concerning treatment, we believe that the bone tumors falling into this category meet the criteria of Merle d'Aubigné [2] for segmental resection, and are of the opinion that in view of their local aggressiveness and recurring pattern of growth simple en bloc excision would fall short of an adequate surgical resection.

Case Report

Patient D.O.C. (Hosp. no. 38.336) is a 10-year-old boy, who was referred from an outside hospital with the pathologic diagnosis of "heterotopic ossification of muscle mass, paraosteal, upper third of right femur." Upon admission to hospital the patient recalled that one year previously he received a kick on the right gluteal region with a subsequent fall upon his knees. Thereafter he always complained of a low intensity, dull pain over the right inguinal region. X-rays at this time were reported to be normal. Clinically the patient also reported malaise and claudication of the right lower extremity.

Clinical examination revealed a scar 1 cm in length, probably corresponding to the previous biopsy, over the adductor muscles of the right hip. There were no local inflammatory signs. There was tenderness on palpation of the adductor muscles and of the ischiopubic bone. Passive hip mobilization was not painful and showed a full range of motion. At this time x-ray films showed mottled dense areas over the inner aspect of the femur, below the trochanter minus. This change corresponded to an apparent tumor mass which was attached to the bone, but with sharp demarcation line that seemed to separate it from the underlying cortex (Figs. 1 and 2). The cortical bone next to the tumor mass was much thickened. It had different opacity in areas, and a tendency to fashion vertical lines. A pyrophosphate 99mTc bone scan showed activity change at the level of the proximal portion of the femur, which was entirely involved by the tumor (Fig. 3).

Clinically the differential diagnosis was posed among a number of conditions, ie, myositis ossificans, osteogenic sarcoma, and parosteal sarcoma. To rule out metastatic disease a complete x-ray and bone scan series were done. Laboratory tests showed normal values.

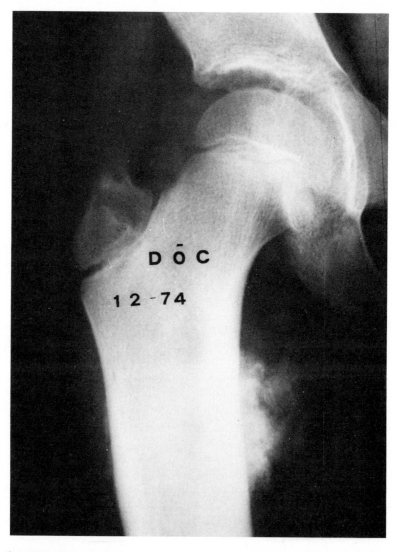

Fig. 1. Anteroposterior radiograph of right femur. There is a tumor mass below the trochanter minus.

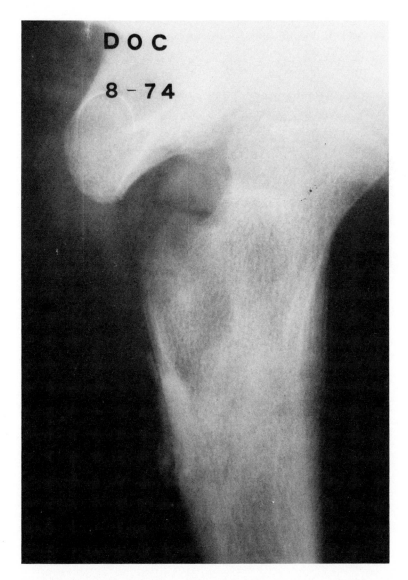

Fig. 2. Axial radiograph of proximal portion of right femur. There is tumor involvement of the bone, but with a faint interphase line of tumor-bone.

A biopsy from the tumor mass was taken. This consisted of several bony frag-ments, the largest measuring 4 × 3.5 × 3 cm, which were placed in decalcification solution after formalin fixation. The microscopic sections showed broad, mature lamellar bone trabeculae forming sclerotic bone and leaving narrow, irregular marrow spaces, which occasionally contained haversian-line channels. In other areas there was intermixing with apposition of woven-type bone. The bone marrow was fibrolipomatous in some areas and loose fibrous in others. There was some

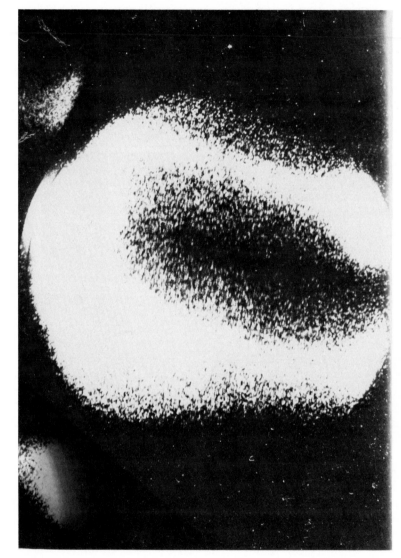

Fig. 3. Bone scan with 99mTc pyrophosphate. Pathologic activity at the level of the upper third of right femur.

resorption–appositional activity with predominating osteoblastic change and resulting osteoid seams. The osteoblastic elements were delicate and showed mature nuclei without mitotic activity. The bone trabeculae were not arranged in an orderly, directional structure. No atypical changes were noted. The pathologic diagnosis was parosteal osteoma, upper third of right femur.

A surgical approach was contemplated. Two possibilities were considered: local excision with a sharp dissection from the underlying bone cortex; and segmental resection, which seemed to be the better choice. The technique consists essentially in the removal of the tumor together with the bone segment on which it is implanted, ie, with interruption of the bone continuity. An amputation was also considered, but was disregarded because it was thought to be too drastic an operation for this kind of tumor.

A detailed operative report follows, because we think the method should be more frequently used in the treatment of the "semimalignant" bone tumors. Previously spongiosa bone chips for grafting were obtained from the right iliac crest, and four 6 × 0.5 cm cortical bone grafts were removed subperiosteally from the middle third of the right fibula. The surgical approach was initiated via dissection of the tensor of the fascia lata and sartorius muscles. This provided good maneuvering space for blunt dissection of the tumor and en bloc removal together with the transected 5 cm of bone shaft that included the tumor. Then the cortical bone grafts were inserted into the femoral shaft ends, using them as a bridge, and the bone chips were applied, providing for the missing tumorous bone. In addition, the femur was stabilized in its outer aspect by means of a Muller type right plate which was screwed onto the cortex. The extremity was immobilized with a cast in a position of hip abduction. No complications occurred during the postoperative period.

After three months it was considered that there was already sufficient consolidation to allow the patient to stand and initiate stepping and walking. The last follow-up check was done 15 months after the operation. The x-rays at this time showed upward displacement of the top plate screw (Figs. 4 and 5), due to the bone growth at the femoral neck with subsequent breaking of the screw tip, but the bone showed better consolidation than at the previous follow-up check done five months earlier (Fig. 6). The filling defect, as seen in the radiographs, had been reduced from 3 × 2.5 × 2 cm in this previous follow-up down to 1 × 1 cm in the last one 15 months after the operation (Fig. 5). This provides proof that bone remodeling and consolidation were far advanced.

The resected tissue was submitted for pathologic diagnosis. It consisted of several irregularly shaped, rather firm fragments, the largest of which measured 4.5 cm in maximal dimensions. This showed at one end a grayish-white osseous texture involving the soft tissue with indurated fibrous areas. In addition, a femoral shaft segment 5 cm in length was submitted that had a grayish-white, considerably thickened, eburnated, slightly convex-shaped cortex on the sagittal section (Fig. 7). Figure 8 shows the abovementioned soft tissue portion involved by tumor at one end. Microscopically, the sections showed mature lamellar bone, similar to the pattern seen in the previous biopsy (Figs. 9 to 11). The parosteal new bone was identical to the mature, trabecular bone seen in the tumor involving the adjacent soft tissue.

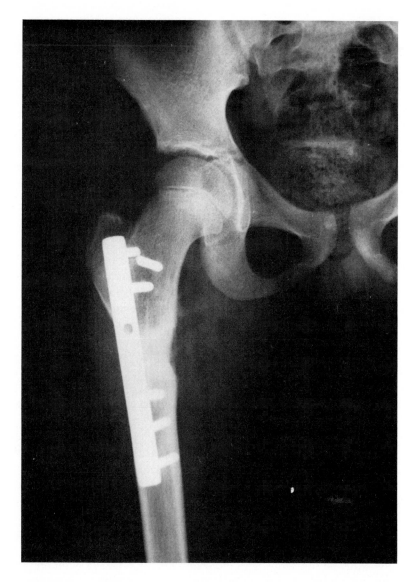

Fig. 4. Anteroposterior radiograph 15 months postoperatively; normal bone axis with well delineated internal cortex.

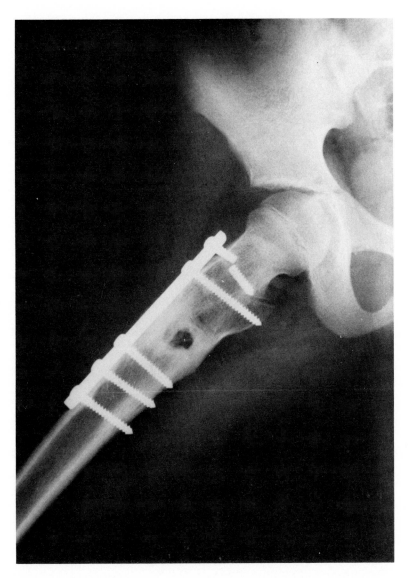

Fig. 5. Axial radiograph 15 months postoperatively. The defect has closed to about 1 × 1 cm.

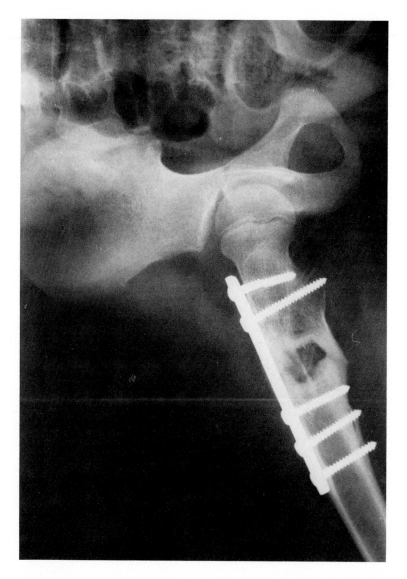

Fig. 6. Axial radiograph of femur, seven months after segmental resection. A fairly large nonossified central defect remains.

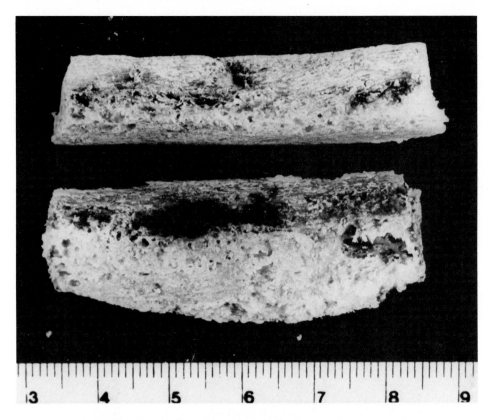

Fig. 7. Segment of femoral shaft involved by tumor; there is infiltration and thickening of the bone cortex and periosteum.

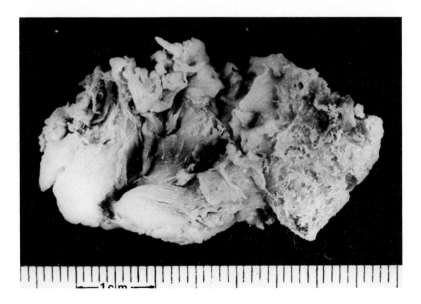

Fig. 8. Tumor involving soft tissue; the osseous texture is more apparent at one end.

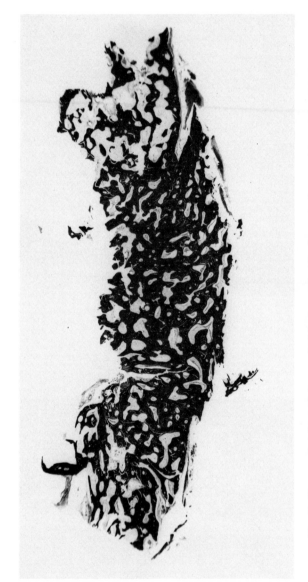

Fig. 9. Panoramic view of tumor fashioning sclerotic bone built up of mature osseous trabeculae. Note convexity of the section corresponding to the gross specimen in Figure 7. Original magnification, × 8.5.

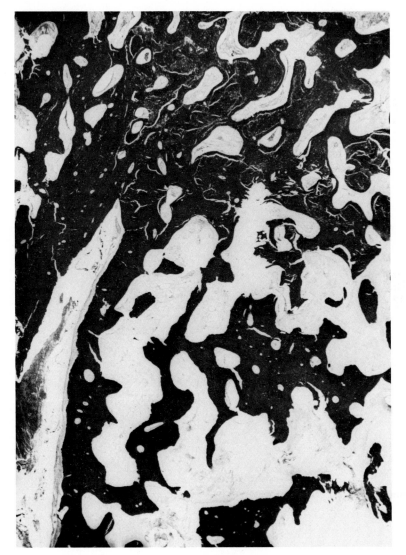

Fig. 10. Irregularly shaped lamellar bone leaving wide marrow spaces. Original magnification, × 34.

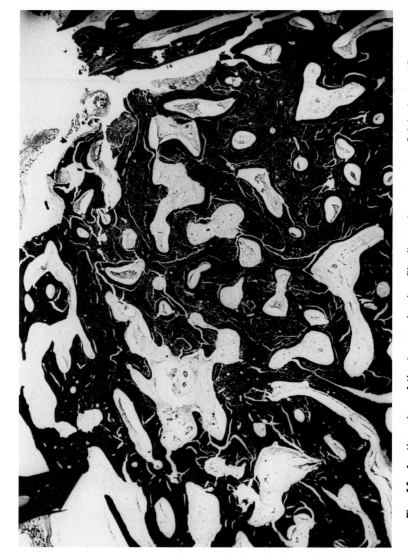

Fig. 11. Another view of the tumor showing fibrolipomatous marrow. Original magnification, × 34.

Discussion

A differential diagnosis should be made of the parosteal osteoma with various tumorous and pseudotumorous conditions. Among these latter the parosteal osseous metaplasia, myositis ossificans, hyperplastic postfracture callus, pseudomalignant osseous tumor of soft tissue,[3] parosteal fasciitis,[4] and the parosteal sarcoma can pose difficulties, unless sarcomatous areas in the latter are obvious. Lichtenstein [5] emphasized the pathologist's responsibility in sampling adequate biopsy material, in order to obtain enough representative tissue to find fusiform cells with hyperchromatic or atypical nuclei to justify a diagnosis of sarcoma. He noted that "not all parosteal growths (on the lower femur posteriorly, for example) develop into sarcomas, although the natural history of many of them indicates that they are potentially malignant. . . ." Most authors mention incidentally the parosteal osteomas when discussing the parosteal sarcomas.[5, 7] Dahlin [6] identified the parosteal osteoma as a separate entity from the parosteal sarcoma, but conceded that a "malignant gradient" exists from the low grade to the highly malignant parosteal sarcomas. Others, among them Spjut et al,[7] included the parosteal osteomas within the group of parosteal sarcomas, warning that the term osteoma suggests benignancy and should not be used in this connection.

Because the parosteal osteoma is made up of mature lamellar bone some nosologic confusion with the parosteal osseous metaplasia is possible. In fact the histogenesis of the latter is not completely clear. However, following the criteria of Willis [8] for the definition of tumor (neoplasm), only the progressive proliferation of mature periosteal new bone can distinguish a neoplastic growth from a simple osseous metaplasia.[5] A point in the differential diagnosis with the myositis ossificans should be made, concerning the so-called zonal phenomenon in which a progressive osseous maturation of this lesion in a centrifugal fashion occurs as contrasted with the uniform growth pattern of the parosteal osteoma. The parosteal osteoma tends to reach a large size; occasionally, as in our case, with involvement of the bone cortex. In other cases [1] the tumor is sharply delineated from the underlying cortex. Growth does not reach beyond the epiphyseal line. The preferred location is, usually, the fossa poplitea, also a usual site of parosteal sarcomas. The sites of occurrence include the proximal metaphysis of the humerus and that of the tibia and fibula. The age of incidence is highest in the third or fourth decades of life. The clinical course is usually protracted, with a tendency to recurrence.

Uehlinger [1] included this tumor among the "semimalignant" new growths, which would meet the following criteria, developed by Zollinger [9]:

1. Local infiltration and destructive growth
2. Characteristic tendency to local recurrence
3. Lack of distant metastases

Since the tendency to local recurrence cannot be anticipated from the histologic pattern of mature lamellar bone growth, a wide excision with interruption of the bone continuity (segmental resection) should be contemplated, representing a more radical surgical approach than simple en bloc resection, yet leaving functional mobility unimpaired.

Although the clinical behavior and biologic growth pattern of both parosteal osteoma and well-differentiated parosteal sarcoma are similar, we feel that these criteria alone could bias a more academic approach to nosologic classification based on the histologic appearance. Leaving aside the point that morphology and biologic behavior may not be absolutely correlated, we feel that well-differentiated parosteal sarcomas are always accompanied by a more or less heavily collagenized stroma, which is rather striking to the pathologist. Such was not the case with the parosteal osteoma we are discussing. In parosteal osteoma it is the mature bone formation with intervening fibrolipomatous or loose fibrous marrow without collagenous stroma that represents the chief distinctive feature. Unni et al [10] acknowledged that parosteal osteomas are very rare tumors indeed. However, they pointed out that "it is the tumefactive bone formation without an active fibrous stroma" that provides a most striking appearance.

By including the parosteal osteoma within the group of the so-called semi-malignant new growths we mean to convey to the orthopedic surgeon a rather disquieting biologic growth behavior which should require a fairly radical therapeutic approach and careful follow-up. If enough representative material from the tumor is examined and the histologic criteria for a well-differentiated parosteal sarcoma, as described by most authors,[5, 7-10] are not met, then the diagnosis of this entity obviously cannot be made on clinical, topographic, or radiographic appearances alone. It is the pathologist's responsibility to harmonize these data with the histology. This is the challenge we must face.

Summary

Parosteal osteomas are rare bone tumors that deserve special consideration regarding their pathologic and clinical behavior. They should be distinguished from among a number of similar tumorous conditions and their nosologic entity as semimalignant growths clearly established. For tumors of this category we propose segmental resection as a safer procedure than simple block excision, following the criteria of Merle d'Aubigné.

References

1. Uehlinger E.: Pathologische Anatomie der Knochengeschwülste unter besonderer Berücksichtigung der semimalignen Formen. Chirurg 45:62, 1974
2. Merle D'Aubigné R: La Réséction dans le Traitement des Tumeurs des Os: Conferences d'Enseignement, 1968. Paris, Expansion Scientific Francaise, 1968, pp 201–22
3. Chaplin DM, Harrison MH: Pseudomalignant osseous tumor of soft tissue. Report of two cases. J Bone Joint Surg [Am] 54B:334, 1972
4. Hutter RVP, Foote Jr FW, Francis KC, Higinbotham NL: Parosteal fasciitis. Am J Surg 104:800, 1962
5. Lichtenstein L: Bone Tumors. St Louis, Mosby, 1965
6. Dahlin DC: Tumores oseos. Barcelona, Toray, 1969. (Transl from the English edition: Bone Tumors. Springfield, Ill, Thomas)
7. Spjut HJ, Dorfman DH, Fechner RE, Ackerman LV: Tumors of bone and

cartilage. Armed Forces Institute of Pathology, fascicle 5, second series. Washington, DC, 1970
8. Willis RA: The Pathology of Tumours, 4th ed. London, Butterworths, 1967
9. Zollinger HU: Geschwulstprobleme. Verh Naturforsch Ges 91:81, 1946
10. Unni KK, Dahlin DC, Beabout JW, Ivins JC: Parosteal osteogenic sarcoma. Cancer 37:3466, 1976

INDEX

Entries in italics refer to figures and tables.